THE STATE OF THE WORLD'S CHILDREN 2011

Acknowledgements

This report was produced with the invaluable guidance and contributions of many individuals, both inside and outside of UNICEF. Important contributions for country panels were received from the following UNICEF field offices: Côte d'Ivoire, Ethiopia, Haiti, India, Jordan, Mexico, Philippines, Ukraine and the US Fund for UNICEF. Input was also received from UNICEF regional offices and the World Health Organization's Adolescent Health and Development Team. Special thanks also to UNICEF's Adolescent Development and Participation Unit for their contributions, guidance and support. And thanks to adolescents from around the world who contributed quotations and other submissions for the print report and the website.

The State of the World's Children 2011 invited adult and adolescent contributors from a variety of stakeholder groups to give their perspectives on the distinct challenges adolescents face today in protection, education, health and participation. Our gratitude is extended to the contributors presented in this report: His Excellency Mr. Anote Tong, President of the Republic of Kiribati; Her Royal Highness Princess Mathilde of Belgium; Her Highness Sheikha Mozah bint Nasser Al Missned; Emmanuel Adebayor; Saeda Almatari; Regynnah Awino; Meenakshi Dunga; Lara Dutta; Maria Eitel; Brenda Garcia; Urs Gasser; Nyaradzayi Gumbonzvanda; Colin Maclay; Cian McLeod; Paolo Najera; John Palfrey; Aown Shahzad; and Maria Sharapova. These essays represent a selection of the full series of Perspectives available at <www.unicef.org/sowc2011>.

Special thanks also to Ayman Abulaban; Gloria Adutwum; Rita Azar; Gerrit Beger; Tina Bille; Soha Bsat Boustani; Marissa Buckanoff; Abubakar Dungus; Abdel Rahman Ghandour; Omar Gharzeddine; Shazia Hassan; Carmen Higa; Donna Hoerder; Aristide Horugavye; Oksana Leshchenko; Isabelle Marneffe; Francesca Montini; Jussi Ojutkangas; and Arturo Romboli for their assistance with the Perspectives essay series and Technology panels. Special thanks also to Meena Cabral de Mello of WHO's Adolescent Health and Development Team for her assistance with the panel on adolescent mental health.

EDITORIAL AND RESEARCH

David Anthony, *Editor;* Chris Brazier, *Principal Writer;* Marilia Di Noia; Hirut Gebre-Egziabher; Anna Grojec; Carol Holmes; Tina Johnson; Robert Lehrman; Céline Little; Charlotte Maitre; Meedan Mekonnen; Kristin Moehlmann; Baishalee Nayak; Arati Rao; Anne Santiago; Shobana Shankar; Julia Szczuka; Jordan Tamagni; Judith Yemane

PRODUCTION AND DISTRIBUTION

Jaclyn Tierney, *Production Officer;* Edward Ying, Jr.; Germain Ake; Fanuel Endalew; Eki Kairupan; Farid Rashid; Elias Salem

TRANSLATION

French edition: Marc Chalamet
Spanish edition: Carlos Perellón

MEDIA AND OUTREACH

Christopher de Bono; Kathryn Donovan; Erica Falkenstein; Janine Kandel; Céline Little; Lorna O'Hanlon

INTERNET BROADCAST AND IMAGE SECTION

Stephen Cassidy; Matthew Cortellesi; Keith Musselman; Ellen Tolmie; Tanya Turkovich

DESIGN AND PRE-PRESS PRODUCTION

Prographics, Inc.

STATISTICAL TABLES

Tessa Wardlaw, *Associate Director*, Statistics and Monitoring Section, Division of Policy and Practice; Priscilla Akwara; David Brown; Danielle Burke; Xiaodong Cai; Claudia Cappa; Liliana Carvajal; Archana Dwivedi; Anne Genereaux; Rouslan Karimov; Rolf Luyendijk; Nyein Nyein Lwin; Colleen Murray; Holly Newby; Elizabeth Hom-Phathanothai; Khin Wityee Oo; Danzhen You

PROGRAMME, AND POLICY AND COMMUNICATION GUIDANCE

UNICEF Programme Division, Division of Policy and Practice, Division of Communication, and Innocenti Research Centre, with particular thanks to Saad Houry, *Deputy Executive Director;* Hilde Frafjord Johnson, *Deputy Executive Director;* Nicholas Alipui, *Director,* Programme Division; Richard Morgan, *Director,* Division of Policy and Practice; Khaled Mansour, *Director,* Division of Communication; Maniza Zaman, *Deputy Director,* Programme Division; Dan Rohrmann, *Deputy Director,* Programme Division; Susan Bissell, *Associate Director,* Programme Division; Rina Gill, *Associate Director,* Division of Policy and Practice; Wivina Belmonte, *Deputy Director,* Division of Communication; Catherine Langevin-Falcon; Naseem Awl; Paula Claycomb; Beatrice Duncan; Vidar Ekehaug; Maria Cristina Gallegos; Victor Karunan; and Mima Perisic.

PRINTING

Hatteras Press

Foreword

Last year, a young woman electrified a United Nations consultation on climate change in Bonn, simply by asking the delegates, "How old will you be in 2050?"

The audience applauded. The next day, hundreds of delegates wore T-shirts emblazoned with that question – including the Chair, who admitted that in 2050 he would be 110, and not likely to see the results of our failure to act. The young woman's message was clear: The kind of world she will live in someday relies both on those who inherit it and on those who bequeath it to them.

The State of the World's Children 2011 echoes and builds on this fundamental insight. Today, 1.2 billion adolescents stand at the challenging crossroads between childhood and the adult world. Nine out of ten of these young people live in the developing world and face especially profound challenges, from obtaining an education to simply staying alive – challenges that are even more magnified for girls and young women.

In the global effort to save children's lives, we hear too little about adolescence. Given the magnitude of the threats to children under the age of five, it makes sense to focus investment there – and that attention has produced stunning success. In the last 20 years, the number of children under five dying every day from preventable causes has been cut by one third, from 34,000 in 1990 to around 22,000 in 2009.

Yet consider this: In Brazil, decreases in infant mortality between 1998 and 2008 added up to over 26,000 children's lives saved – but in that same decade, 81,000 Brazilian adolescents, 15–19 years old, were murdered. Surely, we do not want to save children in their first decade of life only to lose them in the second.

This report catalogues, in heart-wrenching detail, the array of dangers adolescents face: the injuries that kill 400,000 of them each year; early pregnancy and childbirth, a primary cause of death for teenage girls; the pressures that keep 70 million adolescents out of school; exploitation, violent conflict and the worst kind of abuse at the hands of adults.

It also examines the dangers posed by emerging trends like climate change, whose intensifying effects in many developing countries already undermine so many adolescents' well-being, and by labour trends, which reveal a profound lack of employment opportunities for young people, especially those in poor countries.

Adolescence is not only a time of vulnerability, it is also an age of opportunity. This is especially true when it comes to adolescent girls. We know that the more education a girl receives, the more likely she is to postpone marriage and motherhood – and the more likely it is that her children will be healthier and better educated. By giving all young people the tools they need to improve their own lives, and by engaging them in efforts to improve their communities, we are investing in the strength of their societies.

Through a wealth of concrete examples, *The State of the World's Children 2011* makes clear that sustainable progress is possible. It also draws on recent research to show that we can achieve that progress more quickly and cost-effectively by focusing first on the poorest children in the hardest-to-reach places. Such a focus on equity will help all children, including adolescents.

How can we delay? Right now, in Africa, a teenager weighs the sacrifices she must make to stay in the classroom. Another desperately tries to avoid the armed groups that may force him to join. In South Asia, a pregnant young woman waits, terrified, for the day when she will give birth alone.

The young woman who asked the question in Bonn, along with millions of others, waits not only for an answer, but for greater action. By all of us.

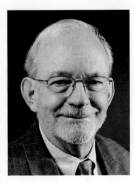

Anthony Lake
Executive Director, UNICEF

CONTENTS

Adolescence: An Age of Opportunity

Essays

PERSPECTIVES

ADOLESCENT VOICES

Figures

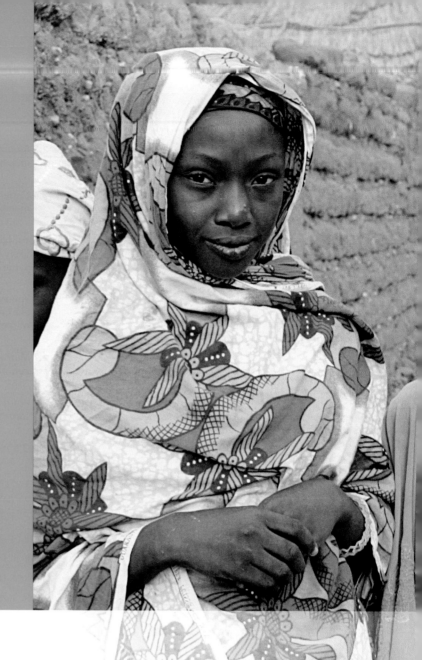

A keener focus on the development and human rights of adolescents would both enhance and accelerate the fight against poverty, inequality and gender discrimination. *Hawa, 12 (second from left), recently re-enrolled in school following the intervention of the National Network of Mothers' Associations for Girls, which advocates for girls' education, Cameroon.*

CHAPTER 1

The Emerging Generation

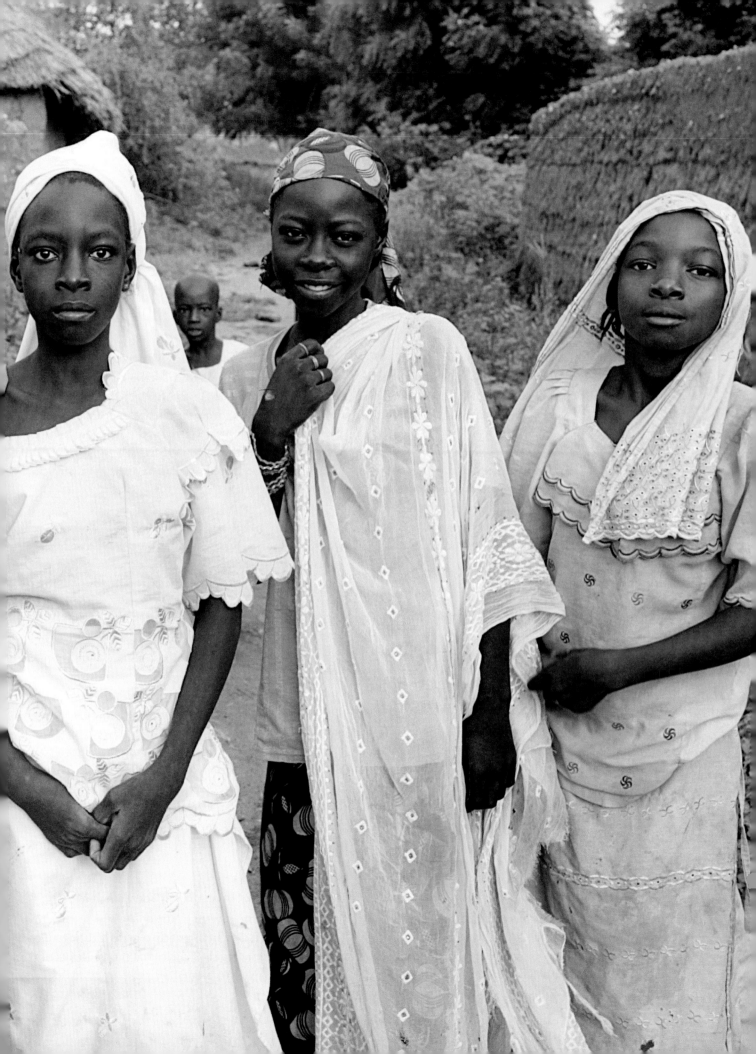

Adolescence is an age of opportunity for children, and a pivotal time for us to build on their development in the first decade of life, to help them navigate risks and vulnerabilities, and to set them on the path to fulfilling their potential.

The world is home to 1.2 billion individuals aged 10–19 years.[1] These adolescents have lived most or all of their lives under the Millennium Declaration, the unprecedented global compact that since 2000 has sought a better world for all.

Many of their number have benefited from the gains in child survival, education, access to safe water, and other areas of development that stand as concrete successes of the drive to meet the Millennium Development Goals, the human development targets at the core of the Declaration. But now they have arrived at a pivotal moment in their lives – just as the world as a whole is facing a critical moment in this new millennium.

In just three years, confidence in the world economy has plummeted. Unemployment has risen sharply, and real household incomes have fallen or stagnated. At the time of writing, in late 2010, the global economic outlook remains highly uncertain, and the possibility of a prolonged economic malaise, with negative implications for social and economic progress in many countries, developing and industrialized alike, still looms.

This economic turmoil and uncertainty have raised the spectre of fiscal austerity, particularly in some industrialized economies, resulting in a more stringent approach to social spending and overseas development assistance. In developing countries, too, public finances have tightened, and social spending, including investments in child-related areas, has come under greater scrutiny.

> "I want to participate in developing my country and promoting human rights for people all over the world."
>
> Amira, 17, Egypt

In this context, the conventional wisdom might dictate that most resources be devoted to children and young people in the first decade of their lives. After all, that is when they are most vulnerable to death, disease and undernutrition; when the effects of unsafe water and poor sanitation pose the greatest threat to their lives; and when the absence of education, protection and care can have the most pernicious lifetime implications.

In contrast, adolescents are generally stronger and healthier than younger children; most have already benefited from basic education; and many are among the hardest and, potentially, most costly to reach with essential services and protection. It hardly seems judicious, in these fiscally straitened times, to focus greater attention on them.

Such reasoning, though seemingly sound in theory, is flawed for several reasons, all stemming from one critical notion: Lasting change in the lives of children and young people, a critical underlying motivation of the Millennium Declaration, can only be achieved and sustained by complementing investment in the first decade of life with greater attention and resources applied to the second.

The imperative of investing in adolescence

The arguments for investing in adolescence are fivefold. The first is that it is right in principle under existing human rights treaties including the Convention on the Rights of the Child, which applies to around 80 per cent of adolescents,

OPPORTUNITIES

and the Convention on the Elimination of All Forms of Discrimination against Women, which applies to all adolescent females.

Second, investing in adolescence is the most effective way to consolidate the historic global gains achieved in early and middle childhood since 1990. The 33 per cent reduction in the global under-five mortality rate, the near-elimination of gender gaps in primary school enrolment in several developing regions and the considerable gains achieved in improving access to primary schooling, safe water and critical medicines such as routine immunizations and antiretroviral drugs – all are testament to the tremendous recent progress achieved for children in early and middle childhood.[2]

But the paucity of attention and resources devoted to adolescents is threatening to limit the impact of these efforts in the second decade of an individual's life. Evidence from around the world shows just how precarious that decade can be: In Brazil, more adolescents die from violence than do children under five from disease and ill health.[3] Global net attendance for secondary school is roughly one third lower than for primary school.[4] Worldwide, one third of all new HIV cases involve young people aged 15–24.[5] And in the developing world, excluding China, 1 in every 3 girls gets married before the age of 18.[6] When confronted with these facts, it is hard to avoid the question: Are our efforts in support of children's rights and well-being limited by a lack of support for adolescents?

Third, investing in adolescents can accelerate the fight against poverty, inequity and gender discrimination. Adolescence is the pivotal decade when poverty and inequity often pass to the next generation as poor adolescent girls give birth to impoverished children. This is particularly true among adolescents with low levels of education. Almost half the world's adolescents of the appropriate age do not attend secondary school.[7] And when they do attend, many of them – particularly those from the poorest and

most marginalized households and communities – fail to complete their studies or else finish with insufficient skills, especially in those high-level competencies increasingly required by the modern globalized economy.

This skills deficit is contributing to bleak youth employment trends. The global economic crisis has produced a

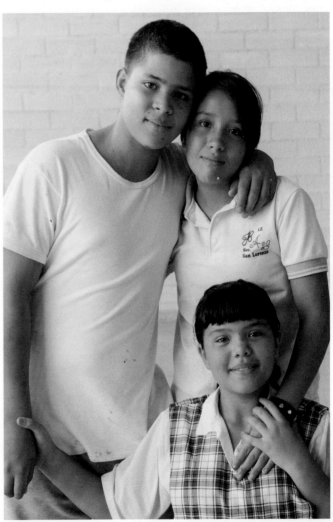

A stronger focus on the second decade of life is imperative to meeting international commitments to children and creating a more peaceful, tolerant and equitable world. *Young students in a secondary school that promotes gender equality, diversity, a culture of peace and respect for human rights; improves social and study skills and self-esteem among students; and encourages the participation of parents and other community members, Colombia.*

large cohort of unemployed youth, which in 2009 stood at around 81 million worldwide.[8] For those who are employed, decent work is scarce: In 2010, young people aged 15 24 formed around one quarter of the world's working poor.[9] In a recent survey of international companies operating in developing countries, more than 20 per cent considered the inadequate education of workers to be a significant obstacle to higher levels of corporate investment and faster economic growth.[10]

The intergenerational transmission of poverty is most apparent among adolescent girls. Educational disadvantage and gender discrimination are potent factors that force them into lives of exclusion and penury, child marriage and domestic violence. Around one third of girls in the developing world, excluding China, are married before age 18; in a few countries, almost 30 per cent of girls under 15 are also married.[11]

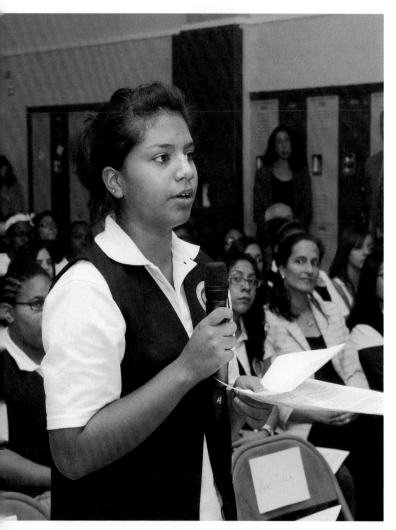

The well-being and the active participation of adolescents are fundamental to the effectiveness of a life-cycle approach that can break the intergenerational transmission of poverty, exclusion and discrimination. *A girl asks a question at a special assembly held at the Young Women's Leadership School of East Harlem, New York City, USA.*

The poorest adolescent girls are also those most likely to be married early, with rates of child marriage roughly three times higher than among their peers from the richest quintile of households. Girls who marry early are also most at risk of being caught up in the negative cycle of premature childbearing, high rates of maternal mortality and morbidity and high levels of child undernutrition. And there is firm evidence to suggest that undernutrition is among the foremost factors that undermine early childhood development.[12]

Adopting a life-cycle approach to child development, with greater attention given to the care, empowerment and protection of adolescents, girls in particular, is the soundest way to break the intergenerational transmission of poverty. Time and again, evidence shows that educated girls are less likely to marry early, less likely to get pregnant as teenagers, more likely to have correct and comprehensive knowledge of HIV and AIDS and more likely to have healthy children when they eventually become mothers. When it is of good quality and relevant to children's lives, education empowers like nothing else, giving adolescents, both female and male, the knowledge, skills and confidence to meet the global challenges of our times.

The urgent need to confront these challenges is the fourth reason for investing in adolescence. Rich and poor alike, adolescents will have to deal with the intergenerational implications of the current economic turmoil, including the structural unemployment that may persist in its wake. They will have to contend with climate change and environmental degradation, explosive urbanization and migration, ageing societies and the rising cost of health care, the HIV and AIDS pandemic, and humanitarian crises of increasing number, frequency and severity.

Far more so than adults, adolescents are disproportionately represented in countries where these critical challenges are likely to be most pressing: those with the lowest incomes, the highest levels of political instability and the fastest rates of urban growth; those most exposed to civil strife and natural disasters and most vulnerable to the ravages of climate change. The adolescents of these countries will need to be equipped with the skills and capacities to address such challenges as they arise throughout the century.

The fifth and final argument for investing in adolescence relates to the way adolescents are portrayed. This quintile of the global populace is commonly referred to as the 'next

Building back better together with young people

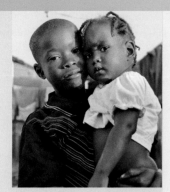

Stanley carries his 2-year-old cousin, Marie Love, near their family's makeshift tent shelter in the Piste Aviation neighbourhood of Port-au-Prince, Haiti.

"A notable aspect of the rebuilding process so far has been the significant role played by young people."

On 12 January 2010, the central region of Haiti was devastated by the strongest earthquake the country had experienced in more than 200 years. Over 220,000 people were killed, 300,000 were injured and 1.6 million were displaced and forced to seek shelter in spontaneous settlements. Children, who make up nearly half the country's total population, have suffered acutely in the earthquake's aftermath. UNICEF estimates that half of those displaced are children, and 500,000 children are considered extremely vulnerable and require child protection services.

Almost a quarter (23 per cent) of Haiti's population is between the ages of 10 and 19, and their situation was extremely difficult even before the earthquake. As the poorest nation in the Western Hemisphere, Haiti lagged well behind the rest of Latin America and the Caribbean in many indicators, and even behind other least developed countries throughout the world. For example, net secondary school attendance in 2005–2009 stood at just 20 per cent (18 per cent for boys and 21 per cent for girls), compared to around 70 per cent for the region as a whole and roughly 28 per cent for the world's least developed countries. Adolescent marriage and pregnancy rates are substantially higher than in other countries in the region. Among 20- to 24-year-old women surveyed in 2005–2006, nearly one third had married by age 18 and 48 per cent by age 20; 30 per cent gave birth for the first time before the age of 20.

These poor education, health and protection outcomes are a direct result of lack of access to services and basic necessities such as water and food due to poverty, political instability, violence and gender-based discrimination. Natural disasters have been a recurring challenge, but the recent earthquake destroyed infrastructure and lives on an unprecedented scale.

The Government has developed an Action Plan for National Recovery and Development of Haiti, with the goal of addressing both short-term and long-term needs. Working with international partners, who pledged US$5.3 billion in the first 18 months following the earthquake and nearly $10 billion over the next three years, the Government is committed to rebuilding the country to be better than its pre-earthquake state. The plan focuses on all aspects of redevelopment, from physical infrastructure and institution-building to cultural preservation, education and food and water security. It prioritizes the needs of pregnant women as well as children's education and health.

A particularly notable aspect of the rebuilding process so far has been the significant role played by young people. Youth groups were critical as responders in search and rescue, first aid and essential goods transport immediately following the earthquake. Since then, they have been important community-based helpers, imparting health information and building infrastructure. The Ecoclubes group, with chapters in the Dominican Republic and Haiti, has been using Pan American Health Organization/World Health Organization materials to provide information on malaria prevention to low-literacy communities. The Water and Youth Movement initiated a campaign to raise $65,000 to train and equip six poor communities with water pumps.

In addition, UNICEF, Plan International and their partners facilitated the voices of 1,000 children in the Post Disaster Needs Assessment (PDNA) process. Child-friendly focus group discussions were held throughout nine of the country's departments. Adolescents and youth who took part raised issues of gender, disability, vulnerability, access to services, disaster risk reduction, and participation in decision-making and accountability mechanisms for the PDNA.

Through partnerships that include young people, programmes have been initiated to vaccinate children, facilitate their return to school, raise awareness of HIV and AIDS, encourage holistic community development and promote sanitation. However, these and future efforts will require continued financial and moral commitment to overcome the host of challenges still to be tackled. One of these is meeting the pressing needs of the most disadvantaged, such as those who lost limbs in the earthquake.

Going forward, it will be critical to listen and respond to the voices of Haiti's young people of all ages, in order to meet their needs, enable them to make the transition to adulthood in such turbulent times – regardless of their poverty status, urban or rural location, gender or ability – and rebuild a stronger, more equitable Haiti.

See References, page 78.

Early and late adolescence

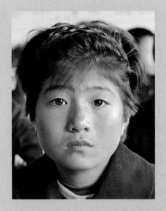

Rim Un Jong, 10, sits in a fourth-grade mathematics class at Jongpyong Primary School in the eastern province of South Hamgyong, Democratic People's Republic of Korea.

The manifest gulf in experience that separates younger and older adolescents makes it useful to consider this second decade of life as two parts: early adolescence (10–14 years) and late adolescence (15–19 years).

Early adolescence (10–14 years)

Early adolescence might be broadly considered to stretch between the ages of 10 and 14. It is at this stage that physical changes generally commence, usually beginning with a growth spurt and soon followed by the development of the sex organs and secondary sexual characteristics. These external changes are often very obvious and can be a source of anxiety as well as excitement or pride for the individual whose body is undergoing the transformation.

The internal changes in the individual, although less evident, are equally profound. Recent neuroscientific research indicates that in these early adolescent years the brain undergoes a spectacular burst of electrical and physiological development. The number of brain cells can almost double in the course of a year, while neural networks are radically reorganized, with a consequent impact on emotional, physical and mental ability.

The more advanced physical and sexual development of girls – who enter puberty on average 12–18 months earlier than boys – is mirrored by similar trends in brain development. The frontal lobe, the part of the brain that governs reasoning and decision-making, starts to develop during early adolescence. Because this development starts later and takes longer in boys, their tendency to act impulsively and to be uncritical in their thinking lasts longer than in girls. This phenomenon contributes to the widespread perception that girls mature much earlier than boys.

It is during early adolescence that girls and boys become more keenly aware of their gender than they were as younger children, and they may make adjustments to their behaviour or appearance in order to fit in with perceived norms. They may fall victim to, or participate in, bullying, and they may also feel confused about their own personal and sexual identity.

Early adolescence should be a time when children have a safe and clear space to come to terms with this cognitive, emotional, sexual and psychological transformation – unencumbered by engagement in adult roles and with the full support of nurturing adults at home, at school and in the community. Given the social taboos often surrounding puberty, it is particularly important to give early adolescents all the information they need to protect themselves against HIV, other sexually transmitted infections, early pregnancy, sexual violence and exploitation. For too many children, such knowledge becomes available too late, if at all, when the course of their lives has already been affected and their development and well-being undermined.

Late adolescence (15–19 years)

Late adolescence encompasses the latter part of the teenage years, broadly between the ages of 15 and 19. The major physical changes have usually occurred by now, although the body is still developing. The brain continues to develop and reorganize itself, and the capacity for analytical and reflective thought is greatly enhanced. Peer-group opinions still tend to be important at the outset, but their hold diminishes as adolescents gain more clarity and confidence in their own identity and opinions.

Risk-taking – a common feature of early to middle adolescence, as individuals experiment with 'adult behaviour' – declines during late adolescence, as the ability to evaluate risk and make conscious decisions develops. Nevertheless, cigarette smoking and experimentation with drugs and alcohol are often embraced in the earlier risk-taking phase and then carried through into later adolescence and beyond into adulthood. For example, it is estimated that 1 in 5 adolescents aged 13–15 smokes, and around half of those who begin smoking in adolescence continue to do so for at least 15 years. The flip side of the explosive brain development that occurs during adolescence is that it can be seriously and permanently impaired by the excessive use of drugs and alcohol.

Girls in late adolescence tend to be at greater risk than boys of negative health outcomes, including depression, and these risks are often magnified by gender-based discrimination and abuse. Girls are particularly prone to eating disorders such as anorexia and bulimia; this vulnerability derives in part from profound anxieties over body image that are fuelled by cultural and media stereotypes of feminine beauty.

These risks notwithstanding, late adolescence is a time of opportunity, idealism and promise. It is in these years that adolescents make their way into the world of work or further education, settle on their own identity and world view and start to engage actively in shaping the world around them.

See References, page 78.

generation' of adults, the 'future generation' or simply 'the future'. But adolescents are also firmly part of the present – living, working, contributing to households, communities, societies and economies.

No less than young children do they deserve protection and care, essential commodities and services, opportunities and support, as well as recognition of their existence and worth. Indeed, in some contexts – particularly with regard to child protection risks such as child marriage, commercial sexual exploitation and children in conflict with the law – adolescents, out of all children, may have the greatest needs. Yet these are precisely the areas where investment and assistance for children are often most lacking and where the least attention is paid, in some cases as a result of political, cultural and societal sensitivities. Given the strong link between protection, education and child survival, it is clear that investing in adolescents, and particularly adolescent girls, is imperative to addressing violence, abuse and exploitation of children and women in earnest.

These facts point to an undeniable truth: Both now and in the coming decades, the fight against poverty, inequality and gender discrimination will be incomplete, and its effectiveness compromised, without a stronger focus on adolescent development and participation.

This truth is known and accepted by many. In the push to meet the Millennium Development Goals and other aspects of the Millennium Declaration, however, there is a risk that the needs of adolescents are not being given sufficient consideration. And their voices, though heard, are rarely heeded.

Adolescents have long demanded that we keep the promise made in the 2000 Millennium Declaration to create a world of tolerance, security, peace and equity – a world fit for children, adolescents, young people – indeed for all of us.

In recent months, UNICEF has begun to refocus its work towards achieving the Goals by redoubling its efforts in pursuit of equity for children, giving priority to those most disadvantaged within countries and communities. While much of the initial drive of the refocus has centred on promoting greater equity in young child survival and

> "Children should not feel afraid or in danger at home or in school."
>
> Victor, 11, Mexico

development, addressing inequity in adolescence is equally important and challenging.

It is in this phase of life, the second decade, that inequities often appear most glaringly. Disadvantage prevents the poorest and most marginalized adolescents from furthering their education with secondary schooling, and it exposes them, girls in particular, to such protection abuses as child marriage, early sex, violence and domestic labour – thus curtailing their potential to reach their full capacity.

If denied their rights to quality education, health care, protection and participation, adolescents are very likely to remain or become impoverished, excluded and disempowered – increasing, in turn, the risk that their children will also be denied their rights.

For these reasons, and in support of the second International Year of Youth, which began on 12 August 2010, UNICEF has dedicated the 2011 edition of its flagship report *The State of the World's Children* to adolescents and adolescence.

The report begins with a brief discussion of the concept of adolescence and explains why a stronger focus on the second decade of life is imperative to meeting international commitments to children and creating a more peaceful, tolerant and equitable world. It then explores the historical context of adolescence, underscoring the growing international recognition of its relative social importance.

The second chapter presents an in-depth appraisal of the global state of adolescents, exploring where they live and the particular challenges they face in survival and health, education, protection and equality.

The third chapter assesses the risks to their present and future well-being posed by emerging trends in economics and employment, by climate change, demographic shifts, juvenile crime and violence, and threats to peace and security.

In its final chapter, *The State of the World's Children 2011* explores ways of empowering adolescents and young people, preparing them for adulthood and citizenship and investing in their well-being, holistic development and active participation. Disaggregated data from international household surveys, supplemented where appropriate by national sources, provide a rich vein of hitherto little used information on adolescents – mostly those in late adolescence (15–19 years) – that constitutes a central feature of the report. The voices of adolescents offering their own perspectives on the state of their world permeate the entire report.

The complexities of defining adolescence

Adolescence is difficult to define in precise terms, for several reasons. First, it is widely acknowledged that each individual experiences this period differently depending on her or his physical, emotional and cognitive maturation as well as other contingencies. Reference to the onset of puberty, which might be seen as a clear line of demarcation between childhood and adolescence, cannot resolve the difficulty of definition.

Puberty occurs at significantly different points for girls and boys, as well as for different individuals of the same sex. Girls begin puberty on average 12–18 months earlier than boys; the median age of girls' first period is 12 years, while boys' first ejaculation generally occurs around age 13. Girls, however, can experience the menarche as early as 8 years old. Evidence shows, moreover, that puberty is beginning earlier than ever before – the age of puberty for both girls and boys has declined by fully three years over the past two centuries, largely due to higher standards of health and nutrition.[13]

This means that girls in particular, but also some boys, are reaching puberty and experiencing some of the key physiological and psychological changes associated with adolescence before they are considered adolescents by the United Nations (defined as individuals 10–19 years old). By the same token, it is not uncommon for boys to enter puberty at the age of 14 or even 15, by which point they will have been effectively treated as adolescents within a school year group for at least two years, associating with boys and girls who are much bigger physically and more developed sexually.[14]

The second factor that complicates any definition of adolescence is the wide variation in national laws setting minimum age thresholds for participation in activities considered the preserve of adults, including voting, marriage, military participation, property ownership and alcohol consumption. A related idea is that of the 'age of majority': the legal age at which an individual is recognized by a nation as an adult and is expected to meet all responsibilities attendant upon that status. Below the age of majority, an individual is still considered a 'minor'. In many countries, the age of majority is 18, which has the virtue of being consonant with the upper threshold of the age range for children under Article 1 of the Convention on the Rights of the Child.

In other countries, this threshold varies widely. One of the lowest national ages of majority is applied to girls in Iran, who reach this threshold at just 9 years old, compared with 15 for Iranian boys.[15] For those countries with ages of majority below 18, the Committee on the Rights of the Child, the monitoring body for the Convention, encourages States parties to review this threshold and to increase the level of protection for all children under 18.

The age of majority is not, however, the only complicating factor in defining adolescence with regard to different national jurisdictions, as it often bears no relation to the

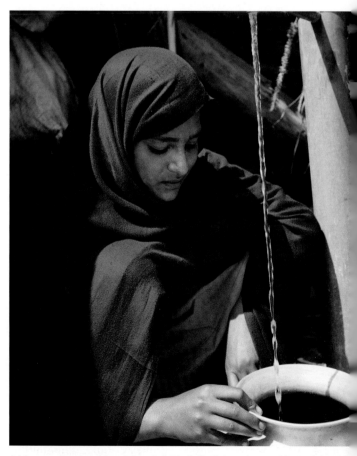

Adolescence is a pivotal decade in an individual's life that requires special attention and protection. *A 12-year-old girl collects water. Since a tap was installed at the doorstep of her family's house, she says that she has more time to do her homework, Pakistan.*

Adult responsibility:
Listen to adolescents' voices

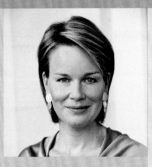

*by Her Royal Highness
Princess Mathilde of
Belgium, Honorary Chair
of UNICEF Belgium and
UNICEF and UNAIDS
Special Representative
for Children and AIDS*

"Adolescents
do not consider
themselves as
'future adults';
they want to be
taken seriously
now."

In the 20 years since the Convention on the Rights of the Child entered into force, the global community has pledged to safeguard children's rights in education, health, participation and protection. These rights entail moral and legal obligations. Governments the world over are held accountable through the Committee on the Rights of the Child for the welfare of their children.

Considerable progress has been made across the world in reducing mortality, improving access to basic health care and ensuring schooling for children during their first decade of life. These accomplishments have paved the way for promising strides in adolescence. We have seen increased secondary school enrolment, albeit from a low base; a decline in early marriage and female genital mutilation/cutting; and an increase in knowledge of HIV transmission. Thanks to global and local efforts to raise awareness, encourage dialogue and build policy, adolescents are better protected from abuse and exploitation. Still, for millions of adolescents, daily life remains a struggle.

A happy upbringing – with opportunities to learn, play and feel safe – is still a distant prospect for many. Instead, millions of teenagers face hazardous employment, early pregnancy and participation in armed conflict. Burdened with adult roles and deprived of their rights as children, adolescents are exposed to protection abuses. Denying this age group their childhood heightens their risk of exploitation in labour, social isolation associated with early marriage, and mortality or morbidity for adolescent girls from pregnancy- and childbirth-related complications. The enormous challenge of protecting adolescents at this vital time in their lives should not be underestimated – and adults have a crucial part to play in meeting it.

Adolescents currently make up 18 per cent of the world's population, but they receive far less attention on the world stage than their numbers merit. Parents, family members and local communities bear a responsibility to promote and protect adolescent development. Implementing laws and pursuing concrete objectives such as the Millennium Development Goals are important ways of building momentum towards investment in adolescents. But if we really want these initiatives to be effective, we must invite young people to be part of the solution and ensure their voices are heard.

Adolescents do not consider themselves as 'future adults'; they want to be taken seriously now. Article 13 of the Convention stipulates that children are free to express their ideas and opinions, through any channel of their choice. Exercising this right not only cultivates self-confidence but also helps prepare them for the active role of citizen.

Equally important, education encourages children to communicate and make their voices heard. Parents, friends and family members play an essential part in stimulating adolescents' educational growth, as learning extends beyond the classroom. A parent's role as mentor should not be underestimated; it deserves more support and appreciation.

I am heartened to hear young peoples' responses to UNICEF Belgium's What Do You Think? project. This effort sheds light on marginalized children: those who are disabled, live in institutions and hospitals, and suffer from poverty. I discovered during my visits with these children that their stories are not, as one might expect, expressions of despair. On the contrary, many articulate extraordinary hope for the future and eagerness to participate in the shaping of their world.

Listening to adolescents is the only way we will understand what they expect from us. This is a critical time in a person's growth. Let us pay close attention to the particular needs and concerns of adolescents. Let us create opportunities for them to participate in society. Let us allow them freedom and opportunity to mature into healthy adults. As the 2015 deadline for the Millennium Development Goals draws near, every effort must be made to ensure the equal well-being of children worldwide. Their hopes and dreams are still very much alive. It is up to us to enable adolescents to reach their full potential. Let us work together with them to make life a positive adventure.

Her Royal Highness Princess Mathilde of Belgium is especially committed to children affected by and living with HIV. In her roles as Honorary Chair of UNICEF Belgium and UNICEF and UNAIDS Special Representative for Children and AIDS, HRH Princess Mathilde has undertaken field trips to Africa and Asia to promote the well-being of vulnerable people and generate awareness of children's rights.

age at which individuals are legally able to perform certain tasks that might be associated with adulthood. This 'age of licence' may vary from activity to activity, and there is certainly no internationally applicable standard. In the United States, for example, where the age of majority is 18, adolescents can legally drive a car at 16 in most states. In contrast, young US adults are generally unable to purchase alcoholic drinks until they are 21.[16]

The age at which marriage is first possible may also diverge significantly from the age of majority. In many countries, a distinction is drawn between the age at which anyone may legally marry and an earlier age at which it is only possible to marry with parental or court permission. This is the case, for example, in Brazil, Chile, Croatia, New Zealand and Spain, where the marriageable age is normally 18 but can be reduced, with parental or court permission, to 16. Many other nations have set a different marriageable age for males and females, normally allowing girls to marry at a younger age than boys. In the world's two most populous countries, for example, the marriageable age for men is higher than that for women – 22 for men and 20 for women in China, and 21 for men and 18 for women in India. In other countries, such as Indonesia, minors are no longer bound by the age of majority once they get married.[17]

The third difficulty in defining adolescence is that, irrespective of the legal thresholds demarcating childhood and adolescence from adulthood, many adolescents and young children across the world are engaged in adult activities such as labour, marriage, primary caregiving and conflict; assuming these roles, in effect, robs them of their childhood and adolescence. In practice, the legal age of marriage is widely disregarded, normally to allow men to marry girls who are still minors. In many countries and communities, child marriage (defined by UNICEF as marriage or union before age 18), adolescent motherhood, violence, abuse and exploitation can in effect deprive girls especially, but also boys, of any adolescence at all. Child marriage in particular is associated with high levels of violence, social marginalization and exclusion from protection services and education. A similar situation occurs with child labour, in which an estimated 150 million children aged 5–14 are engaged.[18]

Weak national birth registration complicates efforts to enforce minimum age thresholds; just 51 per cent of children in the developing world (excluding China) were registered at birth for the period 2000–2009.[19] Without such registration, which is a right under the Convention on the Rights of the Child, it is almost impossible to fully protect

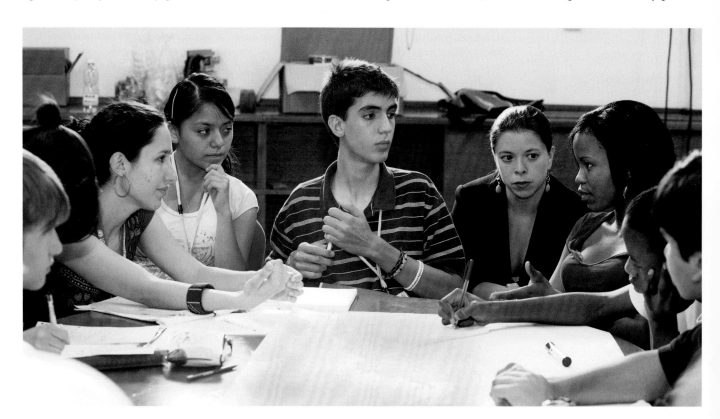

Young people can be instrumental in addressing pressing issues and sharing their recommendations with the global community. *On 6 July 2009, youth delegates discuss global issues during a working group session at the J8 Summit in Rome, Italy.*

Keeping the flame alive:
Indigenous adolescents' right to education and health services

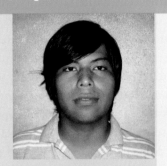

*by Paolo Najera, 17,
Indigenous Térraba,
Costa Rica*

"We just ask for respect for our basic human rights – the respect that every human being deserves in this world."

When I look at the prospects my Térraba people face, my heart sinks for our dying land and drying river. While I do not know much of the world, I know what is right and wrong, and I know this harsh reality is not their fault. The flame of resistance passed on from my great-grandfather to my grandfather, to my father and to me, symbolizes our desire to keep our community alive. My hope is that our indigenous culture and language will endure.

The problem is, my brothers are afraid to live as Térraba Indians. Outside pressures, like teasing, discrimination and disregard for our basic rights have nearly brought our centuries-old struggle for survival to its breaking point. In addition, the country's eight indigenous communities,* including mine, have not been given adequate schools or proper health centres, nor has the integrity of our land been respected.

We want our lifestyle to be protected and our territory not to be invaded by industrial companies that destroy the harmony we have preserved – harmony paid for with the bloodshed our people have suffered. This, however, does not mean we want to be excluded from the world. We just ask for respect for our basic human rights – the respect that every human being deserves in this world. We ask to be seen and listened to.

Thanks to my beloved Térraba school, I am proud to be one of the first and few of my indigenous group to attain higher education and attend university in my country. The education system in Costa Rica is insufficient, and it is worse still for indigenous communities. Inequality is pervasive in the classroom, and the system seeks to preserve neither our identity nor our existence as Indians. I see the Government's lack of investment in indigenous culture reflected in teachers giving lessons using outdated materials or teaching under a tree. I think the Government does not see the assets education can bring to our country, nor the benefit of investing in education for indigenous youth.

In order to provide quality education, our teachers must be provided with proper classrooms and new textbooks. If only the children in my village could access the world through a computer as do children elsewhere. I feel sad that they have been denied their right to education and to achieve their full potential.

Skin tone matters in Costa Rica. If equity existed here, girls in my village would have the same opportunities as the girls from other regions of the country – like better access to technology and secondary school. They would be equipped to promote and protect our culture.

I hope for a time when people will be truly interested in listening to and providing for indigenous people, a time when I would not be one of the few indigenous youth to write an essay such as this one, hoping that it be read and understood. With real equity we would have permanent health centres in indigenous territories, and our secondary education would include lessons in our own culture and language as part of the core curriculum. In spite of being pushed to forget our language and to be ashamed of our way of life, we hold on to our dreams and our will to be indigenous Térraba.

Paolo Najera was recently forced to leave school because of the effects of the economic crisis on his community and family. Paolo's aim is to work in development in order to improve life for indigenous communities, such as his own, in Costa Rica.

*Costa Rica has eight officially recognized indigenous peoples – the Bribris, Cabécares, Brunkas, Ngobe or Guaymi, Huetares, Chorotegas, Malekus and Teribes or Térrabas – about half of whom live in 24 indigenous territories. They make up an indigenous population of 63,876 (1.7 per cent of the country's total population). The Térraba, descendants of Teribes from the Atlantic coast of Panama forced by missionaries to migrate to Costa Rica in the late 17th century, are the second-smallest of these groups, with a population of 621 according to the national census of 2000. Their territory is located in the Boruca-Terre reserve, in the canton of Buenos Aires, in the southern part of Costa Rica.

the rights of adolescents or to prosecute cases of unlawful premature entry into adult roles such as marriage, labour and military service, when the exact age of the child or adolescent plaintiff cannot be determined.

Adolescents and adolescence in the international arena

Although there is no internationally accepted definition of adolescence, the United Nations defines adolescents as individuals aged 10–19: in effect, those in the second decade of their lives.[20] This is the definition that applies to much of the analysis and policy advocacy presented in this report. While the term 'adolescents' is not mentioned in international conventions, declarations or treaties, all adolescents have rights under the Universal Declaration of Human Rights and other major human rights covenants and treaties. Most of them are also covered under the Convention on the Rights of the Child, and adolescent girls are also protected under the Convention on the Elimination of All Forms of Discrimination against Women (CEDAW), the Beijing Platform for Action, and regional instruments such as the Protocol to the African Charter on Human and People's Rights on the Rights of Women in Africa.

Defining adolescence as the second decade of an individual's life makes it possible to collect age-based data for the purpose of analysing this transitional period. Today, it is widely acknowledged that adolescence is a phase separate from both early childhood and adulthood, a period that requires special attention and protection. This was not the case for most of human history.

Widespread acceptance of the importance of adolescence is relatively recent. Indeed, many societies and communities still barely demarcate the line between childhood and adulthood. Adolescents, and often even younger children, are expected to work, pay their own way and even bear arms. In this sense, they are regarded as smaller, less-developed adults.

In other societies, however, the transition from childhood to adulthood has been, or still is, marked by some rite of passage, acknowledging the moment when the individual is expected to assume the independence, responsibilities, expectations and privileges attached to full adulthood. Integral to the notion of a rite of passage is the sense that childhood is a separate space and time from the rest of human life, one that needs to be treated with special care and consideration.

Such precepts were first expressed in the international arena in the first half of the 20th century, through treaties that sought to protect children from exploitative and harmful labour. The first conventions drawn up by the International Labour Organization after the First World War had the goal of protecting child labourers, most of whom were over the age of 10. These included the International Labour Office (ILO) Convention No. 6, Night Work of Young Persons (Industry) Convention of 1919, and ILO Convention No. 10, the Minimum Age (Agriculture) Convention of 1921. The first convention cited here stipulated 16 as the age limit for work in specified hazardous industrial settings, while the second placed clear limits on children's participation in public and private work settings. Most other international legislation introduced between the world wars did not, however, explicitly specify rights for children or adolescents as distinct from those of adults.

After the Second World War, the burgeoning movement for children's rights focused its attention on gaining special recognition for children and adolescents within the newly formed United Nations. This was achieved in 1959 with the Declaration of the Rights of the Child, which was significant in establishing legal provisions to safeguard children's well-being rather than presuming that this could simply be met under the general principles of the major human rights instruments. Children's welfare, rather than their political, economic, civic and social rights, was the principal motivation behind the push for the Declaration.

Two decades later, the UN declared 1979 to be the International Year of the Child, and this was swiftly followed by the first International Youth Year, in 1985. These initiatives raised the profile of global efforts to promote and protect the interests of children and young people. At the same time, advocates for children were busy drawing up an overarching human rights treaty for children by which all States parties would be bound. The Convention on the Rights of the Child, a decade in the drafting, was finally adopted by the United Nations General Assembly on 20 November 1989.

The treaty fulfilled all those hopes with its comprehensiveness and far-sightedness. The rights of all young children and adolescents under age 18 were expressed in such a way as to not only protect their welfare but also give them a central place as rights holders, providing an ethical basis for their active participation in all aspects of their lives.

Ensuring productive work for youth

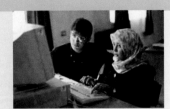

Adolescents attend a computer-skills training session at a social centre for youth in Amman, Jordan.

"Almost 60 per cent of the job seekers in Jordan are below the age of 25."

Jordan is a lower-middle-income country with an average gross national income per capita in 2009 of US$3,740. Owing to the country's limited natural resources, its economy is dominated by commerce and services, which account for more than 70 per cent of gross domestic product (GDP) and more than 75 per cent of jobs. Over the past decade, the country has enjoyed unprecedented growth, with real GDP growth averaging 6.4 per cent yearly between 2003 and 2007. This has been accompanied by improvements in social development indicators, particularly health and education.

Nevertheless, Jordan still faces some key challenges. There is significant income disparity: Almost 14 per cent of the population lives below the poverty line, and between 1995 and 2007 the lowest 40 per cent of income earners earned less than a fifth (18 per cent) of the total income in the country. There are also high rates of unemployment, particularly among the young. While Jordan's overall unemployment rate is 15 per cent, the rate among young people is almost 32 per cent. Nearly 70 per cent of the population is under the age of 30, and adolescents accounted for almost 22 per cent of the total population in 2009. With an annual growth rate of 3.3 per cent between 2000 and 2009, Jordan's population is one of the fastest growing in the world.

According to a 2005 study by the European Training Foundation, almost 60 per cent of the job seekers in Jordan are below the age of 25. The main causes of youth unemployment are lack of career guidance counselling, lack of opportunities to find satisfying work following graduation, the difficulty of obtaining jobs compatible with qualifications, the mismatch between the skills of graduates and the needs of employers, social and cultural obstacles to the full integration of women into the labour market and the wider international economic situation. The risk of being unemployed is greater for women, despite their higher educational achievements. Currently, less than 12 per cent of women participate in the economic sector, putting Jordan close to the bottom of the list of Arab countries in female economic participation.

The Government of Jordan has engaged in a number of policy initiatives to address these challenges.

For instance, the National Social and Economic Development Plan for 2004–2006 aimed at reducing poverty and unemployment. Section I of the plan emphasized the need to address human resource development, including public education, higher education, vocational and technical training and youth care. Its successor, the National Agenda for 2006–2015, focuses on reforming institutional frameworks. The Government has also strengthened collaborative efforts with partner and donor agencies. One example is the development of an Internet-based labour market information system with the support of the Canadian International Development Agency. Managed by the National Centre for Human Resources Development, the project links employers with job seekers and also has a professional career-counselling component.

Partner agencies have also taken steps to increase employment opportunities among young people. For instance, Mustaqbali ('My Future' in Arabic) was launched jointly by UNICEF and Save the Children in 2009 to increase opportunities for adolescents between the ages of 15 and 19 to learn and develop skills that will ultimately enable them to improve their livelihoods and household economic security. It delivers an integrated package of career exploration and preparedness activities to adolescents at various youth and women's centres, and also includes a community awareness component specifically for parents of adolescents, as well as sensitization sessions with private sector employers. The project has been implemented in a number of regions, as well as at the Jerash camp for Palestinian refugees (known locally as the Gaza camp), and has reached more than 250 adolescents, half of them girls. Currently, discussions are ongoing with various stakeholders, including the Government, to scale up the programme at a national level.

Addressing unemployment and poverty remains a critical concern for Jordan. A key part of any solution to this problem will be increasing the participation of women in the labour market. Preparing young people for employment and creating opportunities in the public and private sectors will have both economic and social returns.

See References, page 78.

The Convention was sufficiently inspiring and all encompassing that in merely two decades from its adoption it has been ratified by all but two of the world's nations, becoming the most widely supported human rights treaty in history. Its two Optional Protocols, both adopted by the United Nations in 2000, sought to further strengthen the rights of children by specifying provisions to protect them from involvement in situations of armed conflict and from trafficking, slavery, prostitution and pornography.

Adolescent participation in key international forums has increased steadily in recent decades

Prior to the adoption of the Convention, adolescents' participation in international development and human rights forums was almost non-existent. The 1990 World Summit for Children provided an opportunity to dispel the notion that adolescents are incapable of making a contribution to the international development agenda in general on issues related to them specifically. At this global event, adolescents made their voices and opinions heard on issues affecting them and were instrumental in the formulation of the final outcome document.

This participatory process was replicated during the 2002 UN General Assembly Special Session on Children, which brought more than 400 adolescents from 150 countries to New York to exchange experiences and make demands of world leaders in a three-day Children's Forum. Five years later, adolescents participated in the follow-up to the Special Session, and they also made presentations at the commemorative event celebrating the 20th anniversary of the Convention on 20 November 2009.

TECHNOLOGY

Digital natives and the three divides to bridge

by John Palfrey, Urs Gasser and Colin Maclay of the Berkman Center for Internet & Society, Harvard University, and Gerrit Beger of UNICEF.

While we use the term 'digital natives' to describe the generation born after roughly 1980, not all young people fall into this category. Digital natives share a common global culture defined less by age than by their experience growing up immersed in digital technology. This experience affects their interaction with information technologies and information itself, as well as the ways they relate with one another, other people and institutions.

Reaping the benefits of digital tools, therefore, means more than just being born in a certain period or having access to a laptop. For adolescents to realize the full promise of new technologies, three divides must be bridged. The first has to do with basic access to these technologies and related infrastructure, such as electricity; the second involves the skills needed to use the technologies once they become accessible; and the third stems from our limited understanding of how young people navigate the online world. Each of these divides exists in every society, but their effects are felt most acutely in the developing world.

Over the past decade, access to the Internet, mobile devices and digital media has increased at a rapid rate. Approximately a quarter of the world's 6.8 billion people have access to the Internet, and 86 per cent can connect to the world's communications networks through mobile devices. Yet such access remains highly inequitable, with rates in Africa, for instance, far below those in Europe.

There are signs that committed investment may shrink the access divide. For example, Botswana is developing one of the highest rates of technology penetration in sub-Saharan Africa; the Communications Ministry stated in 2010 that there was "over 100 per cent" mobile coverage (though broadband household Internet access continues to lag behind). Meanwhile, President Paul Kagame of Rwanda has committed to making his country a leader in economic development through investment in new technologies and Internet infrastructure.

While necessary, such efforts are not sufficient. There is also a participation gap between those with sophisticated skills in using digital media and those without. In the developing world, many youth rely on mobile devices rather than fixed line connections with faster speeds. Basic literacy is also an issue.

Digital literacy – the ability to navigate a digitally mediated world – further separates youth who are likely to benefit from digital technologies from those who are not. Young people who do not have access to the Internet at home or in schools – and who lack the support that comes from teachers and parents equipped with strong digital skills – will not develop the necessary social, learning and technical skill sets

Over the past two to three decades, the international community has paid increasing attention to the particular needs of adolescents. This reflects a keener understanding of participation as a right of all children and especially of adolescents. It also underscores a growing acknowledgement that advances in health and education achieved in early and middle childhood must be consolidated in adolescence so as to effectively address the intergenerational transmission of poverty and inequality. In part, this sharper focus has been forced by the global challenges – such as the AIDS pandemic, massive global youth unemployment and underemployment, demographic shifts and climate change – that have emerged as major threats to the present and future for millions of adolescents and young people.

The world is now waking up to the central importance of the rights of adolescents – and to humanity's need to harness the idealism, energy and potential of the emerging generation. But even existing international commitments will not be met unless there is a much greater concentration of resources, strategic planning and political will towards the cause of adolescent rights.

Adolescents are as worthy of care and protection as young children, and as worthy of consideration and participation as adults. Now is the moment for the world to recognize both what it owes to them and the singular dividends that investing in this age of opportunity can generate – for the adolescents themselves and for the societies in which they live.

for success in a wired global economy. Without the opportunity to become familiar with electronic media, adolescents may have trouble navigating social interactions in online communities or recognizing biased, unreliable information.

The third divide is the lack of knowledge about how young people use digital media across societies. In some countries – such as the United Kingdom, the United States and parts of East Asia – both quantitative and qualitative data exist about the ways in which young people use new technologies, and these data have begun to reveal how electronic media are changing practices among youth. Beyond basic information on access, however, such data are scarce in most parts of the world. One challenge is that youth technology practices have only recently become subjects of research, especially outside of a few parts of the world.

It is clear, however, that engagement with digital technologies is transforming learning, socializing and communication among youth who are able to access and use them. For these individuals, activities like content generation, remixing, collaboration and sharing are important aspects of daily life. Many of these activities are 'friendship-driven', serving to maintain relationships with people already known offline. Others are 'interest-driven', allowing youth to develop expertise in specialized skill sets such as animation or blogging. In either context, the casual,

frequent use of new media contributes significantly to the development of both technological and social skills. Electronic media also provide an opportunity for intense, self-directed, interest-driven study.

The benefits of far-reaching digital technologies extend beyond learning to promoting creativity, entrepreneurship and activism. Adolescents and young people are using these technologies to express themselves through videos, audio recordings and games. They are creating inspiring political movements, watchdog groups and new modes of organizing that combine the online and the offline. As they become young adults, some of them are inventing new businesses and technologies that create jobs and opportunities. They teach one another as they build out into the global cyber environment.

Our challenge as a global society is to design and build online experiences for adolescents that help them seize the opportunities – while mitigating the challenges – of life that are partially mediated by digital technologies. If the three divides of digital access can be bridged, new interfaces and experiences will expand adolescents' minds, connect them to people around the world and enable them to participate in the making and sharing of knowledge in the information economy.

" Our challenge as a global society is to design and build online experiences for adolescents and young people that help them seize the opportunities – while mitigating the challenges – of life that are partially mediated by digital technologies."

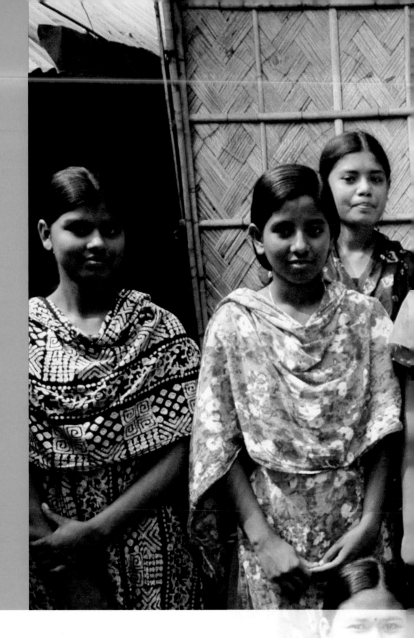

Adolescents are often considered the next generation of actors on the social and economic stage; therefore all societies would benefit from harnessing their energy and skills. *A 16-year-old girl leads an adolescent girls' hygiene-monitoring group that is transforming the slum neighbourhood she lives in, Comilla, Bangladesh.*

CHAPTER 2

Realizing the Rights of Adolescents

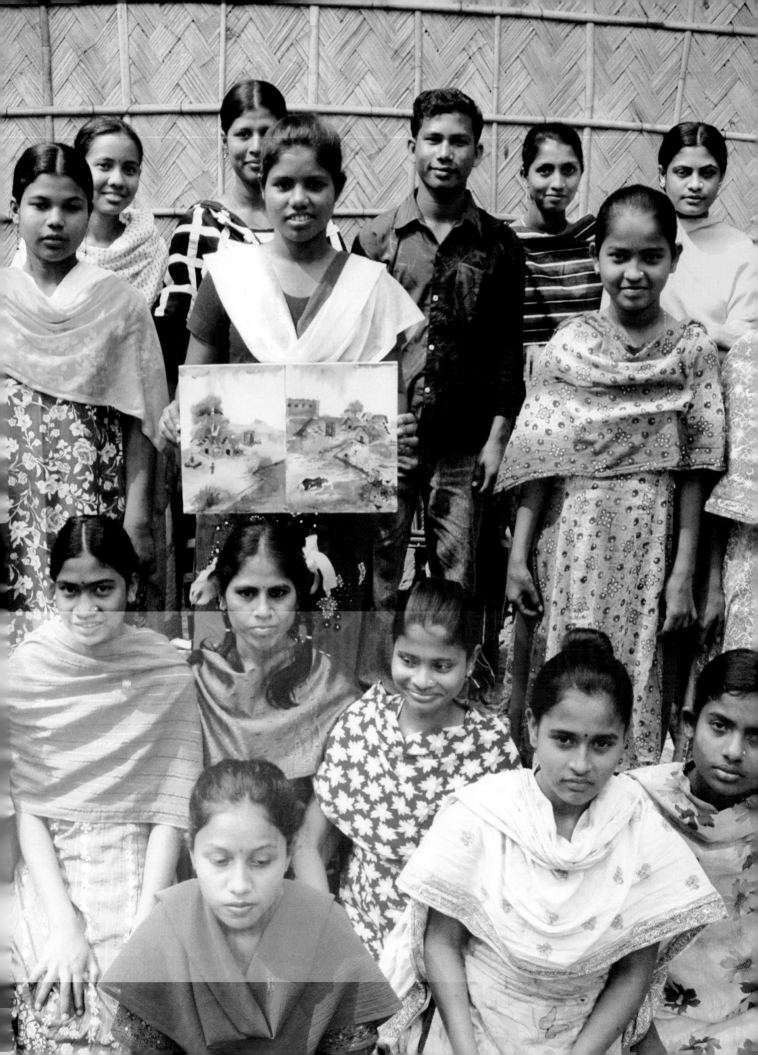

Realizing the rights of adolescents and advancing their development requires a keen understanding of their current circumstances. Using the latest available data from international surveys, supplemented by national sources and research studies where appropriate, this chapter examines the state of adolescent health and education before looking at gender and protection issues.

At the international level, the evidence base on middle childhood (5–9 years) and adolescents (10–19 years) is considerably thinner than it is for early childhood (0–4 years). This relative paucity of data derives from several factors. The survival and health care of children under five years – the time of greatest mortality risk for individuals – has been at the cornerstone of international efforts to protect and care for children for more than six decades. In recent decades, vast leaps have taken place in the collection of health data, driven by the child survival revolution of the 1980s, the 1990 World Summit for Children, the Convention on the Rights of the Child and the push for the MDGs. Consequently, national and international health information systems for children mostly focus on the early years, concentrating on such indicators as neonatal deaths, infant immunization and underweight prevalence among under-fives.

Health information on adolescents, by contrast, is not widely available in many developing countries apart from indicators on sexual and reproductive health collected by major international health surveys, particularly in the context of HIV and AIDS. Where health data on adolescence are available, it is often not disaggregated by sex, age cohort or other factors that could give much-needed details on the situation of adolescents.

Education presents a similar story. The decades-long international drive for universal primary education and, more recently, for early childhood development has fostered the development of indicators and analysis of education in the first decade of life. This is most welcome, and it reflects the growing and sustained commitment of international and national stakeholders to education, increasingly for girls as well as boys.

The evidence base at the international level on secondary education, is far narrower. Sufficient data do not exist to determine the share of secondary-school-age children who complete education at this level globally, or to assess the quality of the education they receive. And as with health, not many developing countries can provide comprehensive disaggregated data on key quantitative and qualitative indicators.

Child protection is the third field in which the availability of data is fundamental to understanding how vulnerable adolescents are to violence, abuse, exploitation, neglect and discrimination. It is heartening that since UNICEF and others began to adapt the 1980s concept of 'children in especially difficult circumstances' into the more holistic concept of child protection, we now have many more key protection indicators. Thanks to the USAID-supported Demographic and Health Surveys (DHS) and the UNICEF-supported Multiple Indicator Cluster Surveys (MICS) in particular – but also to national systems – data are available on child labour, child marriage, birth registration and female genital mutilation/cutting. More recently, through both expanded household surveys and targeted studies, data have emerged on other child protection concerns such as violence.

But the scope for more and better information on child protection remains vast. Many aspects of this most vulnerable of areas for adolescents are still hidden from view, partly owing to intractable difficulties associated with the collection of such information in circumstances often involving secrecy and illegality. Furthermore, the international household surveys from which much of the data on adolescents is derived do not, by definition, capture adolescent males and females living outside the household – in institutions, for example, or on the streets, in slums or in informal peri-urban settlements where records do not exist.

Oft-quoted estimates of the number of children associated with or affected by armed conflict and child trafficking and of those in conflict with the law – to name but three areas – are outdated, not fully reliable and generally believed to vastly underestimate the true scope of the abuse.

This pattern of data collection is beginning to change. Enhanced national surveys and censuses, along with international household surveys such as MICS and DHS, are providing an increasingly rich vein of evidence on the situation of adolescents and young people on a wide range of issues. Recent work by the UNESCO Institute of Statistics, the Education for All Initiative and other mechanisms are providing a stronger evidence base on education than before. Analysis of this new data is enriching our understanding of the state of adolescents worldwide and will enhance the international community's ability to realize their rights.

Health in adolescence
Healthier adolescents today, despite lingering risks

Despite popular perceptions to the contrary, adolescents across the world are generally healthier today than in previous generations. This is in large measure a legacy of greater attention to and investment in early childhood, higher rates of infant immunization and improved infant

> "Adolescents need the opportunity to assert themselves, express themselves, to flourish."
>
> Mamadou, 19, Senegal

nutrition, which yield physiological benefits that persist into adolescence.

Those children who reach adolescence have already negotiated the years of greatest mortality risk. While the survival of children in their earliest years is threatened on many fronts – for example, by birth complications, infectious diseases and undernutrition – mortality rates for adolescents aged 10–14 are lower than for any other age cohort. Rates for young people aged 15–24, while slightly higher, are still relatively low. Girls have lower rates of mortality in adolescence than boys, though the difference is much more marked in industrialized countries than in developing countries.[1]

Yet in 2004 almost 1 million children under age 18 died of an injury.[2] Risks to adolescent survival and health stem from several causes, including accidents, AIDS, early pregnancy, unsafe abortions, risky behaviours such as tobacco consumption and drug use, mental health issues and violence. These risks are addressed below, with the exception of violence, which is tackled later on in the section on gender and protection.

Survival and general health risks
Accidents are the greatest cause of mortality among adolescents

Injuries are a growing concern in public health in relation to younger children and adolescents alike. They are the leading cause of death among adolescents aged 10–19, accounting for almost 400,000 deaths each year among this age group. Many of these deaths are related to road traffic accidents.[3]

Fatalities from injuries among adolescents are highest among the poor, with low- and middle-income countries experiencing the greatest burden. Road traffic accidents

Demographic trends for adolescents:
Ten key facts

Figure 2.1: Adolescent population (10–19 years) by region, 2009

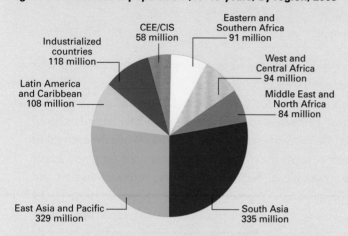

Source: United Nations, Department of Economic and Social Affairs, Population Division, *World Population Prospects: The 2008 Revision,* <www.esa.un.org/unpd/wpp2008/index.htm>, accessed October 2010.

Figure 2.2: Trends in the adolescent population, 1950–2050

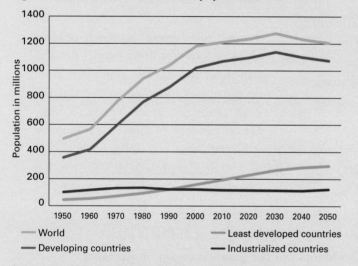

Source: United Nations, Department of Economic and Social Affairs, Population Division, *World Population Prospects: The 2008 Revision,* <www.esa.un.org/unpd/wpp2008/index.htm>, accessed October 2010.

- In 2009, there were 1.2 billion adolescents aged 10–19 in the world, forming 18 per cent of world population. Adolescent numbers have more than doubled since 1950.

- The vast majority of adolescents – 88 per cent – live in developing countries. The least developed countries are home to roughly 1 in every 6 adolescents.

- More than half the world's adolescents live in either the South Asia or the East Asia and Pacific region, each of which contains roughly 330 million adolescents.

- On current trends, however, the regional composition of adolescents is set to alter by mid-century. In 2050, sub-Saharan Africa is projected to have more adolescents than any other region, marginally surpassing the number in either of the Asian regions.

- India has the largest national population of adolescents (243 million), followed by China (207 million), United States (44 million), Indonesia and Pakistan (both 41 million).

- Adolescents account for only 12 per cent of people in the industrialized world, reflecting the sharp ageing of Europe and Japan in particular. In contrast, adolescents account for more than 1 in every 5 inhabitants of sub-Saharan Africa, South Asia and the least developed countries.

- Adolescent boys outnumber girls in all regions with data available, including the industrialized countries. Parity is closest in Africa, with 995 girls aged 10–19 for every 1,000 boys in Eastern and Southern Africa and 982 girls per 1,000 boys in West and Central Africa, while the gender gap is greatest in both Asian regions.

- At the global level, adolescents' share of the total population peaked in the 1980s at just over 20 per cent.

- Although adolescent numbers will continue to grow in absolute terms until around 2030, adolescents' share of the total population is already declining in all regions except West and Central Africa and will steadily diminish all over the world through 2050.

- One trend that will continue to intensify in the coming decades is that ever more adolescents will live in urban areas. In 2009, around 50 per cent of the world's adolescents lived in urban areas. By 2050, this share will rise to almost 70 per cent, with the strongest increases occurring in developing countries.

See References, page 78.

are a regular threat in urban areas, and rising affluence – with attendant increases in traffic volume – may account for the higher road fatalities recently seen in Asia and the eastern Mediterranean. Boys are more prone than girls to injury and death from such accidents as well as from violence stemming from chance encounters or organized gang conflict. Because the rate of urbanization is most rapid in the poorest regions of sub-Saharan Africa and South Asia – which are also the areas with the greatest share of adolescents in the population – averting injuries in the second decade of life must become a major international health objective.[4]

Tobacco consumption and drug and alcohol use are growing health risks for adolescents

In part, injuries arise from a propensity to take risks that is a common feature of adolescence, connected with the psychological need to explore boundaries as part of the development of individual identity. Such readiness to take risks leads many adolescents to experiment with tobacco, alcohol and other addictive drugs without sufficient understanding of the potential damage to health or of other long-term consequences of addiction, such as being drawn into crime to pay for a habit.

The most common addiction is cigarette smoking, a habit that almost all tobacco users form while in their adolescent years.

It is estimated that half the 150 million adolescents who continue smoking will in the end die from tobacco-related causes.[5] Risky behaviours often overlap: A 2007 UNICEF report on child poverty in Organisation for Economic Co-operation and Development (OECD) countries indicated that adolescents who smoke are three times more likely to use alcohol regularly and eight times more likely to use cannabis.[6]

Nutritional status

Adolescent females are more prone to nutritional difficulties than adolescent males

In early childhood (0–4 years), the available international evidence suggests that differences in nutritional status between girls and boys are statistically negligible in all regions except South Asia.[7] As the years pass, however, girls run a greater risk than boys of nutritional difficulties, notably anaemia. Data from 14 developing countries show a considerably higher incidence of anaemia among female adolescents aged 15–19 as compared to their male counterparts in all but one country.[8]

In nine countries – all, aside from India, in West and Central Africa – more than half of girls aged 15–19 are anaemic.[9] India also has the highest underweight prevalence among adolescent girls among the countries with available data, at 47 per cent. The implications for adolescent girls in this

Figure 2.3: Anaemia is a significant risk for adolescent girls (15–19) in sub-Saharan Africa and South Asia

Prevalence of anaemia among adolescent girls aged 15–19 in a subset of high-prevalence countries with available data*

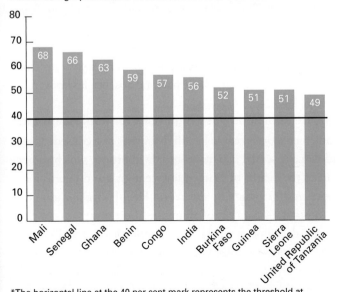

*The horizontal line at the 40 per cent mark represents the threshold at which anaemia is considered a severe national public health issue.
Source: DHS and national surveys, 2003–2009.

Figure 2.4: Underweight is a major risk for adolescent girls (15–19) in sub-Saharan Africa and South Asia

Percentage of adolescent girls aged 15–19 who are underweight* in a subset of high-prevalence countries with available data

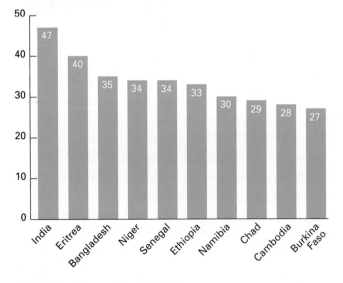

* Defined as a body mass index of 18.5 or less.
Source: DHS and other national surveys, 2002–2007.

country are particularly serious, given that in the period 2000–2009, around 47 per cent of Indian women aged 20–24 were married by age 18.[10] Adolescent pregnancy is a regular consequence of child marriage, and underweight mothers have a higher risk of maternal death or morbidity.

Obesity is a growing and serious concern in both industrialized countries and the developing world. Data from a subset of 10 developing countries show that the percentage of girls aged 15–19 who are overweight (i.e., those with a body mass index above 25.0) ranges between 21 and 36 per cent.[11] Among the OECD countries, the highest levels of obesity in 2007 were found in the four southern European countries of Greece, Italy, Spain and Portugal, together with the mainly Anglophone nations of Canada, the United Kingdom and the United States.[12]

Sexual and reproductive health matters

Girls are more likely to have engaged in early sex in adolescence but also less likely to use contraception

Investing in sexual and reproductive health knowledge and services for early adolescents is critical for several reasons. The first is that some adolescents are engaging in sexual relations in early adolescence; international household survey data representative of the developing world, excluding China, indicate that around 11 per cent of females and 6 per cent of males aged 15–19 claim to have had sex before the age of 15.[13]

Latin America and the Caribbean is the region with the highest proportion of adolescent females claiming to have had their sexual debut before age 15, at 22 per cent (there are no equivalent figures for young men for this region). The lowest reported levels of sexual activity for both boys and girls under 15 occur in Asia.[14]

The second reason concerns the alarming and consistent disparity in practice and knowledge of sexual and reproductive health between adolescent males and adolescent females. Adolescent males appear more likely to engage is risky sexual behaviour than adolescent females. In 19 selected developing countries with available data, males aged 15–19 were consistently more likely than females to have engaged in higher-risk sex with non-marital, non-cohabiting partners in the preceding 12 months. The data also suggest, however, that boys are more likely than girls to use a condom when they engage in such higher-risk sex – despite the fact that girls are at greater risk of sexually transmitted infections, including HIV. These findings underscore the importance of making high-quality sexual and reproductive health services and knowledge available to adolescent girls and boys alike from an early age.[15]

Early pregnancy, often as a consequence of early marriage, increases maternity risks

The third challenge is empowering adolescent girls in particular with the knowledge of sexual and reproductive health, owing to the gender-related protection risks they face in many countries and communities. Child marriage, often deemed by elders to protect girls – and, to a much lesser extent, boys – from sexual predation, promiscuity and social ostracism, in fact makes children more likely to be ignorant about health and more vulnerable to school dropout. Many adolescent girls are required to marry early, and when they become pregnant, they face a much higher risk of maternal mortality, as their bodies are not mature enough to cope with the experience.

The younger a girl is when she becomes pregnant, whether she is married or not, the greater the risks to her health. In Latin America, for example, a study shows that girls who give birth before the age of 16 are three to four times times more likely to suffer maternal death than women in their twenties. Complications related to pregnancy and childbirth are among the leading causes of death worldwide for adolescent girls between the ages of 15 and 19.[16]

For girls, child marriage is also associated with an increased risk of sexually transmitted infections and unwanted pregnancies. Research suggests that adolescent pregnancy is related to factors beyond girls' control. One study undertaken in Orellana, an Ecuadorian province in the Amazon basin, where nearly 40 per cent of girls aged 15–19 are or have been pregnant, found that the pregnancies had much less to do with choices made by the girls themselves than with structural factors such as sexual abuse, parental absence and poverty.[17]

Unsafe abortions pose high risks for adolescent girls

A further serious risk to health that arises as a consequence of adolescent sexual activity is unsafe abortion, which directly causes the deaths of many adolescent girls and injures many more. A 2003 study by the World Health Organization estimates that 14 per cent of all unsafe abortions that take place in the developing world – amounting to 2.5 million that year – involve adolescents under age 20.[18] Of the unsafe abortions that involve adolescents, most are conducted by untrained practitioners and often take place in hazardous circumstances and unhygienic conditions.[19]

Risks and opportunities for the world's largest national population of adolescent girls

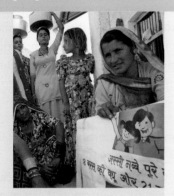

Khamma Devi, an advocate for women in the community, explains the ill effects of child marriage to girls and women in Himmatpura Village, India.

"Ensuring the nutritional, health and educational needs of its adolescent population, particularly girls, remains a key challenge for India."

India is home to more than 243 million adolescents, who account for almost 20 per cent of the country's population. Over the past two decades, rapid economic growth – with real gross domestic product averaging 4.8 per cent between 1990 and 2009 – has lifted millions of Indians out of poverty; this, combined with government programmes, has led to the improved health and development of the country's adolescents. However, many challenges remain for India's youthful population, particularly for girls, who face gender disparities in education and nutrition, early marriage and discrimination, especially against those belonging to socially excluded castes and tribes.

India ranked 119 out of 169 country rankings in the United Nations Development Programme's gender inequality index (GII) in 2010. While the country has made significant progress towards gender parity in primary education enrolment, which stands at 0.96, gender parity in secondary school enrolment remains low at 0.83. Adolescent girls also face a greater risk of nutritional problems than adolescent boys, including anaemia and underweight. Underweight prevalence among adolescent girls aged 15–19 is 47 per cent in India, the world's highest. In addition, over half of girls aged 15–19 (56 per cent) are anaemic. This has serious implications, since many young women marry before age 20 and being anaemic or underweight increases their risks during pregnancy. Anaemia is the main indirect cause of maternal mortality, which stood at 230 maternal deaths per 100,000 live births in 2008. Such nutritional deprivations continue throughout the life cycle and are often passed on to the next generation.

Although the legal age for marriage is 18, the majority of Indian women marry as adolescents. Recent data show that 30 per cent of girls aged 15–19 are currently married or in union, compared to only 5 per cent of boys of the same age. Also, 3 in 5 women aged 20–49 were married as adolescents, compared to 1 in 5 men. There are considerable disparities depending on where girls live. For instance, while the prevalence of child marriage among urban girls is around 29 per cent, it is 56 per cent for their rural counterparts.

The Government of India, in partnership with other stakeholders, has made considerable efforts to improve the survival and development of children and adolescents. One such effort is the adolescent anaemia control programme, a collaborative intervention supported by UNICEF that began in 2000 in 11 states. The main objective of the programme is to reduce the prevalence and severity of anaemia in adolescent girls through the provision of iron and folic acid supplements (weekly), deworming tablets (bi-annually) and information on improved nutrition practices. The programme uses schools as the delivery channel for those attending school and community Anganwadi Centres, through the Integrated Child Development Services programme, for out-of-school girls. The programme currently reaches more than 15 million adolescent girls and is expected to reach 20 million by the end of 2010. Attention has also been given to child protection issues. In 2007, the Government enacted the Prohibition of Child Marriage Act, 2006 to replace the earlier Child Marriage Restraint Act, 1929. The legislation aims to prohibit child marriage, protect its victims and ensure punishment for those who abet, promote or solemnize such marriages. However, implementation and enforcement of the law remain a challenge.

Non-governmental organizations such as the Centre for Health Education, Training and Nutrition Awareness (CHETNA) work closely with the Government and civil society to improve the health and nutrition of children, youth and women, including socially excluded and disadvantaged groups. CHETNA also works to bring awareness of gender discrimination issues to communities, particularly to boys and men, and provides support for comprehensive gender-sensitive policies at state and national levels.

Ensuring the nutritional, health and educational needs of its adolescent population, particularly girls, remains a key challenge for India. Widening disparities, gender discrimination and the social divide among castes and tribes are also among the barriers to advancing the development and protection rights of young people. Increased investment in the country's large adolescent population will help prepare them to be healthy and productive citizens. As these young people reach working age in the near future, the country will reap the demographic dividend of having a more active, participatory and prosperous society.

See References, page 78.

Gathering accurate data on adolescent abortions is almost impossible given the level of secrecy and shame surrounding the procedure, but the number has been estimated at 1 million–4 million per year.[20] Many of the girls and women who seek abortions do so because they have had insufficient control over their own fertility, whether because of poverty, ignorance, problems with male partners or lack of access to contraception.

HIV and AIDS

HIV and AIDS are life-threatening challenges for adolescents in high-prevalence countries

Preventing the transmission of HIV is one of the most important challenges for adolescent survival and health. Although AIDS is estimated to be only the eighth leading cause of death among adolescents aged 15–19, and the sixth leading cause among 10–14-year-olds, it takes a disproportionately high toll in high-prevalence countries.[21] It is the sheer scale of the AIDS epidemic in Eastern and Southern Africa that

makes this disease a prominent cause of death for women aged 15–29 worldwide, as well as one of the leading causes of death for men in this age group.[22]

Many new HIV cases worldwide involve young people aged 15–24. In four of the world's seven regions, young females are more likely to be living with HIV than young males – around twice as likely. In Eastern and Southern African countries with adult HIV prevalence of 10 per cent or higher, prevalence among girls and women aged 15–24 is two to three times higher than it is for their male peers.[23]

The risk of HIV infection is considerably higher among adolescent girls than adolescent boys

Adolescent girls are at far greater risk of contracting HIV than boys, as data from six countries in Eastern and Southern Africa show. In Lesotho, for example, population based survey data show that HIV prevalence among males aged 15–19 was around 2 per cent in 2004, compared with 8 per cent for girls of the same age. The risks of HIV preva-

Figure 2.5: Young males in late adolescence (15–19) are more likely to engage in higher risk sex than females of the same age group

Percentage of young people aged 15–19 who had higher-risk sex with a non-marital, non-cohabitating partner in the last 12 months in selected countries

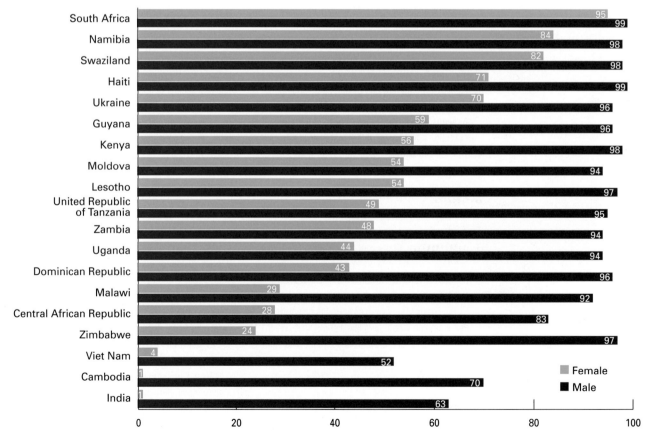

Source: DHS, MICS and national surveys, 2003–2009.

lence for both sexes continue to rise for the following two five-year cohorts (20–24 years and 25–29 years).[24]

The higher incidence of the virus among girls and women is not solely a result of their greater physiological susceptibility. In many settings, adolescent girls and young women face a high risk of sexual violence and rape, both inside and outside of marriage. Child marriage, though often intended by families to shield girls and young women from physical and sexual risks, often fails to protect them from HIV and other sexually transmitted diseases because condom use tends to be lower in long-term relationships. Moreover, the available evidence indicates that adolescent girls in child marriages, and women in general, have less say than their partners over the use of contraception or over whether sex takes place at all.

Enhancing HIV services and knowledge is essential to empowering and protecting adolescents

Investment in HIV prevention and treatment is critical to reversing the spread of HIV in adolescence. Offering adolescents and young people high-quality reproductive health services, and ensuring that they have sound knowledge of sexually transmitted infections, empowers them in their choices and behaviours. Making such services and knowledge available in early adolescence, particularly for girls, is imperative; by late adolescence, the risk of infection for young people in high-prevalence countries is already considerable.

Encouragingly, efforts to enhance knowledge of HIV across the developing world are beginning to bear fruit. Analysis of 11 developing countries with available trend data shows that in 10 countries adolescent girls were more likely to know where to go for an HIV test in the latter half of the 2000s than they were in the early years of the decade.[25] Testing remains low, however, among both sexes. In contrast to testing, when it comes to comprehensive knowledge about HIV prevention, adolescent males consistently edge ahead of their female counterparts; and closing this divide is a particular challenge. For both

Figure 2.6: Young women in late adolescence (15–19) are more likely to seek an HIV test and receive their results than young men of the same age group

Percentage of young people aged 15–19 years who have been tested for HIV in the last 12 months and received results in selected countries

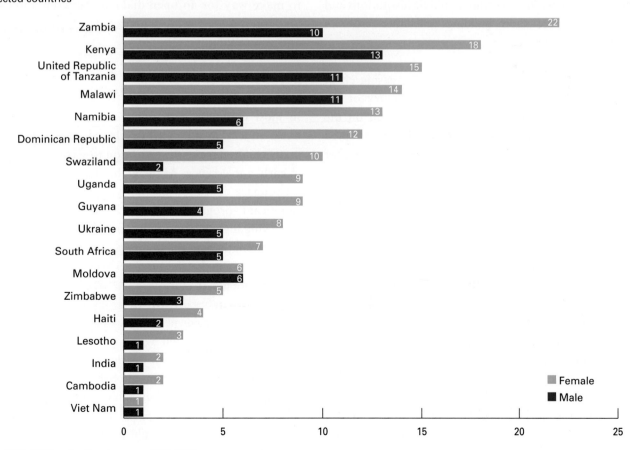

Source: DHS, MICS and national surveys, 2003–2009.

sexes, there is still a considerable gap between knowing about HIV and actually changing practices; this stems partly from the difficulty of addressing social and cultural mores.

Disability in adolescence

Nobody knows how many adolescents are affected by physical or mental disability. Adolescents with disabilities are likely to suffer forms of discrimination, exclusion and stigmatization similar to those endured by younger children. Disabled adolescents are often segregated from society and regarded as passive victims or objects of charity. They are also vulnerable to physical violence and abuse of all kinds. They are substantially less likely to be in school, and even if they are, they may suffer below-average transition rates. This lack of educational opportunities may contribute to long-term poverty.

An equity-based approach to disability – together with the assertive campaigning of disability-rights organizations – has led to a sharp change in perceptions. This approach, founded on human rights, emphasizes the barriers and bottlenecks that exclude children and adolescents living with disabilities. Such barriers include retrograde attitudes, government policies, the structure of public institutions and lack of access to transport, buildings and other resources that should be available to all.

This evolution of attitudes is having an increasing effect on policy and practice in almost every country of the world. A seal was set on it by the Convention on the Rights of Persons with Disabilities, which was adopted by the United Nations General Assembly in December 2006.[26]

Nevertheless, adolescents with disabilities still all too often suffer discrimination and exclusion. Disability issues cannot be considered in isolation but must factor into all areas of provision for adolescents.

Adolescent-friendly health services

Adolescents face health challenges that paediatric and adult physicians alike are often ill-equipped to handle. Rapid physical and emotional growth, as well as the frequently conflicting and influential cultural messages they receive from the outside world, account for the unique nature of their health concerns. Without proper education and support, adolescents lack the knowledge and confi-

dence to make informed decisions about their health and safety – decisions that may have life-long consequences. In order to protect young people from health threats such as disease, sexually transmitted infections, early and unwanted pregnancy, HIV transmission and drug and alcohol abuse, communities must address their particular needs, and governments must invest in establishing adolescent-friendly health care services in hospitals, clinics and youth centres.

Studies show that adolescents avoid health care services – effectively nullifying preventive care – and distrust staff. They can be put off by the long waits, distance to health facilities or unwelcoming services, or they may feel too ashamed to ask for the money to cover the cost of their visit. Creating a welcoming, private space, where adolescents feel comfortable and are able to obtain prescriptions and counselling, is crucial to realizing their right to adequate health care services. Adolescent-friendly health facilities should be physically accessible, open at convenient times, require no appointments, offer services for free and provide referrals to other relevant services. In addition, cultural, generational and gender-specific barriers must be broken down to make way for an open dialogue between adolescents and trained staff who can provide effective treatment and counselling.

Education in adolescence

In most countries with universal or near-universal primary education and well-developed education systems, many children make the transition to secondary education in early adolescence. At the global level, however, universal primary education has not yet been achieved, despite significant progress towards it over the last decade. Achieving higher rates of primary education is fundamental to strengthening the numbers of early adolescents who are ready to make the jump to secondary school at the appropriate age.

Net primary enrolment in developing countries stood at 90 per cent for boys and 87 per cent for girls in the period 2005–2009, with much lower levels of 81 per cent and 77 per cent respectively in sub-Saharan Africa, the most disadvantaged region.[27] Many millions of adolescents across the world have not completed a full course of quality primary education that would prepare them to participate in secondary education.

Adolescent mental health: An urgent challenge for investigation and investment

It is estimated that around 20 per cent of the world's adolescents have a mental health or behavioural problem. Depression is the single largest contributor to the global burden of disease for people aged 15–19, and suicide is one of the three leading causes of mortality among people aged 15–35. Globally, an estimated 71,000 adolescents commit suicide annually, while up to 40 times as many make suicide attempts. About half of lifetime mental disorders begin before age 14, and 70 per cent by age 24. The prevalence of mental disorders among adolescents has increased in the past 20–30 years; the increase is attributed to disrupted family structures, growing youth unemployment and families' unrealistic educational and vocational aspirations for their children.

Unassisted mental health problems among adolescents are associated with low educational achievement, unemployment, substance use, risk-taking behaviours, crime, poor sexual and reproductive health, self-harm and inadequate self-care – all of which increase the lifetime risk of morbidity and premature mortality. Mental health problems among adolescents carry high social and economic costs, as they often develop into more disabling conditions later in life.

"Mental health problems account for a large proportion of the disease burden among young people in all societies."

The risk factors for mental health problems are well established and include childhood abuse; family, school and neighbourhood violence; poverty; social exclusion and educational disadvantage. Psychiatric illness and substance abuse in parents, as well as marital violence, also place adolescents at increased risk, as does exposure to the social disruption and psychological distress that accompany armed conflict, natural disasters and other humanitarian crises. The stigma directed towards young people with mental disorders and the human rights violations to which they are subjected amplify the adverse consequences.

In many countries, only a small minority of young people with mental health problems receive basic assessment and care, while most suffer needlessly, unable to access appropriate resources for recognition, support and treatment. Despite the substantial progress in developing effective interventions, most mental health needs are unmet, even in wealthier societies – and in many developing countries, the rate of unmet need is nearly 100 per cent.

Mental health problems in young people thus present a major public health challenge worldwide. Preventive efforts can help forestall the development and progression of mental disorders, and early intervention can limit their severity. Young people whose mental health needs are recognized function better socially, perform better in school and are more likely to develop into well-adjusted and productive adults than those whose needs are unmet. Mental health promotion, prevention and timely treatment also reduce the burden on health-care systems.

Greater public awareness of mental health issues and general social support for adolescents are essential to effective prevention and assistance. Safeguarding adolescent mental health begins with parents, families, schools and communities. Educating these critical stakeholders about mental health can help adolescents enhance their social skills, improve their problem-solving capacity and gain self-confidence – which in turn may alleviate mental health problems and discourage risky and violent behaviours. Adolescents themselves should also be encouraged to contribute to debates and policy-making on mental health.

Early recognition of emotional distress and the provision of psychosocial support by trained individuals – who need not be health workers – can mitigate the effects of mental health problems. Primary health-care workers can be trained to use structured interviews to detect problems early on and provide treatment and support. Psycho-educational programs in schools, supportive counselling and cognitive-behavioural therapy, ideally with the involvement of the family, are all effective in improving the mental health of adolescents, while the complex needs of young people with serious mental disorders can be addressed through stepped referrals to specialist services.

At the international level, a number of instruments and agreements are in place to promote the health and development of adolescents, most notably the Convention on the Rights of the Child and the Convention on the Rights of Persons with Disabilities. The integration of mental health into primary health-care systems is a major endeavour to reduce the treatment gap for mental health problems. To that end, the World Health Organization and its partners have developed the 4 S Framework, which provides a structure for national initiatives to gather and use strategic information; develop supportive, evidence-informed policies; scale up the provision and utilization of health services and commodities; and strengthen links with other government sectors. Such integration will increase the accessibility of services and reduce the stigma attached to mental disorders.

One of the most urgent tasks in addressing adolescent mental health is improving and expanding the evidence base, particularly in resource-constrained countries. Systematic research on the nature, prevalence and determinants of mental health problems in adolescents – and on prevention, early intervention and treatment strategies – will be pivotal to ensuring adolescents' rights to health and development in these settings.

See References, page 78.

Facing the challenge:
Reproductive health for HIV-positive adolescents

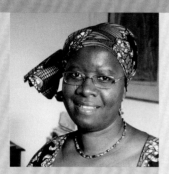

by Nyaradzayi Gumbonzvanda, General Secretary, World Young Women's Christian Association

"Most adolescents living with HIV struggle for recognition, rights, protection and support."

In recent years, the global community has also made great strides to protect children and facilitate access to education and health services for HIV-positive children and orphans. Organizations such as UNICEF, faith-based organizations and women's networks such as the World Young Women's Christian Association (YWCA) have directed resources to train caregivers in social protection policies and to defend children's rights to information and dignity.

Many of those living with HIV are adolescents. These young people do not fit any one model: They are in school, out of school, living with foster parents, in stable families, heading families or seeking employment. But all of them deserve a nurturing environment and coherent support to make informed decisions about their particular condition. In the last two years, the World YWCA conducted a series of dialogues with HIV-positive adolescent girls on the particular issues they face. We discovered three key challenges that adolescents living with HIV contend with: disclosure, education and developing relationships.

First, in terms of disclosure, many children and young people are not informed of their HIV-positive status. Caregivers may not be prepared to tell them for a variety of reasons. Parents may feel an overwhelming guilt for unintentionally 'infecting' their child, for example, or they may dread answering questions about how HIV is transmitted. They may also wonder whether their child will be able to live a 'normal' life, knowing she or he is HIV-positive, or have fulfilling relationships (sexual or otherwise) in the future. Counselling for both caregiver and child is indispensable when handling disclosure.

Some adolescents know their status but do not disclose it to others because they fear rejection or exclusion. Both circumstances put young people at risk of transmitting HIV to others. In order to stop the spread of this virus, we must counteract prevailing stigma. It is imperative that policies and programmes – especially those established by governments – provide safe spaces for adolescents to feel comfortable disclosing their status, secure in the knowledge that they will be supported.

The second challenge is that comprehensive information on reproductive health for HIV-positive adolescents is still scarce. Health-care systems and family support networks lack the means to break down such information to show its relevance to a particular age group or gender. "Aunt, should I stop taking the medicine now that I have started my period?" asks 15-year-old Tendai from Zimbabwe. Tendai was born HIV-positive and worries that taking medication during her period could result in side effects or adversely affect the chance of her having a child later in life. Local health-care workers and caregivers need training to provide answers to such questions about the fertility risks for HIV-positive adolescents. Providing education and accessible information to people living with HIV is pivotal to eliminating the epidemic.

The third challenge is developing relationships. Whether with friends or family, relationships are fraught with difficulty for young people living with HIV. UNICEF recently organized a dialogue with HIV-positive adolescents in Zimbabwe. These wonderful, bright voices brought painful and piercing messages. Conscious of their HIV status, adolescents fear they may never experience a sustainable romantic relationship. If they are blessed with a loving and understanding partner, will the partner's family accept them? If so, how do they go about conceiving a child? In such resource-poor countries, what are the risks and options?

It is the duty of governments to make sure medication and services such as counselling are available to all those living with HIV, including young people. International organizations such as Save the Children and community groups such as Rozaria Memorial Trust must join hands to enable HIV-positive adolescents to enjoy all their rights, especially their right to sexual and reproductive health. Most adolescents living with HIV struggle for recognition, rights, protection and support. They seek advice and information, not judgement. The sooner these adolescents' questions are answered, the sooner they will be empowered with the confidence that only knowledge can provide.

As World YWCA General Secretary, Nyaradzayi Gumbonzvanda leads a global network of women in 106 countries, reaching 25 million women and girls. She previously served as Regional Director for the United Nations Development Fund for Women (UNIFEM) and as a human rights officer with UNICEF in Liberia and Zimbabwe.

More than 70 million adolescents of lower secondary age are out of school, with sub-Saharan Africa the most affected region

The overwhelming focus on achieving universal primary education by 2015 may have led to the educational challenge for adolescents being understated. Reports repeatedly talk about the 'number of children out of school' but refer only to the number of children of primary age who are out of school – currently 69 million.[28] Yet there are virtually equal numbers of adolescents of lower secondary age – almost 71 million,[29] which is around one in five of that total age group – who are also out of school, either because they have not completed their primary schooling or because they have been unable to make the transition to lower secondary school – or because they have simply dropped out of secondary education. Taking account of adolescents, therefore, doubles the worldwide problem of children out of school. Of these out-of-school adolescents, 54 per cent are girls. The region most affected in this respect is sub-Saharan Africa, with 38 per cent of adolescents out of school.[30]

There is a growing need to focus on the transition from primary to lower secondary school, which often proves particularly difficult in developing countries. Some children are not transitioning to secondary school at typical ages while other children drop out entirely. For example, of lower-secondary-age adolescents in sub-Saharan Africa, 39 per cent are still in primary school, repeating earlier grades or catching up after a late start. In sub-Saharan Africa, 64 per cent of primary school students transition to secondary school.[31] Of those adolescents who do transition to secondary school, many do not make it to the upper secondary. For developing countries, the upper secondary gross enrolment ratio stood at just 48 per cent in 2007, compared with 75 per cent at the lower secondary level.[32]

As more sub-Saharan African countries are reaching universal primary education, they are expanding their education goals to universal basic education, which includes an element of lower secondary as well as primary schooling. Ghana, for example, in 2007 established basic education to include 11 years of schooling, including two years of kindergarten, six years of primary school and three years of junior high school.[33]

The barriers to school attendance at secondary level are largely similar to those at the primary level, but often even more entrenched. The cost of secondary schooling is often higher than the cost of primary schooling and therefore more difficult for families to afford; secondary schools are further from home, often requiring transportation; and the conflict between educational aspirations and the potential income that could be earned by a working adolescent is greater.

Across the developing world, girls still lag behind boys in secondary school attendance

At the global level, girls still lag behind boys in secondary school participation, with net enrolment at 53 per cent for boys and 48 per cent for girls for the period 2005–2009. Although girls lag behind boys generally, their disadvantage is not wholesale. Girl disadvantage is highest in the least developed countries, particularly in sub-Saharan Africa and South Asia. However, in the East Asia and Pacific and the Latin America and Caribbean regions, net attendance in secondary school is higher for girls than boys.[34]

Adolescent girls and boys face different challenges to school attendance. Girls, especially poor girls, are less likely to attend secondary school due to the compounding forms of disadvantage and discrimination they face, including domestic labour, child marriage, ethnic or social exclusion and early pregnancy.[35] Boys may face psychosocial challenges to school attendance. Adolescent boys tend to report lower satisfaction with school than girls.[36] Studies show that teenage boys tend to spend less time in academic activities than girls, while lack of family involvement and the influence of their peer group may also adversely affect boys' levels of satisfaction and adjustment to school.

Secondary education is critical to adolescent empowerment, development and protection

Girls' secondary education remains critical to their development. The existence of secondary schools tends to improve not only enrolment and completion in primary schools but also the quality of the education they provide. Secondary education contributes to greater civic participation and helps to combat youth violence, sexual harassment and human trafficking. It results in a range of long-term health benefits, including lower infant mortality, later marriage, reduced domestic violence, lower fertility rates and improved child nutrition. It functions as a long-term defence against HIV and AIDS, and also acts to reduce poverty and foster social empowerment.[37]

Many countries in the developing world have made significant progress in enrolling more girls in secondary school since 1990, though the goal of gender parity remains

Inequality in childhood and adolescence in rich countries –
Innocenti Report Card 9: The children left behind

In comparison with those in the rest of the world, children in the wealthiest countries enjoy a very high standard of living – but not all benefit equally from the relative prosperity of their nations.

Over the past decade, the UNICEF Innocenti Research Centre's Report Card series on child well-being in the Organisation for Economic Co-operation and Development (OECD) countries has emphasized the importance of measuring the well-being of children in industrialized countries. The latest in the series, Report Card 9, asks, *How far behind are the least advantaged children being allowed to fall?*

Analysing three dimensions of the lives of adolescents – material well-being, education and health – the report ranks 24 OECD countries according to how successfully they practice the 'no child left behind' ethos. Denmark, Finland, the Netherlands and Switzerland appear at the top of the league table, while Greece, Italy and the United States are shown to have the highest levels of inequality for children.

> "Poverty and disadvantage in childhood are closely and consistently associated with many practical costs and consequences."

By measuring economically advanced countries against one another, the Report Card creates a meaningful comparison, revealing the real potential for improvement to reach the standards of other OECD countries.

The cost of inequality

Allowing a child to suffer avoidable setbacks in the most formative stages of development is a breach of the most basic principle of the Convention on the Rights of the Child – that every child has a right to develop to his or her full potential.

According to the report, poverty and disadvantage in childhood are also closely and consistently associated with many practical costs and consequences. These include poorer health outcomes, including a greater probability of low birthweight, obesity, diabetes, chronic asthma, anaemia and cardiovascular disease. Early disadvantage is linked to inadequate nutrition and compromised physical development as well as impaired cognitive and linguistic progress.

The least advantaged children are also more likely to experience food insecurity and parental stress (including lack of parental time), and to have higher allostatic loads due to recurrent stress. Further on in life, there is a greater probability of behavioural difficulties, lower skills and aspirations, lower levels of education and reduced adult earnings. Other risks include a higher incidence of unemployment and welfare dependence, teenage pregnancy, involvement with the police and courts, and alcohol and drug addiction (see adjacent column for full list).

Risks and consequences of inequality in the OECD

Efforts to prevent children from falling behind are right in principle, as they meet the basic tenet of the Convention that every child has the right to develop to her or his full potential. But they are also right in practice; based on hundreds of studies in OECD countries, the costs of young children and adolescents falling behind are grave, and include the greater likelihood of:

- low birthweight
- parental stress and lack of parental time
- chronic stress for the child, possibly linked to long-term health problems and reduced memory capacity
- food insecurity and inadequate nutrition
- poor health outcomes, including obesity, diabetes, chronic asthma, anaemia and cardiovascular disease
- more frequent visits to hospitals and emergency wards
- impaired cognitive development
- lower educational achievement
- lower rates of return on investments in education
- reduced linguistic ability
- lower skills and aspirations
- lower productivity and adult earnings
- unemployment and welfare dependence
- behavioural difficulties
- involvement with the police and courts
- teenage pregnancy
- alcohol and drug dependence.

Source: UNICEF Innocenti Research Centre, *Report Card 9, The children left behind – A league table of inequality in child well-being in the world's rich countries,* UNICEF IRC, Florence, 2010, p. 26.

Many families succeed in overcoming the odds and raising children who do not fall into any of the above categories. But Report Card 9 demonstrates that, on average, children who fall far behind their peers in their early years are likely to find themselves at 'a marked and measurable disadvantage' – through no fault of their own. And a society that aspires to fairness 'cannot be unconcerned that accidents of birth should so heavily circumscribe the opportunities of life'.

Principle and practice argue as one, concludes Report Card 9. Preventing millions of individual children from falling behind in different dimensions of their lives will not only better fulfil their rights, but also enhance the economic and social prospects of their nations. Conversely, when large numbers of children and young people are allowed to fall well below the standards enjoyed by their peers, both they and their societies pay a heavy price.

See References, page 78.

elusive. The gender gap is widest in sub-Saharan Africa and South Asia.[38]

The global economy's increasing emphasis on knowledge-based skills means that the educational experience of adolescents in the developing world is coming more under the microscope. The foundation for providing young people with the skills they need to make the most of the opportunities in the modern economy remains basic education. Such education, however, needs to teach students how to think and how to solve problems creatively rather than simply passing on knowledge. Technical and vocational education also needs to be improved, and not treated as a second-best option for the less academic. It is also vital to extend the opportunity to participate first in basic education and subsequently in technical and vocational courses to adolescents from marginalized groups within society. Flexible 'catch-up' programmes can often reach these adolescents, especially if these are incorporated into national poverty reduction initiatives.[39]

This equitable dimension is fundamental. The most vulnerable adolescents – those affected, for example, by poverty, HIV and AIDS, drug use, disability or ethnic disadvantage – are unlikely to be reached by the 'standard' offer of secondary schooling.[40] They will need to be approached through a range of strategies, including non-formal education, outreach and peer education, and the sensitive provision of education within a context of treatment, care and support.

Gender and protection in adolescence

Many of the key threats to children from violence, abuse and exploitation are at their height during adolescence. It is primarily adolescents who are forced into conflict as child combatants, or to work in hazardous conditions as child labourers. Millions of adolescents are subjected to exploitation, or find themselves in conflict with criminal justice systems. Others are denied their rights to protection by inadequate legal systems or by social and cultural norms that permit the exploitation and abuse of children and adolescents with impunity.

Threats to adolescent protection rights are exacerbated by gender discrimination and exclusion. Genital mutilation/cutting, child marriage, sexual violence and domestic servitude are four abuses estimated to affect a far greater number of adolescent females than adolescent males. But there are also human rights abuses that largely befall adolescent boys because of assumptions about their gender; it

is primarily boys, for example, who are forcibly recruited as child combatants or who are required to perform the most physically punishing forms of child labour.

Any examination of, or action on child protection – particularly in relation to the adolescent years – must consider the gender dimension. The other side of the coin is that addressing violence, abuse and exploitation of adolescents is vital to promoting gender equality and challenging the underlying discrimination that perpetuates it.

Violence and abuse

Violence and sexual abuse, particularly against girls, are commonplace and too frequently tolerated

Acts of violence take place within the home, at school, and in the community; they can be physical, sexual or psychological. The full scale of violence against adolescents is impossible to measure, given that most abuses occur in secret and remain unreported. Data from 11 countries with available estimates show a wide variation in levels of violence against adolescent females aged 15–19; in every country assessed, however, it remains an important problem.[41]

In addition to enduring violence from adults, however, adolescents are also much more likely to encounter violence from their peers than at any other stage in life. Acts of physical violence reach a peak during the second decade of life, with some adolescents using it to gain the respect of their peers or to assert their own independence. Most of this violence tends to be directed towards other adolescents.

For many young people, the experience of physical violence, whether as victim or as perpetrator, is largely confined to the teenage years and diminishes as they enter adulthood. Certain groups of adolescents are particularly vulnerable to physical violence, including those with disabilities, those living on the streets, those in conflict with the law, and refugee and displaced children.

Sexual violence and abuse occur in many different forms and may happen anywhere: at home, in school, at work, in the community or even in cyberspace. Although boys are also affected, studies show that the majority of the victims of sexual abuse are girls. Adolescents may be lured into commercial sexual exploitation under the pretence of being offered education or employment, or in exchange for cash. Or they may become involved due to family pressure, or the need to support their families, themselves, or both.

Act responsibly:
Nurse our planet back to health

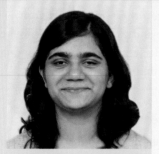

by Meenakshi Dunga, 16, India

"We have to wake up and realize that we are accountable not only to ourselves but also to Mother Nature and future generations."

What can I say about climate change that hasn't already been written, read or discussed? In school we learn about global warming daily from our textbooks; we attend lectures and presentations. The earth is a sick patient whose temperature is slowly rising. Her condition is worsening. So what can I – a 16-year-old who can't decide what to have for lunch – say or do to make a difference? You might be surprised.

Although we are the caretakers of the planet, we have become too engrossed in our personal lives and our desire to succeed. Oblivious to the wounded world around us, we neglect our duties and responsibilities to the environment. We are quick to remember money owed to us and easily recall when the teacher was away, but we can't be bothered to unplug appliances to save energy or plant a tree. We can climb Mount Everest, cure illnesses and land on the moon, but we can't remember to turn off the light when we leave a room or to throw trash in the bin or separate it for recycling.

Many wake-up calls later, we remain asleep – or perhaps we choose not to be roused, thinking that other people will deal with the problem. But they won't. Gandhi said, "We need to be the change we wish to see in the world." This is our planet, and it is up to us to care for it. Nursing our planet back to health is our responsibility, for the greater good.

My brother and I fight every morning because I insist he take a five-minute shower, using 10–25 gallons of water, instead of a 70-gallon bath. As in the butterfly effect, our daily actions – even minute ones – have far-reaching consequences. They determine whether life on Earth will perish or flourish. Closing the tap while we brush our teeth saves up to 30 litres of water per day. Biking or walking just twice a week can reduce CO_2 emissions by 1,600 pounds per year. Properly insulating our houses, thereby using less energy to heat and cool them, also makes a tremendous difference.

These small steps will help the earth, a patient who is struggling and who, I think, is eager to get well soon. We have to wake up and realize that we are accountable not only to ourselves but also to Mother Nature and future generations. Adolescents: Be more alert, active and engaged. I will continue to spread awareness to family members, friends and neighbours. We must respect our environment and keep it clean and safe. Who knows? One day, our patient might be cured, begin to thrive and become a greener, more beautiful place to live.

Meenakshi Dunga lives in Dwarka, New Delhi. Following her graduation, she plans to study medicine in India and become the best surgeon she can be. Meenakshi also enjoys singing, listening to music and caring for the environment.

Poverty, social and economic exclusion, low educational level and lack of information about the risks attached to commercial sexual exploitation, increase adolescents' vulnerability to sexual abuse. The driving factor behind commercial sexual exploitation of children, however, is demand. While foreign tourists are often involved, research shows that the vast majority of the demand is actually local.

The gender dimension of protection abuses in adolescence is pronounced

The gender dimensions of violence and abuse – physical, sexual and psychological – against adolescents are critical. Girls experience higher rates of domestic and sexual vio-lence than boys; these abuses reinforce male dominance in the household and community, and concurrently impede female empowerment. Evidence from 11 developing countries with available data show a broad spread of experi-ence of sexual or physical violence against adolescent females aged 15–19, reaching a height of 65 per cent in Uganda.[42]

The widespread acceptance of spousal violence as a normal feature of life, particularly by young women, is a grave cause for concern. The latest international household data for 2000–2009 show that on average more than 50 per cent of adolescent females aged 15–19 in the developing world (excluding China) consider that a husband is justified in hitting or beating his wife under certain circumstances, such as if she burns the food or refuses to have sex.[43]

Similar attitudes are prevalent among adolescent males of the same age cohort. In two thirds of the 28 countries with available data on this indicator, more than one third of adolescent males aged 15–19 considered a husband justified in hitting or beating his wife under certain circumstances.[44] Prevailing notions of masculinity and feminity reinforce these attitudes.

Adolescent marriage

Most adolescent marriages take place after age 15 but before age 18

Adolescent marriage – defined here as a marriage or union where one or more of the spouses is age 19 or younger – is most common in South Asia and sub-Saharan Africa. New figures from 31 countries in these two regions show that most adolescent marriages take place between the ages of 15 and 18. In three countries – Bangladesh, Chad and the Niger – around one third of women aged 20–24 were married by the age of 15.[45]

While the impact of child marriage on girls' health and education has been noted earlier in this report, the psychosocial effects are also enormous. Girls are likely to find themselves in a position of powerlessness within the household of their husband's family, with no clear access to friends of the same age or other sources of support. This powerlessness means they are more vulnerable to abuse and may also have to bear an excessive burden of domestic work.

Female genital mutilation/cutting

The prevalence of female genital mutilation/cutting (FGM/C), though declining, is still widespread in 29 countries

More than 70 million girls and women aged 15–49 have undergone female genital mutilation/cutting (FGM/C), usually by the onset of puberty.[46] Of the 29 countries where FGM/C prevalence is higher than 1 per cent, only Yemen is outside the African continent.[47] Such cutting is extremely dangerous, especially when – as is common – it takes place in an unsanitary environment. It can do significant long-term damage and heightens the risk of complications during childbirth for both mother and baby. It also reduces girls' capacity to enjoy normal, healthy sexual development.

The prevalence of FGM/C is declining – it is measurably less common among younger women than older, and among daughters compared with their mothers. But progress is slow, and millions of girls remain threatened by the practice.

Child labour

Child labour is declining, but still affects a large number of adolescents

Around 150 million children aged 5–14 are currently engaged in child labour, with incidence highest in sub-Saharan Africa.[48] Adolescents who work excessive hours or in hazardous conditions are unlikely to be able to complete their education, severely curtailing their ability to escape from poverty. The evidence shows that the prevalence of child labour has been falling in recent years, and that the incidence of hazardous child labour is declining sharply.[49] But it continues to blight the life chances and well-being of adolescents in much of the developing world.

Better data have revealed the extent to which lower rates of school enrolment and attainment in the developing world relate to child labour. The data also show the gender discrimination prevalent in child labour, especially domestic labour by adolescents. Although aggregate numbers suggest that more boys than girls are involved in child labour, it is estimated that roughly 90 per cent of children involved in domestic labour are girls.[50]

Adolescents are also victims of trafficking

The extent to which adolescents, especially females, are vulnerable to protection abuses is being increasingly documented through household surveys and targeted studies. Nonetheless, many forms of protection risk remain largely invisible, owing either to their clandestine nature or to the difficulty encountered by adolescents in reporting these issues.

Trafficking is such an illegal and clandestine activity that statistics purporting to show the number of children and adolescents affected are likely to be unreliable. Adolescents may be trafficked into forced labour, marriage, prostitution or domestic work. They may be transported across borders, though it is more common for the trafficking to take place within countries. The number of countries with specific anti-trafficking laws has more than doubled over the past decade, though not all of them have actually brought prosecutions against offenders.[51]

Initiatives on gender and protection

Experience shows that programmes that cut across sectors, promote discussion, debate and broad participation and successfully, over time, generate consensus around human rights principles and corresponding social change, can lead to a decrease in harmful practices that predominantly affect women and girls. This directly results in greater equality between men and women, reduced child mortality and improved maternal health.

In Uganda, for example, Raising Voices and the Centre for Domestic Violence Prevention supported community initiatives designed to challenge gender norms and prevent violence against women and children. Their activities included raising awareness on domestic violence, building networks of support and action within the community and professional sectors, supporting community activities such as discussions, door-to-door visits and theatre, and using media such as radio, television and newspapers to promote women's rights.[52]

In Senegal, a community empowerment programme supported by Tostan, a non-governmental organization that engages local facilitators to lead sensitization and awareness-raising sessions in villages, led to a 77 per cent decrease in

the prevalence of FGM/C. The community sensitization initiative also involves raising awareness of the negative implications of child marriage.[53]

In Ethiopia, as a result of the Kembatta Mentti Gezzima-Tope (KMG) programme, which facilitated community dialogue and collective community decisions around FGM/C and alternatives, most families in the zone abandoned FGM/C. Whereas before the programme, which took place in 2008, 97 per cent of villagers were in favour of FGM/C, after it 96 per cent accepted that it should be abandoned. Just as vitally, 85 per cent of villagers believed that uncut girls were no longer "despised" in their communities.[54]

Around 60 per cent of programmes combating child marriage are based on community sensitization of this kind. Other programmes aim to educate girls directly about the disadvantages of early marriage and offer incentives not to engage in it. The Government of Bangladesh, for example, has since 1994 been offering secondary school scholarships to girls who postpone marriage,[55] while in the Indian state of Maharashtra, girls' participation in a life-skills education course has been demonstrated to delay their marriage by a year.[56]

In other Indian states – Andhra Pradesh, Haryana, Karnataka, Madhya Pradesh, Punjab, Rajasthan and Tamil Nadu – both girls and their families are offered financial incentives to delay marriage until the age of 18.[57]

Figure 2.7: Marriage by age of first union in selected countries with available disaggregated data

Percentage of women aged 20–24 who were first married or in union by ages 15, 18 or 20

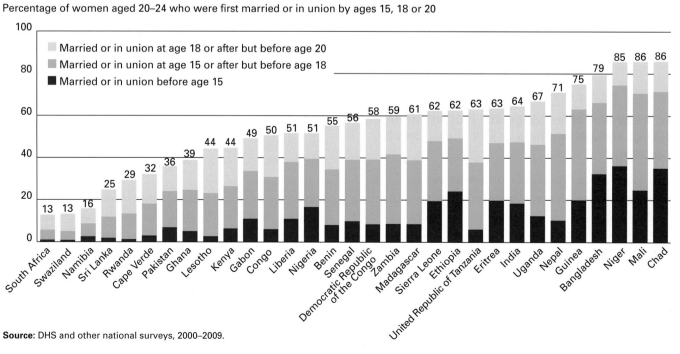

Source: DHS and other national surveys, 2000–2009.

Gender, poverty and the challenge for adolescents

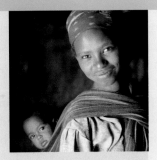

A woman carrying her baby daughter on her back stands in her home, Ethiopia. Nurse Midwife Association and health extension workers are integrating the abandonment of FGM/C into existing maternal and child health clinics and programmes.

"Ethiopia's population is young; over 50 per cent was under 18 in 2009."

Although Ethiopia remains one of the poorest countries in the world, its economy has been growing, and many programmes to improve the health and education of children have shown success. The country is on track to reach Millennium Development Goals 4 and 5 to reduce child mortality and improve maternal health. Enrolment rates in primary school increased from 2008 to 2009, and girls' participation in education has improved. In the global economic recession, the Government has taken steps to maintain budget allocations for the benefit of the poor. Yet environmental challenges such as drought and subsequent water shortages, along with poverty and violence against girls and women, present obstacles to development and threaten to reverse the progress that the nation has made.

Ethiopia's population is young; over 50 per cent was under 18 in 2009. It is one of seven countries worldwide that account for half of all adolescent births (the others are Bangladesh, Brazil, the Democratic Republic of the Congo, India, Nigeria and the United States). In a country where most people survive on subsistence agriculture, children are valued for their labour as well as for the emotional and physical support they give parents, and many rural communities perceive large numbers of children as a social and religious boon. In urban areas, however, fertility levels have dropped due to a number of factors including decreasing poverty and improved access to medical services, including contraception.

The Population Council has found that 85 per cent of adolescents in Ethiopia live in rural areas, where education levels tend to be much lower, particularly for girls. Some regions have very high rates of early marriage, and almost 70 per cent of young married girls interviewed in the Amhara region had experienced sexual debut before they began menstruation. A substantial number of adolescents do not live with their parents, especially in urban areas; one third of girls between 10 and 14 in cities live with neither parent. Nationally, there are between 150,000 and 200,000 children living and working on the streets, where the girls among them face sexual abuse by adults, rape, unwanted pregnancy, early motherhood and the risk of HIV infection.

Programmes tend not to reach the most vulnerable children – rural youth, married girls and out-of-school adolescents. Rather, older, unmarried boys who live in cities and attend school are the most likely to benefit from development initiatives. A survey conducted in Addis Ababa in 2004 that asked boys and girls aged 10–19 about their use of reproductive health programmes found that boys in the city's poorer sections were significantly more likely than girls to be in school or to live with one or both parents; they also enjoyed greater mobility and better access to services. Although older boys and girls were more likely to use programmes than their younger counterparts, younger boys were more likely than older girls to use them, showing that age did not correct for gender disparity. A major obstacle for girls was their heavier workload, particularly in domestic settings, as compared to boys who worked in manual labour or trades.

The Ethiopian Ministry of Youth and Sport, working with regional and local governments as well as international partners, initiated the Berhane Hewan ('Light for Eve' in Amharic) programme in 2004 to prevent early marriage and support married adolescent girls by focusing on three areas: mentorship by adult women, continuation of school, and livelihood training for out-of-school girls. Over the course of two years the programme, which targeted girls aged 10–19 in the Amhara region, increased girls' friendship networks, school attendance, age at marriage, knowledge of reproductive health and contraceptive use. The intervention owed its success in large part to its attention to the complex social and economic drivers of girls' isolation and disadvantage. Following an 18-month pilot period, the project is being expanded to other parts of the region.

Further programmes need to be designed with an understanding of local cultural perceptions and social dynamics, especially those that create multiple forms of disadvantage for Ethiopia's adolescent girls and rural youth. Many of the basic needs and rights of adolescents are not being met, and when economic and environmental constraints combine, the situation worsens. A recent study of food insecurity in the Jimma region, for example, found that girls in food-insecure households suffered more than boys. It is clear that investments must be targeted and should begin with efforts to ensure a decent standard of living for all the country's girls and boys, no matter their ethnic origin, place of residence or class.

See References, page 78.

Yet other initiatives against child marriage take a legal route. In Ethiopia, for example, the organization Pathfinder International takes action against proposed child marriages that come to its notice, employing a network of local partners to try to persuade the parents concerned not to go ahead. If this strategy is unsuccessful, the organization joins with the Ethiopian Women Lawyers' Association in launching legal action aimed at stopping the ceremony.[58]

Initiatives to counter violence and sexual abuse cannot confine themselves to legal protection. Much of the sexual violence experienced by adolescent girls is at the hands of their male partner and may not therefore come to the notice of the police or other authorities. In addition, tak-

ing punitive legal action without addressing the underlying causes of the violence may have unintended consequences, such as pushing the problem further underground.

For this reason it is essential to take steps to raise the awareness of boys and men about gender relations and power. Program H, developed by four Latin American non-governmental organizations, trains facilitators to help young men consider the drawbacks attached to traditional gender roles and the unhealthy behaviour attached to them. The aim of the programme is to foster more equitable relationships between men and women, and an evaluation of its effects in Brazil indicated that it had been successful in encouraging such gender-equitable behav-

TECHNOLOGY

Young people, mobile phones and the rights of adolescents

by Graham Brown,
Co-founder, mobileYouth

With only five years left to meet the Millennium Development Goals, much remains to be done to ensure equitable access to technological advances in underserved and hard-to-reach communities, especially among young people. Working at mobileYouth, I have seen how adolescents are using mobile technology in new and groundbreaking ways. Emerging markets dominate the growth of this technology. Alongside the throng of street urchins and trinket sellers in Chennai, India – to take just one example – local schoolchildren surround a makeshift stall. You might mistake it for an ice cream vendor, but this stall is actually selling mobile phones. In a country where the average gross domestic product per capita is around $225 a month and Internet access via personal computers (PCs) is the exception, it is no coincidence that youth (defined here as those aged 5–29) have gravitated towards mobile phones, which cost as little as $10 and offer call rates that approach zero.

Three of the five markets with the highest numbers of mobile accounts among young people are developing countries: Brazil, China and India (Japan and the United States are the other two). By 2012, the number of subscribers below the age of 30 in South Asia is projected to rise by 30 per cent, to 380 million, sub-Saharan Africa is expected to have 108 million subscribers under 30, and Latin America, 188 million. This increased connectivity offers an opportunity for young people to access knowledge and fulfil their right to information.

Although it was long thought that low-cost laptops would unlock the world of cheap mass communications for youth in developing markets, the mobile phone has become the de facto access channel to the Internet in places where there is low PC penetration. In South Africa, for example, mobile phone subscriptions among youth outstrip PC ownership by as much as 123 per cent.

Back in 1996, nobody imagined that Short Message Service (SMS), a format that limits messages to 160 characters, could be of any use apart from receiving a simple test signal from your mobile carrier. How wrong we were. By experimenting with and exploiting the medium, young people evolved the format before returning it to the commercial world. While we struggled to conceive of a successor to SMS, investing heavily in picture messaging (MMS) and similar services, youth once again arrived at the answer without industry intervention. They adopted, adapted and converted services originally intended for business – such as BlackBerry Messenger – into their own medium, not only to communicate among themselves but also to advance social campaigns.

Young people are keen to take up new content formats, with adolescents in particular having the time to explore and exploit new technologies. SMS, in turn, is being challenged by mobile Instant Messaging (IM), which is becoming the platform of choice owing to the increasing number of users, iour and attitudes in young men aged 14–25 as compared with a control group.[59]

As this suggests, gender equality is not only about women and girls. Adolescent boys and young men are often at risk of protection abuses on the basis of gender. Gender equality requires the committed participation of all – men and boys, women and girls – to eradicate discrimination based on sex and age. A world in which adolescent girls and boys are adequately protected will also be a world that has seriously confronted the entrenched gender discrimination that is at the root of so much abuse.

lower costs, popularity in emerging markets and the widespread growth of mobile Internet everywhere. Brazil has 18 million mobile IM users, representing 23 per cent of the country's mobile youth. In India, 87 million – 31 per cent of mobile youth – claim to be mobile IM users.

In the slums of Cape Town, South Africa, against a backdrop of gang violence, social entrepreneurs like Marlon Parker – founder of the non-profit Reconstructed Living Labs (RLabs) – show how technology can empower adolescents to change their lives. For example, Jason, aged 19, has spent the last four years transforming himself from petty thief to community role model using mobile chat, Facebook and texting. In conjunction with Drug Awareness Week in South Africa, RLabs and Mxit – South Africa's leading mobile social network – recently launched a live Drug Counselling Portal called Angel, which offers young people 24-hour mobile access to information and support. Since its inception, the portal has attracted more than 23,000 users, filling a gap in social services important for young people and children.

The landscape has shifted significantly in less than a generation. We can no longer rely on specific organizations to be the sole agents of change; the speed at which issues arise and crises strike requires that we supplement more traditional modes of organizing with the kinds of youth-led grass-roots movements made possible through mobile phone technology. Directed onto the right track, such movements could create cost-effective and easily deployed platforms for social change. Imagine, for example, the millions of girls under 18 living in rural India: How many of them – if armed with a mobile phone and supported by youth non-governmental organizations – have the potential to become advocates who proclaim an alternative message of hope? The world's mobile youth will not only change the nature of mobile markets; they will also transform the development community's outreach to promote social change and realize adolescents' rights.

Graham Brown is one of the founders of mobileYouth <www.mobileyouth.org/>, the the world's largest aggregator of data on youth mobile phone use. He hosts the youth marketing stream on Upstart Radio and mobileYouth's own TV channel. A widely published writer on issues related to young people and mobile technology, Mr. Brown is also a judge on the Mobile Marketing Association's Award Panel and an advisor to the Global Youth Marketing Forum held in India in 2010.

" The mobile phone has become the de facto access channel to the Internet in places where there is low PC penetration."

Chernobyl 25 years later:
Remembering adolescents in disaster

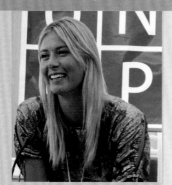

by Maria Sharapova, professional tennis player and Goodwill Ambassador for the United Nations Development Programme

"We believe in your ability and your right to realize your full potential, and we pledge our support as you move into adulthood."

In 2011, the world marks the 25th anniversary of the disaster at Chernobyl, the worst nuclear power plant accident in history. The region, however, has yet to fully recover from this catastrophe. While adolescents currently living in Belarus, Ukraine and the Russian Federation – the three countries most affected by the fallout – were not yet born when parts of the nuclear power station exploded, they bear the scars of the tragedy.

Although we may never know the full extent of the harm done, approximately 5,000 cases of thyroid cancer have since been diagnosed among those who were under 18 years old at the time of the blast, and around 350,000 people – including my family – were uprooted from their towns and villages. Emergency workers risked their lives in responding to the accident, and millions were left traumatized by lingering fears about their health and livelihood. Young people, in particular, now face limited opportunities and suffer from mental health problems that threaten their social and economic welfare.

Even 25 years later, the psychological impact manifests itself in the residents' belief in a shortened life expectancy, in radiophobia (fear of radiation as a psychological consequence of a traumatic experience) and in a lack of initiative resulting from their designation as 'victims' rather than 'survivors'. In turn, young people lead unhealthy lifestyles, resort to drugs and alcohol and suffer from a lack of confidence in their ability to succeed and excel.

I have always wanted to contribute to the recovery of this region – a place to which I have a deep and personal connection. As a global community, we must provide the region's young people with the tools they need to reach their full potential, and we must help its communities get back on their feet and overcome the stigma that hangs over the area. Providing adolescents with educational and social opportunities and positive reinforcement is one way to move forward.

Organizations such as the International Atomic Energy Agency, the World Health Organization, UNICEF and the United Nations Development Programme (UNDP) have teamed up with the

International Chernobyl Research and Information Network to provide the affected population with information on how to pursue healthy and productive lives. Psychosocial support has been particularly important for young people. In my capacity as UNDP Goodwill Ambassador, I have focused on seven UNDP initiatives in the three Chernobyl-affected countries, aiming to improve young people's self-confidence, to restore a sense of hope and to encourage them to take control of their lives.

We opened music schools in rural areas of Belarus. Children from the city of Chechersk took up community activities such as cleaning springs, making bird feeders and planting bushes. A newly established 'Fairytale Room' at the Chechersk Central Rayon Hospital now provides therapy in the form of healing and inspirational activities like interactive games and mini-circuses. In the Russian Federation, a modern sports facility was built at the Novocamp summer camp to boost the physical and mental well-being of adolescents. A network of rural youth centres was established in Ukraine to bring computer skills to rural teens. We also launched a Scholarship Programme in Belarus that enables students to pursue higher education at the Belarusian State Academy of Arts and the Belarusian State University.

I have great faith in the young people of this area. My goal is to impart a message of optimism to adolescents who suffer from the consequences of the Chernobyl fallout and to help restore a healthy and productive environment. I would also like to tell young people in this and other regions affected by disasters, whether natural or human-made – such as Hurricane Katrina, the Indian Ocean tsunami, the earthquake in Haiti and, most recently, the oil spill in the Gulf of Mexico – that the world has not forgotten you or your struggle. We believe in your ability and your right to realize your full potential, and we pledge our support as you move into adulthood.

Maria Sharapova is a professional Russian tennis player who has won 3 Grand Slam titles. She was named Goodwill Ambassador for UNDP in 2007 and has focused specifically on the Chernobyl Recovery and Development Programme.

Protecting unaccompanied migrant adolescents

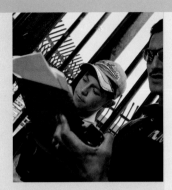

A Mexican immigration officer questions a repatriated migrant child in Tijuana, Mexico.

"Protecting adolescents from discrimination based on nationality or migration status and from administrative detention will be pivotal."

Mexico is the fifth largest country in the Americas and ranks eleventh in the world in terms of population. Given it's location between the United States of America and the rest of Latin America, it is a point of origin, transit and destination for migrants, experiencing both internal (rural to urban) and external (cross-border) migration. In 2009, around 78 per cent of Mexicans were living in urban areas. Increased urbanization has been spurred by migration to the northern border states, where the rapid growth of the maquila industry has attracted workers, and to tourist centres such as Cancun on the Caribbean coast. Large numbers of Mexicans have also crossed borders, most notably to the United States, where an estimated 10.3 million first-generation Mexican immigrants were living in 2004.

Recently, ensuring the rights of young people in the context of migration has become a challenge for Mexico. Children and adolescents migrating alone make up one of the least visible faces of migration. These young people, the majority of whom are adolescents aged 12–17, are on the move for various reasons, seeking to reunite with their families, to earn income or to escape violence and exploitation. During their journeys, adolescents are vulnerable to exploitation by unscrupulous persons and may fall prey to trafficking for labour or sexual purposes or be subjected to physical and sexual abuse. They are regularly exposed to humiliating and confusing situations that can leave deep scars. Within the last two years, over 58,000 adolescents and children – close to 34,000 of whom were unaccompanied – were repatriated from the United States to Mexico. Mexico, in turn, repatriated almost 9,000 adolescents and children to their countries of origin.

The Government of Mexico has taken determined steps to address issues related to migrant adolescents and children. The Inter-Institutional Panel on Unaccompanied Child and Adolescent Migrants and Migrant Women, set up in March 2007, has been instrumental in advancing this agenda. The panel brings together some 17 institutions, ranging from public authorities such as the National Family Development System, the Ministry of Foreign Affairs and the National Migration Institute, to international agencies such as UNICEF, the Inter-

national Organization for Migration (IOM), the United Nations Development Fund for Women and the United Nations Refugee Agency. It develops public policies and coordinates programmes oriented to the protection of this highly vulnerable population.

Such efforts have resulted in the development of a new model for the protection of unaccompanied migrant adolescents and children, and in 2009 the Mexican Congress increased the national budget allocation for its implementation. The Government, in partnership with UNICEF and other stakeholders, has also made considerable efforts to ensure that the rights of adolescents and children in migration are taken up in international forums. Consequently, regional guidelines for the protection of unaccompanied migrant children were approved in 2009 at the Regional Conference on Migration. The guidelines are applicable in 11 countries of North and Central America as well as the Dominican Republic.

Specific actions have also been taken to respond to the immediate needs of repatriated adolescents and children, such as setting up special care units in the northern border areas of Mexico. Bilateral efforts are also under way between Mexico, as the transit and destination country, and countries of migrant origin, such as Guatemala.

Globally, considerable challenges still remain in the endeavour to ensure the rights of migrant adolescents and children. Overall, a fundamental challenge is the general absence of a child perspective within migration laws and policies and the corresponding lack of a migrant perspective within childhood policies. Specific issues such as access to justice, family reunification and international special protection still need to be addressed. Protecting adolescents from discrimination based on nationality or migration status and from administrative detention will be pivotal. Lastly, the migratory circuit must be dealt with in a more comprehensive way in order to tackle the root causes of migration and to ensure that adolescents do not see themselves as forced to migrate, but instead are able to make choices that serve their best interests.

See References, page 78.

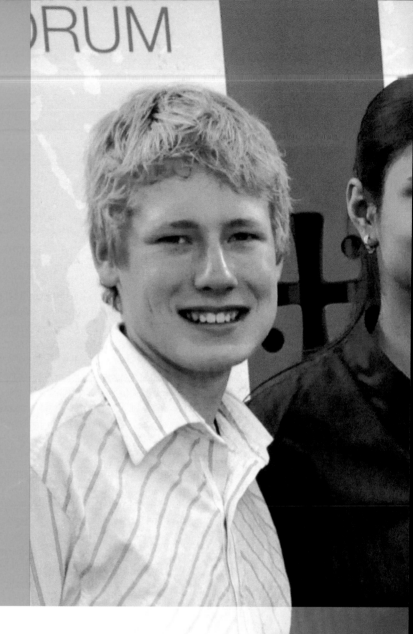

Adolescents are deeply concerned about climate change and should be encouraged to be integral partners along with adults in decision-making. *On 4 December 2009, youth delegates held up a copy of their finalized Declaration during the closing ceremony of the Children's Climate Forum in Copenhagen, Denmark.*

CHAPTER 3

Global Challenges for Adolescents

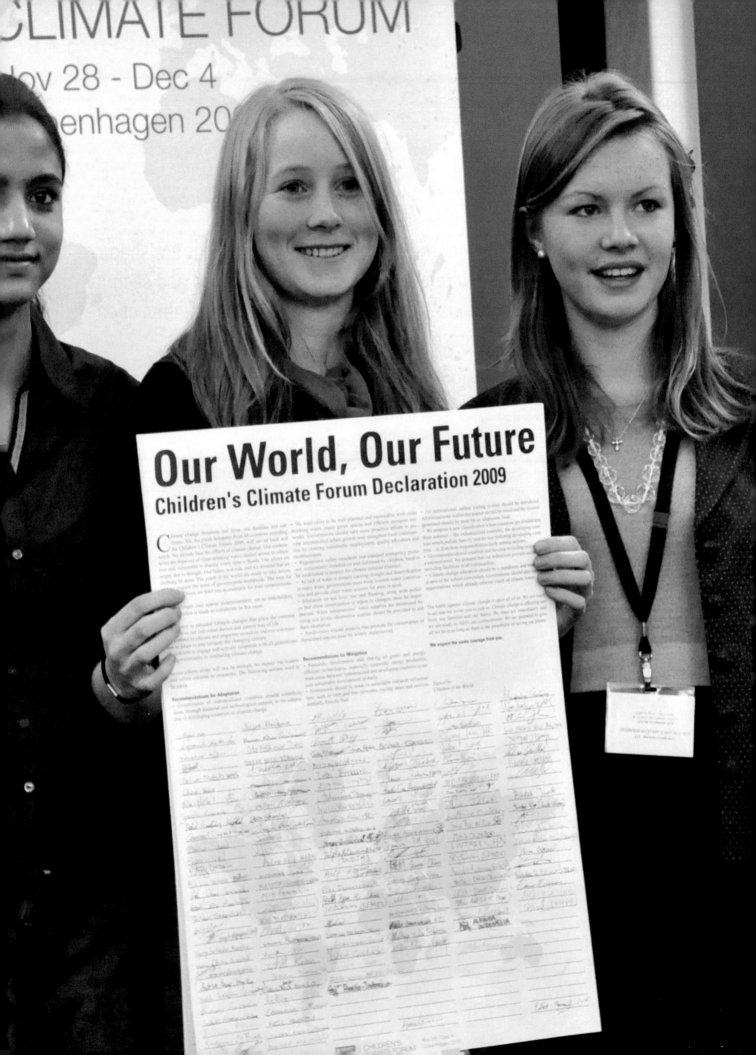

This chapter considers some of the key global challenges that are shaping today's world – including environmental sustainability, peace and security, and key economic and social trends – and assesses their potential impact on and relevance for adolescents.

Climate change and the environment

Along with severe pollution and loss of biodiversity, climate change is the most urgent and alarming threat to the environment. Contributing to environmental degradation, loss of vital natural resources and the conditions that undermine food and water security, it disrupts the very context in which adolescents live and develop.

Climate change and increased frequency and severity of humanitarian crises have the potential to adversely impact not only young people's health and nutrition, but also their

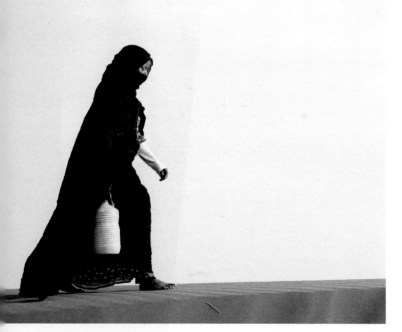

If water, food and fuel insecurity intensify as a result of climate change, adolescents, most often girls, can expect to bear the brunt of the additional time it will take to acquire drinking water. *A 16-year-old girl carries a jug of water across the sand towards her family's nomadic compound in the Sahara Desert, Morocco.*

education and development. For instance, families who lose their livelihood to drought may no longer be able to afford sending children to school or paying for health care.[1]

Climate change is not just an 'environmental' issue. It requires collective action that brings together sustainable development, energy security, and actions to safeguard children's health and well-being. While children and young people are most seriously affected by the accelerating deterioration of the environment, they can become effective agents of change for the long-term protection and stewardship of the earth if they are provided with knowledge and opportunity. Some community-based monitoring and advocacy activities already involve young people in efforts to improve living conditions in their environments.

Natural disasters are increasingly frequent, and they most severely effect those developing countries that lack the resources to restore 'normality' quickly. At times of crisis, children and adolescents are most vulnerable. While the youngest are most likely to perish or succumb to disease, all children and young people suffer as a result of food shortages, poor water and sanitation, interrupted education and family separation or displacement.[2]

Two other facts are clear. The first is that this generation of adolescents will bear a major portion of the burden and cost of mitigating and adapting to climate change. Adolescents will be harder hit than adults simply because 88 per cent of them live in developing countries, which are projected to suffer disproportionately from the effects of rising global average temperatures. An estimated 46 developing and transition countries are considered to be at high risk of climate change worsening already existing problems and heightening the possibility of conflict; a further 56 countries face a lower but still marked risk of climate-exacerbated strife.

Adolescents are deeply concerned about climate change

The second is adolescents' passionate concern for the issue. Adolescents are extremely conscious that their own future, as well as future generations, will be severely jeopardized by climate change. The advent of the United Nations Framework Convention on Climate Change (UNFCCC) has spurred the already vibrant dialogue and advocacy among adolescent and young people across the globe on this issue.

In particular, since the 11th Conference of the Parties (COP) – the governing body of the UNFCCC – held in Montreal in 2005, youth involvement in the UNFCC process has intensified. In 2008, the UN established the Joint Framework Initiative on Children, Youth and Climate Change, which has spurred the integration of efforts for and by adolescents and youth on climate change at the international level.

The year 2009 also saw considerable youth engagement in global climate change issues, with youth officially recognized as a civil society actor in the UNFCCC negotiating process.[3] In that same year, children and youth from some 110 countries participated in a discussion of the challenges of climate change at the TUNZA International Children and Youth Conference organized by the United Nations Environment Programme and held in Daejeon, Republic of Korea.[4]

At the UN Climate Change Talks, held in March–April 2009 in Bonn, a young woman from the United Kingdom caused a stir when she posed the following question to the delegates: "How old will you be in 2050?" Her intervention won a round of applause. By the following day, hundreds of people in Bonn were wearing T-shirts emblazoned with that question – including the Chair himself, who started the next day's session stating that he would be 110 in 2050 but that his children would then be in their fifties. The question encapsulated young people's acute sense that climate change is an issue that demands an intergenerational response involving adolescents as integral partners along with adults in decision-making.[5, 6]

> "To build a green world, we must give priority to tree plantation and eco-living practices."
>
> Abu Bakkor, 10, Bangladesh

Adolescents and young people are calling for urgent action on climate change. At both the 2008 UN Summit on Climate in New York and COP 15, delegations of youth and adolescents appealed to world leaders to act more quickly and comprehensively to stem the rising tide of carbon emissions. An online space, Unite for Climate, has been developed by UN agencies and other international organizations to enable children, young people and experts to collaborate on climate issues. Time and again, their discourse has urged governments to take bold and decisive action.

Consideration of the impact on adolescents and children should be an integral part of all international frameworks and national programmes established to counter climate change. But merely considering the needs and interests of young people is insufficient, since their participation is also urgently required. All national and local initiatives aimed at adapting to climate change or at reducing disaster risks should involve adolescents from the outset.[7] Incorporating adolescents' perspectives and knowledge and encouraging their participation in disaster risk reduction and climate change adaptation strategies is not just a matter of principle – it is an imperative.

Establishing a protective environment for vulnerable children

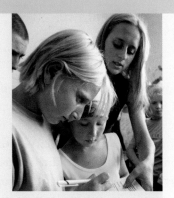

A 17-year-old volunteer helps a girl complete a questionnaire during an HIV/AIDS awareness campaign to promote healthy lifestyles, Ukraine.

"The under-five mortality rate has continued to decline, from 21 deaths per 1,000 live births in 1990 to 15 per 1,000 in 2009."

Ukraine has undergone a period of profound transformation since the collapse of the Soviet Union in 1991. Despite a deep recession in the late 1990s, the country's economic growth between 2001 and 2008 – an average annual 7.5 per cent – was among the highest in Europe. Education and health indicators for children and adolescents continue to be the best in the Central and Eastern Europe and Commonwealth of Independent States (CEE/CIS) region. Literacy is almost universal, and the net secondary enrolment ratio for both girls and boys was almost 85 per cent in 2009. The under-five mortality rate has continued to decline, from 21 deaths per 1,000 live births in 1990 to 15 per 1,000 in 2009.

Yet Ukraine remains one of the poorest countries in Eastern Europe and disparities are widening. As in other transition countries, large families, women and children are the most affected by poverty.

An urgent challenge is the continuing spread of the HIV epidemic and the particular vulnerability of adolescents to HIV infection and other risks. Ukraine has the highest HIV infection level in Europe, with an adult prevalence rate of 1.1 per cent. While injecting drug use remains the primary route of HIV transmission, sexual transmission is growing.

Children and young people – particularly those living on the street, orphans, those in correctional facilities, and those in families or communities where drug use is common – constitute a group whose risk of contracting HIV is particularly high. A recent study indicates that young people account for a significant number of infections among injecting drug users in Ukraine as well as the CEE/CIS in general. Baseline research conducted among young people by UNICEF and partners shows that almost 15.5 per cent of those surveyed reported injecting drugs; almost three quarters had experienced sexual debut (most prior to age 15); roughly half of females reported receiving money, gifts or a reward for sexual intercourse; and condom use was low.

Many Ukrainian adolescents between the ages of 10 and 19 live in unsafe environments. Although official figures are lacking, a large number of most-at-risk adolescents live and work on the streets. This puts them in a particularly risky situation, vulnerable to sexual and labour exploitation and violence, as well as to HIV risk behaviour and infection. Additionally, many adolescents on the streets face a high level of exclusion from education, health care and legal and social services.

Addressing the increasing prevalence of the HIV epidemic and protecting adolescents has become a major concern for Ukraine. Collaborative efforts between the Government and partner agencies are under way. For instance, since 2007 UNICEF has provided assistance to the Government in building an evidence base on most-at-risk adolescents, strengthening the capacity of local research institutions and developing national norms and standards and evidence-based programming on HIV prevention for these young people.

The intervention also supported the integration of most-at-risk adolescents into the National AIDS Programme 2009–2013, which set a national coverage target of 60 per cent for at-risk groups (defined as "injecting drug users, orphans, homeless children, detained or incarcerated children, children from families in crisis, sex workers, men who have sex with men, migrants and other similar groups"). The 2006 State Programme on Homelessness and Neglect of Children also lays out the Government's commitment to protecting children and adolescents and preventing drug abuse among the most-at-risk groups.

Ukraine still has much do to address the critical needs and concerns of its young population and the HIV epidemic in general. Concerted efforts, including a comprehensive HIV and AIDS information, education and communication strategy at the national and sub-national levels, are needed to safeguard the rights of most-at-risk adolescent girls and boys and provide them with access to essential services and protection from violence, abuse and exploitation.

See References, page 78.

Poverty, unemployment and globalization

Adolescents are often seen as the next generation of actors on the social and economic stage. While it is true that the future economic development of nations depends on harnessing their energy and developing their skills, this view does not take account of the social and economic contribution that many adolescents and young people make today. It also fails to acknowledge that many young people are struggling to find adequate employment that can provide them with a safe foothold above the poverty line – and that their prospects of attaining such security have worsened amid the global economic malaise that has taken hold since 2007. Most young people in general are in a better position to take advantage of global development than any previous generation, due in part to improved levels of education and better health. However, many of them remain excluded from the opportunities afforded by globalization.

Lack of appropriate skills and a dearth of work opportunities are denying adolescents and youth a future of stable, productive work

Adolescence is a time when poverty and inequity pass to the next generation. This is particularly true among adolescents with low levels of education. Almost half of the world's adolescents of appropriate age do not attend secondary school. And when they do attend, many of them fail to complete their studies or finish with insufficient skills – especially those high-level competencies that are increasingly required by the modern globalized economy.

This skills deficit is contributing to bleak youth economic employment trends. In August 2010, the International Labour Organization released the latest edition of *Global Employment Trends for Youth*, whose central theme was the impact of the global economic crisis on youth aged 15–24. In its introduction, the report summarized some key long-term trends in youth participation in the labour force between 1998 and 2008. Youth unemployment is a significant concern in almost every national economy. Prior to the crisis, youth unemployment rates were falling and stood at just over 12 per cent in 2008. At the same time, the youth population has grown at a faster pace than the available employment opportunities.

In 2008, youth were almost three times as likely to be unemployed as adults, and suffered disproportionately from a deficit of decent work. This is unfortunate not least because decent work can provide adolescent girls and boys with opportunities to develop and apply skills, responsibilities and resources that will be useful throughout their lives.

Figure 3.1: Word cloud illustrating key international youth forums on climate change

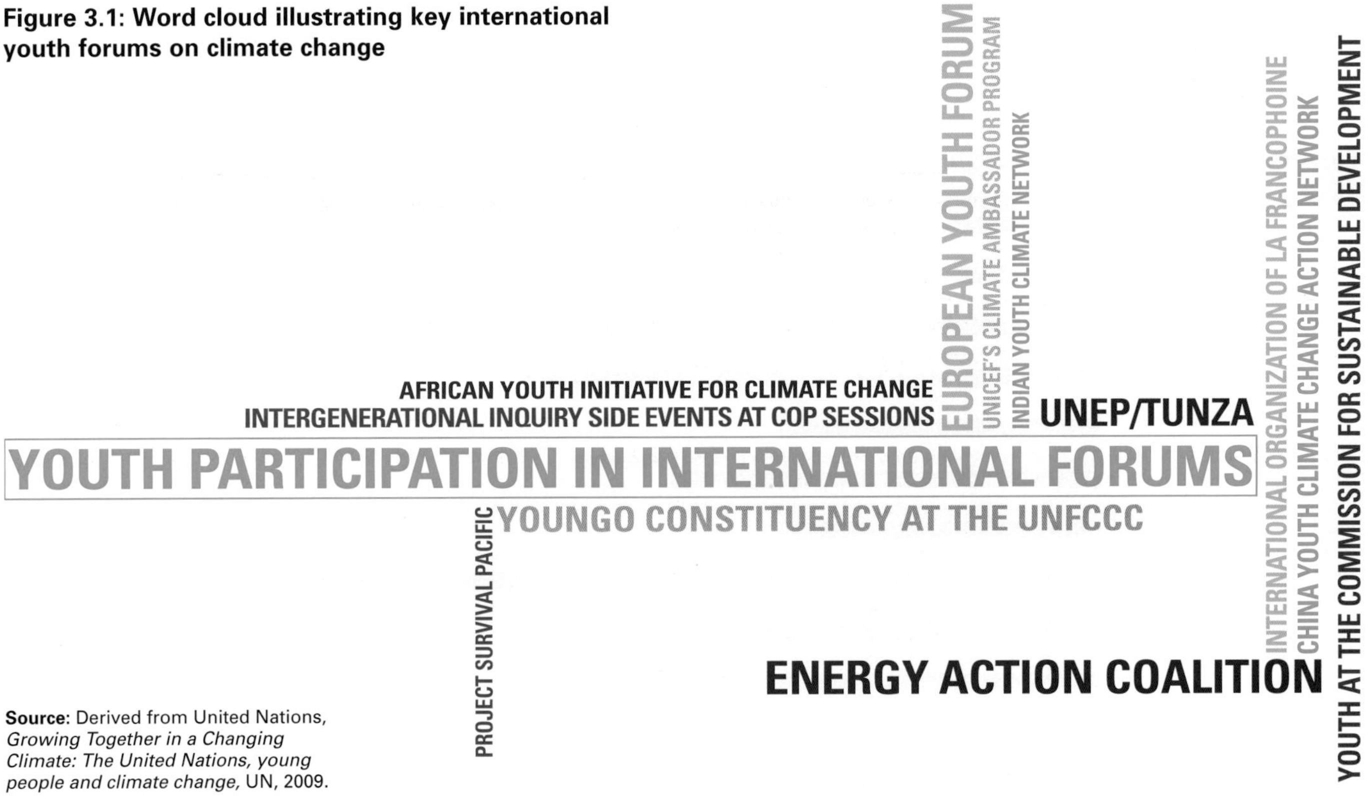

EUROPEAN YOUTH FORUM
UNICEF'S CLIMATE AMBASSADOR PROGRAM
INDIAN YOUTH CLIMATE NETWORK
INTERNATIONAL ORGANIZATION OF LA FRANCOPHOINE
CHINA YOUTH CLIMATE CHANGE ACTION NETWORK
YOUTH AT THE COMMISSION FOR SUSTAINABLE DEVELOPMENT
PROJECT SURVIVAL PACIFIC

AFRICAN YOUTH INITIATIVE FOR CLIMATE CHANGE
INTERGENERATIONAL INQUIRY SIDE EVENTS AT COP SESSIONS
UNEP/TUNZA
YOUTH PARTICIPATION IN INTERNATIONAL FORUMS
YOUNGO CONSTITUENCY AT THE UNFCCC
ENERGY ACTION COALITION

Source: Derived from United Nations, *Growing Together in a Changing Climate: The United Nations, young people and climate change*, UN, 2009.

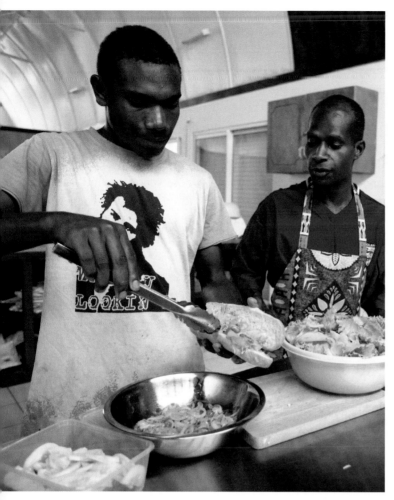

Almost one quarter of the world's working poor were young people in 2008; moreover, these 150-million-plus young poor workers tended to be predominantly engaged in agriculture, which left little time for them to gain the skills and education that could improve their earnings potential and future productivity. While education and demographic trends were easing pressures on youth in regional markets for most of the first decade of this century, the youth labour force continued to expand in the most impoverished regions of sub-Saharan Africa and South Asia. Across the world, however, youth employment trends were fairly bleak, particularly in CEE/CIS and the Middle East and North Africa regions.

The economic crisis has resulted in the largest cohort of unemployed youth ever, estimated at around 81 million worldwide in 2009. Moreover, the ILO report indicated that youth unemployment has proved much more vulnerable to the crisis than adult unemployment. This bodes ill for the new entrants to the global labour market – particularly young women, who typically experience more difficulty than young men in finding work. In most developing regions, the gap between male and female unemployment rates has widened during the crisis. Going forward, youth unemployment rates and numbers are only expected to begin to decline in 2011, but the projected recovery will be slower than for adults.[8]

Throughout the world, a major difficulty in tackling youth unemployment is that many adolescents who have been to school are emerging with insufficient skills – especially those

Vocational training enables adolescents and young people to acquire marketable skills. A 16-year-old boy makes a sandwich while his instructor watches during a cooking class at the Wan Smolbag Theatre Centre in Tagabe, a suburb of Port Vila, Vanuatu.

Figure 3.2: Global trends in youth unemployment

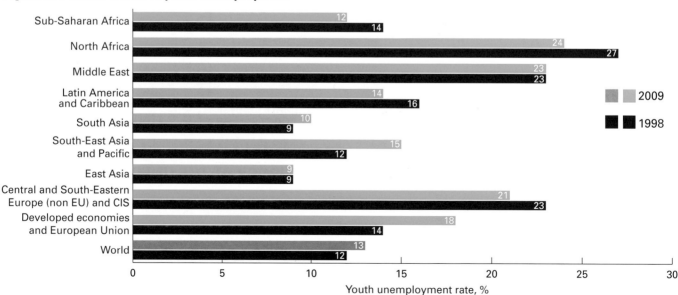

Source: International Labour Organization, *Global Trends in Youth Employment,* ILO, Geneva, 2010, Annex 1, Table A5.

The effects of climate change in Kiribati:
A tangible threat to adolescents

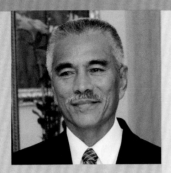

by His Excellency Mr. Anote Tong, President of the Republic of Kiribati

"Climate change is eating away [adolescents'] future and putting their physical and mental development at risk."

For adolescents in the Republic of Kiribati, climate change is not up for debate – it is real and it is happening now. Our young people feel its impact whenever high tides flood their houses; they taste its effects as their drinking water becomes salty. Rising sea levels, which have already brought pools of brackish water to the doorsteps of many homes, are consuming our tiny islets, contaminating our vegetable gardens and poisoning our freshwater wells.

Kiribati is a Pacific island country with a total land area of 811 square kilometres. We have 33 atolls and reef islands, which are home to over 97,000 people – nearly half of whom are children. Global warming will change the lives of our young people in more ways than we can imagine. In 30 to 40 years, their nation, their home may no longer be habitable – it may not even exist. It is time to face facts. We need to act swiftly and decisively to minimize the adverse impact that climate change is having and will continue to have on Kiribati.

Global warming destroys our ability to grow the variety of foods required to provide our children with a balanced and nutritious diet. Resources are diverted away from their education and health as expenses to maintain basic infrastructure increase due to the encroaching sea. Climate change is eating away their future and putting their physical and mental development at risk. Failure to react to climate change now will result in high cultural, social and financial costs. For low-lying countries, such as Kiribati, which are at the frontline of climate change, the threat it poses is real and immediate. The economic disruption could be catastrophic, even requiring the population to relocate to other countries.

While the Convention on the Rights of the Child – the only United Nations Convention to have been ratified by every independent Pacific island country – does not explicitly mention the right to be protected from natural disaster, climate change directly affects children's right to life, survival and development. As the Convention states, every child has the right to a standard of living adequate for her or his physical, mental, spiritual, moral and social development. Our children's right to preserve their identity, including their nationality, and their right to the enjoyment of

the highest attainable standard of health are being threatened. Climate change also jeopardizes the sustainable development agenda established by the Millennium Development Goals.

When I speak with teenagers in Kiribati about global warming and its effects, it is clear that their knowledge of the issue varies significantly depending on where they live. For those who live in remote atolls, limited access to information may lead to confusion and anxiety. We cannot afford this. We need to ensure that every child and adolescent in Kiribati is provided with the means to partake in this vital debate. Investing in information communication technology across the country will enable us to teach, learn and share information on climate change and its related issues much more quickly. As the ones facing the brunt of this global challenge, our children and adolescents must be at the forefront of tackling the problem. Adolescents in particular are often quick to grasp problems and apply great energy and enthusiasm to finding solutions. They are our future and they need to be empowered to take action.

This year, we celebrated 31 years of independence. It is my fervent hope that our children, grandchildren and future generations will be able to celebrate many more years of independence in Kiribati. As a small island developing state (SIDS), we cannot afford the needed investments or solve the issue alone. This is a call to action for families, communities and governments of developed nations to partner with us as we work to give our children and adolescents a chance to have a future. Let us re-examine the impact on our shared environment of what we are all doing right now and determine how we can collectively tackle the challenges of climate change together with our children and adolescents. Let us begin today.

Mr. Anote Tong, President of the Republic of Kiribati since July 2003, is serving his second term. He holds a Master of Science degree from the London School of Economics. His professional experience includes work at the University of the South Pacific and the Pacific Islands Forum Secretariat, as well as senior civil service positions in the Government of the Republic of Kiribati before he went into politics in 1994. From 1994 to 1996, he was the Minister of Natural Resources Development.

Strengthening the participation rights of adolescents

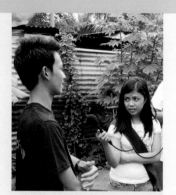

Youth reporters record a segment for Kabataan News Network, Philippines.

"In 2009, the country was home to almost 20 million adolescents between the ages of 10 and 19."

The Philippines lies in the Pacific Ring of Fire, a region of high volcanic and seismic activity, making it one of the most risk-prone countries in the world. Recurrent natural disasters, together with periodic bouts of conflict and social unrest, are among the challenges the country faces in advancing the rights and development of adolescents. Yet the Philippines has made considerable progress towards meeting most of the Millennium Development Goals – in poverty reduction, child mortality, gender equality, combating HIV and AIDS, and access to safe drinking water and sanitary facilities. The net primary school enrolment ratio for girls was 93 per cent in 2008, exceeding that of boys, for whom it was 91 per cent. The Philippines ranked sixth in the world in providing equal opportunities for women according to the World Economic Forum's Gender Gap Index in 2007.

Over the past decades, the country has made the transition from a mainly rural to a predominantly urban society. Around half of the population live in urban areas, with the metropolitan area of Manila, the capital, accommodating the largest share of rural-to-urban migrants. In 2009, the country was home to almost 20 million adolescents between the ages of 10 and 19. Real growth in the gross domestic product averaged 5.8 per cent in 2003–2007, helping to improve the lives of many. Inflows of remittances from Filipinos working overseas have been an important driver of the economy. It is estimated that around 10 per cent of the population live abroad, making the Philippines the third largest migrant-sending country, after China and India.

There are still significant challenges to sustaining and amplifying the advances that have been made. Growing disparities and inequalities are apparent across and within the country's provinces. According to the country's 2009 report under the aegis of UNICEF's ongoing *Global Study on Child Poverty and Disparities*, poverty increased from 24.4 per cent in 2003 to 26.9 per cent in 2009. Two out of three poor people live in rural areas. The other third live in the country's mega-cities, where they face overcrowding, inadequate sanitation and limited access to basic health services.

The Government of the Philippines has taken steps to realize the fundamental rights of children and adolescents and has incorporated the Convention on the Rights of the Child into national laws. For instance, the Special Protection of Children Against Child Abuse, Exploitation and Discrimination Act of 1991 recognizes the 'best interests' principle with explicit reference to the Convention. The Juvenile Justice and Welfare Act of 2006 reaffirms this principle and calls for the participation of children in programme and policy formation and implementation relating to the Act. There is no comprehensive national youth strategy.

The Government has developed a number of policies that support young people's civic engagement, including an article in the Constitution of 1987 and the Youth in Nation Building Act of 1995, along with institutional mechanisms to implement these policies. Youth civic engagement programmes, integrated into school curricula, address a wide variety of issues. These programmes are often run by youth-led organizations. For example, the Sangguniang Kabataan (National Youth Council) provides various incentives and support mechanisms for decentralized youth participation. The representatives, aged 15–21, are elected by other young people at the local level.

Other adolescent participation initiatives are also under way. The Kabataan News Network (KNN), for instance, is a network of young people from around the country, with different ethnic and religious backgrounds, who engage in the media. These young people have produced their own nationwide TV programme, *KNN* – a first for the Philippines. In addition, the Philippines hosted the first ASEAN meeting of adolescents in October 2010, a landmark in young people's participation in South-East Asia.

Progress towards realizing the rights and development of adolescents is encouraging, but more concerted efforts will be critical to increasing their meaningful and positive participation. The country still confronts many challenges – particularly in addressing disparities and inequalities among the regions, and ensuring progressive legislation, such as the Juvenile Justice and Welfare Act, is fully implemented. Maintaining political stability and security throughout the country, including protecting young people from involvement in armed conflict, will be crucial to further improving the lives of adolescents in the years ahead.

See References, page 78

high-level competencies that are increasingly required by the modern globalized economy. In the developing world, while primary enrolment has risen significantly in the developing world, this has not always been matched by attainment levels, and there are still far too few places available in secondary schools, as chapter 2 attests. Standardized tests have shown that many pupils completing primary school in developing countries have not reached the same levels of knowledge and skills as those in industrialized countries, prompting concerns about the quality of the basic education being offered. More than 20 per cent of companies in developing countries surveyed – including Algeria, Bangladesh, Brazil, China and Zambia – consider the inadequate education of workers to be a significant obstacle to higher levels of investment and faster economic growth.[9]

In many developing countries the lack of formal employment opportunities is a long-established reality. In the absence of productive full-time employment, many adolescents and young adults wrestle with underemployment – taking bits and pieces of casual work where they can, or else engaging in the informal economy. This may involve working for low pay in exploitative conditions for employers who do not observe national labour, health and safety standards. Alternatively, it may involve engaging in petty commerce on the street, which entails a precarious day-to-day subsistence and can operate on the margins of more dangerous and illegal activities, from organized crime to prostitution.

Such unemployment or underemployment is a depressing waste of young people's energy and talents. At a time when they should be learning new skills and adapting themselves to the needs of their community and society – while earning themselves a living wage that offers the prospect of a secure future – their first experience of work is all too often one of disillusionment and rejection that locks them into poverty.

This represents a double disadvantage to society. Not only is it failing to make productive use of the capacities of the young, but the failure to do so may foster desperation and disenchantment, which can result in social fracture and political

Young people can use their knowledge and skills to contribute in their homes, schools and communities. *Adolescent girls learn to do embroidery in a home-based school in the Khairkhana neighbourhood of Kabul, Afghanistan.*

protest as well as susceptibility to fundamentalism or crime. The World Programme of Action for Youth in 2007 recognized that while the global economic boom that lasted for much of the 1990s and 2000s had many positive impacts for young people, such as the cross-fertilization of ideas and the internationalization of opportunity for those with the necessary skills, it has excluded many young people in developing countries from its potential benefits. Today many still lack the education or the skills to meet the demands of the global economy and cannot take advantage of either the enhanced information or the economic opportunities that globalization offers.

Now is the time to invest in the skills of adolescents

The need for concerted international action to confront these problems has long been recognized. In 1995, governments focused particularly on youth unemployment in the Copenhagen Declaration and Programme of Action adopted at the conclusion of the World Summit for Social Development. The UN Millennium Declaration in 2000 explicitly committed governments to pursue strategies aimed at providing young people with productive work opportunities.

The Youth Employment Network (YEN) – comprising the UN, the International Labour Organization and the World Bank – was set up to help them fulfil that commitment. In 2001, a team of youth employment experts appointed by the then UN Secretary-General, Kofi Annan, made recommendations in four key policy areas – employability, entrepreneurship, equal opportunities for young men and women, and employment creation – and the YEN is now working with many countries to devise or implement national action plans addressing them.

Countries across the developing world have taken up the challenge of tackling youth unemployment, primarily by establishing initiatives to enhance skills. Using the YEN recommendations, Uganda's Ministry of Education and Sports, the Kampala City Council and Germany's international development agency (GTZ) developed a curriculum to complement formal schooling that teaches young people reading, writing and arithmetic skills while teaching them about their rights and giving them practical skills to improve their employment prospects. In El Salvador, the Ministry of Education and Labour, non-governmental organizations and GTZ targeted young rural women in particular to offer the skills, personal development and vocational and other training needed to promote employment. Among the national strategies adopted elsewhere have been youth entrepreneurship and leadership training, microcredit schemes, the establishment of new careers guidance services and the promotion of information and communication technology (ICT) skills.[10]

Despite the current economic storm clouds, there is no better time than the present to invest in developing the skills of adolescents and job opportunities for young people. The slowing of fertility rates worldwide represents a demographic opportunity for many developing countries. A large number of developing countries, particularly low-income nations, are approaching a period – long past in the industrialized countries and even some middle-income countries – when lower birth rates combine with higher numbers of adolescents and youth than ever before to make the productive workforce an extremely large proportion of the total population. While the number of dependents relative to the working population is falling,

Digital safety for young people:
Gathering information, creating new models and understanding existing efforts

by Colin Maclay,
Gerrit Beger, Urs Gasser
and John Palfrey

One of the most profound changes in the past decade has been the widespread – although uneven – proliferation of information and communications technologies.

Social network sites, mobile phone operators and other private actors are implementing savvy methods designed to appeal to youth in developing countries. The following events are particularly interesting:

- Orkut, Google's social network site, was voted MTV India's Youth Icon of 2007.
- In response to the overwhelming presence of Orkut in India, Facebook made its social network site available in Bengali, Hindi, Malayalam, Punjabi, Tamil and Telugu, to target Indian youth who are not fluent in English.
- Facebook has also been available in Swahili since the summer of 2009, targeting 110 million people in Africa.
- Facebook Zero was launched in May 2010 as a mobile site free of data charges and available in 45 countries – 10 in Africa – where access to the Internet can be slow and costly.
- Other sophisticated information and communication technology innovations include Mxit, the number one social network site in South Africa; and Sembuse, in East Africa, the first mobile network site to allow the cheap sending of messages up to 1,000 characters (compared to only 160 for regular short text messaging).

These developments are exciting and offer possibilities for transforming learning, civic engagement, innovation, entrepreneurship and much more. But they also pose risks.

A growing concern for parents, educators and others involved with the welfare and well-being of children and adolescents is related to young people's ability to use these tools safety and effectively. In addition, the explosive growth of ICT also presents challenges to young people's privacy, freedom of expression and physical and psychological well-being – and there remain fundamental knowledge gaps regarding their impact. Despite agreement that risks for young people exist, these have largely gone both unexamined and unaddressed in developing countries. At the same time, a mixture of genuine concern, powerful anecdote, traditional culture and diverse political forces is driving interventions in the name of child safety and may lead to ineffective or even counterproductive policies.

Effective problem solving begins with the definition and exploration of the problem in question. While it may seem straightforward, a comprehensive and uniform concept of what safety means in the online context is lacking. In addition, the interpretation and relative prevalence of risks varies. In developing nations, for instance, while some forms of aggressive behaviour may be less common, certain sexual risks – whether sex tourism, trafficking of children or production of child pornography – are likely to a window for possible economic development of at least two decades opens, and many developing countries are just about to enter this phase. Some studies indicate that much of the success of East Asian economies in recent years derived from reaping this demographic dividend, which depends nevertheless on investment in human capital at the right time.[11]

Information and communications technology can accelerate skills and knowledge acquisition

ICT offers the potential to remove barriers to education and literacy and to hand adolescents a key to unlock many of the benefits of the modern knowledge economy and not

be left adrift by globalization. The panels on youth and technology presented throughout this report highlight that adolescents and young people are particularly receptive to new technology and adapt to its demands with alacrity when they are given the chance.

The poor in many developing countries, however, remain largely excluded from ICT and its benefits. A vast digital divide continues to exist not only between the industrialized and the developing world – particularly the least developed nations – but also between rich and poor within countries. Access to ICT is also much more problematic for disabled adolescents and those from marginalized communities or

be more pressing. Coming to terms with a uniform concept of safety and arriving at ways to discuss and track the varying risks and behaviours are essential. Refining these risks to children's rights to protection from violence, abuse and exploitation from online sources is essential.

A range of factors – including the setting and means of access, usage patterns, attitudes and skill levels – is important in mapping risks and designing responses. Also important are factors such as age, gender and socio-economic status, as well as peer behaviour and mediation by caregivers. Whether a child accesses the Internet from home, school or a cybercafe, for instance, has significant implications for supervision, just as the speed of access and type of device (i.e., mobile versus computer) affect usage and risks. Information fluency and related digital skills to evaluate online materials and perform research are also the basis for identifying predators, avoiding risky situations and safely sharing personal information. These factors do not exist in isolation but interact with the broader technological, economic, institutional, educational and cultural context.

Current approaches to increasing digital safety for children and young people typically consist of some combination of new or improved national legislation against child pornography and stronger law enforcement; filtering technologies at the individual access point as well as the network level to screen out child sexual abuse images or other forms of pornography

in particular; and awareness-raising and educational campaigns targeted at parents, teachers and children. Within these broad categories, differences exist with regard to the actual design and use of the instruments, including the procedural safeguards that should accompany them.

The transfer of 'solutions' from one context to another calls for a careful analysis of the institutional framework and of the interplay among the factors outlined above, including a comprehensive stakeholder analysis. Addressing knowledge deficits requires more research and capacity-building, both in developing and developed nations, including field experiments and meaningful engagement with young people. Programmes that genuinely try to improve the safety of children and young people in a digital context must be separated from the merely rhetorical, lest policymakers use the cover of protecting children to accomplish other goals such as broadly limiting access to information.

Colin Maclay, Urs Gasser and John Palfrey work at the Berkman Center for Internet & Society, Harvard University, while Gerrit Beger heads the Division of Communications Youth Section at UNICEF. The Berkman Center, which was founded to explore cyberspace and help pioneer its development, represents a network of faculty, students, fellows, entrepreneurs, lawyers and virtual architects working to identify and engage with the challenges and opportunities it offers.

"Effective problem solving begins with the definition and exploration of the problem in question."

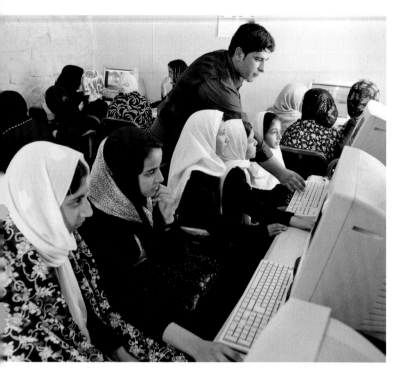

Information and communication technology offers the potential to remove barriers to education and literacy. *Young women who are youth volunteers learn computer skills at a computer and literacy training centre run by the Afghan Red Crescent Society.*

ethnic minorities. And in some societies adolescent girls may also find it more difficult than boys to gain access to the technology itself and the training necessary to harness it, owing to factors similar to those that tend to exclude girls from education and equal participation in household and community life.

Social protection is also a critical area for investment

Another area of necessary investment in adolescents is the provision of social protection, especially child-sensitive social protection. In industrialized countries this is a common mechanism for ensuring that the poorest and most marginalized sectors of the population – and especially their children – receive sufficient support to meet their basic needs. It encompasses social insurance, basic services and labour market regulation.

In developing countries, the social assistance aspect of social protection has a primary, broad role in reducing poverty and is a key component of development policy. In developing countries with the relevant experience, there is increasing evidence that social protection programmes can not only improve children's health, nutrition and educational achievement but also reduce the danger of abuse and exploitation. Social protection is vital if countries are to break the intergenerational cycle of poverty and offer

the economic opportunities so badly needed by adolescents and young people entering the job market.[12, 13]

Juvenile crime and violence

Adolescents are sometimes perceived as a threat to community peace and security. This view is by no means confined to the scaremongering or routine stereotyping of youth in the mass media; the UN High-level Panel on Threats, Challenges and Change, for example, considers that the combination of a booming adolescent population with unemployment and urbanization can raise the risk of civil strife.

The suggestion is that if adolescents are not productively employed or feel disaffected from society, particularly males, they more likely to express their frustrations through violence. But despite the difficulties of making the transition to adulthood, the fact is that the vast majority of young people function as stable members of society going peacefully about their affairs.[14]

In practice, while a small proportion of adolescents develop bad habits of drug abuse, violent behaviour and criminality that adversely condition the course of their adult lives, the overwhelming majority move on to an adulthood in which they accept the prevailing codes of conduct and themselves come to be concerned about the criminal behaviour of later generations. According to the United Nations Guidelines for the Prevention of Juvenile Delinquency (the Riyadh Guidelines), "youthful behaviour or conduct that does not conform to overall social norms and values is often part of the maturation and growth process and tends to disappear spontaneously in most individuals with the transition to adulthood."[15]

As with every other age group in society, adolescents are infinitely varied in their characteristics, life situations and attitudes. In the literature about young people and violence, there is generally a marked absence of material pointing to the positive contributions to society made by adolescents, or reference to the vast majority who do not become involved in violence of any kind.

In today's world, the word 'juvenile' is being seen followed by the word 'delinquency' to a disturbing degree. Clearly adolescence is an uncertain period that can put some young people in conflict with the law and endanger their health and well-being. Moreover, there are global trends that

ADOLESCENT VOICES

Reclaim Tijuana:
Put an end to drug-related violence

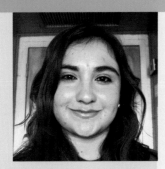

by Brenda Garcia, 17, Mexico

"The drug trafficking trade has the power to silence people."

Growing up in Tijuana, I often heard stories of the time when it was considered the Mexican Promised Land. This frontier city on the Mexico-United States border offered hope to settlers from other parts of the country, like my grandparents, who sought a better standard of living. As it grew, Tijuana turned into one of the most prosperous cities in Mexico. I was told that school attendance and employment rates soared, people felt safe and tourists from the United States would crowd the main shopping street, Avenida Revolución, on weekends.

As I grew up and started reading local newspapers, I realized that bad things were happening. Over the last few years, a wave of violent crime related to drug trafficking has hit Tijuana as well as other Mexican cities. Kidnapping, torture, murder, persecution, threats, military intervention, innocent lives destroyed – all in the place I call home. Tijuana today is one of the most dangerous places in the country. This has ruined the tourism industry and caused a dramatic loss of jobs.

In the last year, we have seen some progress: Key drug cartel leaders have been arrested and the drug trade's influence has diminished. However, with the cartels' activities disrupted, violence has increased and may get worse before it gets better. Confronted with the global economic downturn, and upsurge in violence, some Mexicans have migrated to the United States. While many residents are terrified and avoid leaving their homes, others say it is an issue between gangsters and does not concern them. Yet how can we look the other way when we learn of shootings in hospitals or outside kindergartens?

There is a difference between apathy and ignorance. I was ignorant. I thought Tijuana was a peaceful city and that the media's stories were exaggerations. However, once you learn that your neighbour has been shot or that a close friend has lost his father, you stop and think: How can we end this?

Many residents feel that Tijuana's lack of adequate law enforcement has allowed violence to grow. Consequently, the community has lost faith in its representatives. This makes people – both young and old – feel helpless and discourages them from being active

citizens. The drug trafficking trade has the power to silence people. In my opinion, young people in Tijuana no longer expect change; they have lost hope. It is hard for citizens to trust authority when they hear that part of the police force has been involved in the drug trafficking.

People get used to violence; they end up accepting it. I hear teenagers and parents say that violence in Tijuana is 'normal'. When they hear about a new murder, they say "that is not news." The drug trade even transforms dreams. Some teenage boys are fascinated by the illusion of glamour it offers and call themselves *mangueras*, which means aspiring gangsters. They say their dream is to become a drug dealer so that they have money to attract women and buy cars. What happened to people like my grandparents, who wanted a better, safer life for their children?

I know that we often blame the government when things go wrong, but we must do more than complain or throw up our hands. We need honest law enforcement officials and a responsive criminal justice system. In order to move forward, we need to restore public confidence and hope in the local community. It is time to reclaim the city of Tijuana.

Brenda Garcia grew up in Tijuana, Mexico. She is a university student and speaks Spanish, English, Italian and some Portuguese. She plans to major in international security and conflict resolution.

Advocacy through sports:
Stopping the spread of HIV among young people

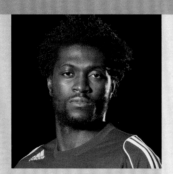

by Emmanuel Adebayor, professional football player and Goodwill Ambassador for the Joint United Nations Programme on HIV/AIDS (UNAIDS)

"Only 1 in 10 adolescents in Togo understands the ways in which HIV can be transmitted."

As a youngster growing up in Lomé, Togo, my passion and love for football were fuelled by my desire to play with my friends, to compete, win and, of course, sometimes lose. Today, my profession gives me the chance to see people of varied backgrounds, religions and faiths come together to watch the exciting game of football. In doing so, they celebrate diversity from all corners of the earth. Sports and games possess the unique virtue of cutting across cultural and generational gaps. While young people may at times find it hard to communicate with adults, engaging in sports allows families, friends and, perhaps, even adversaries a window to put aside differences and cheer in unison.

I am grateful to have a career in football and to participate in top-level clubs. Throughout the time that I have played, however, I have carried with me the awareness that my homeland – while culturally rich and vibrant – was suffering from the effects of poverty, ill health and lack of access to education. I witnessed first-hand the effects of HIV on Africa. I noticed the singular hardships that confront young people living with HIV, especially those who are marginalized, who live a life of poverty and despair, and those most at risk: adolescent girls. In sub-Saharan Africa, girls account for an overwhelming majority of all infections in young people. Their voices often go unheard. These same young people face stigma, discrimination and exclusion.

Motivated by what I had seen, I teamed up with UNAIDS in 2008 to spread global awareness about HIV – particularly to young people, as the majority of our football fans are young. I seized the opportunity to promote a cause in need of special attention. Thanks to UNAIDS, I have the chance to pass on a life-saving message to young people who may not have access to the information I have regarding HIV. We must all do our part.

HIV stands out, not only because of the number of people living with the virus, but because we know how to prevent it. Of the 2.5 million HIV-positive children under age 15 in the world, more than 90 per cent are in sub-Saharan Africa. At last count, there were 120,000 people living with HIV in Togo in a population of just 6.6 million. Many of them were infected at a young age. Only 1 in 7 young women in Togo understands the ways in which HIV can be transmitted.

During my first year as a Goodwill Ambassador, I learned that giving clear and sound information on HIV prevention, treatment, care and support is one thing – but changing peoples' attitudes, beliefs and behaviour towards those who are infected or seen as vulnerable to HIV infection is a much bigger challenge. Many who are living with HIV still encounter discrimination or are reluctant to approach counselling centres, accept advice on preventing mother-to-child transmission or seek antiretroviral treatment for fear of social alienation. In sub-Saharan Africa, 12 million children have been orphaned by AIDS. In Togo alone, 88,000 have lost one or both parents to the epidemic, and 94 per cent of those do not receive any medical, educational or psychological support.

If young people are to have a chance at living up to their full potential, they urgently need to know how to protect themselves from HIV infection and where to find counselling and treatment. This is our only chance to halt the spread of HIV. I hope to inspire adolescents around the world to speak out on the issues surrounding HIV with the same ardour that I and other advocates do.

With the increasing global popularity of football, sports play an important role as a vehicle for change. HIV can be prevented if each person plays his or her part in stopping its spread. I have faced hardships in life, like everyone else, but I have also been fortunate to have enjoyed success on the football pitch. I see the power of young people every time I play. There are more young people on this planet now than ever before. Their energy and dynamism present a tremendous opportunity for change. We owe it to them to overcome HIV, so that future young people can live in an HIV-free world.

Emmanuel Adebayor is a Togolese professional football player titled African Footballer of the Year in 2008. He was named Goodwill Ambassador for the Joint United Nations Programme on HIV/AIDS (UNAIDS) in 2009 and continues to use his popularity to raise awareness about the epidemic globally, particularly the importance of preventing new infections among young people.

are exacerbating those risks, including rapid population growth and urbanization, social exclusion and the rising incidence of drug abuse. Yet juvenile crime or violence is only part of the story. It is important to recall that many adolescents come into contact with the law as victims.

Whatever the circumstances, effective social work with youthful offenders and victims is generally lacking in many national and local settings. Worldwide, UNICEF estimates that at any given moment more than 1 million children are detained by law enforcement officials.[16] And this is likely an underestimate. In the 44 countries with available data, around 59 per cent of detained children had not been sentenced.[17] A 2007 report studying El Salvador, Guatemala, Jamaica, and Trinidad and Tobago found that adolescents 15–18 years old – particularly boys – are the most at risk from armed violence and confirmed that children are much more frequently the victims of armed violence rather than the aggressors.[18] In prisons and institutions across the world, adolescents are often denied the right to medical care, education and opportunities for individual development.[19] Detention also exposes children to serious forms of violence, such as torture, brutality, sexual abuse and rape, as well as poor conditions.[20]

The most disadvantaged adolescents are at greatest risk of coming into conflict with the law

The adolescents most at risk of coming into conflict with the law are often the product of difficult family circumstances that might include poverty, family breakdown, parental abuse or alcoholism. A large number of juvenile offences are actually 'status offences' – actions, such as truancy or running away from home, that would be acceptable behaviour in an adult and are only outlawed on the basis of age. Another very large body of crimes, however, is much more serious and tends to emerge from adolescents' involvement in gangs. At their worst, gangs can act as precursors of adult criminal groups and can effectively involve a 'career choice' of criminality.

Adolescents in gangs, or groups tend to be hierarchically organized but tight-knit, with a rigid internal code of behaviour. Many use violence as a routine mechanism for resolving interpersonal conflict, and this culture of violence is likely to spill over and influence members' behaviour towards people outside the group as well, establishing a pat-

tern or likelihood of criminality. Territorial gang members commit many more crimes than adolescents who do not belong to gangs, with the most frequent offences involving violence and extortion.

Juvenile crime is much more likely to be committed by males than females. In part this is because in some cultures girls are more restricted by their families and the society at large as to what they can do, and many cultures are more tolerant of deviant behaviour among boys than among girls. In addition, aggression is often an established part of the construction of masculine identity in male-dominated societies. Though gang culture often does involve the rejection of some established adult values, it tends uncritically to import and apply very rigid gender roles.

The majority of adolescents who come into conflict with the law are still children, whose rights under the Convention must be protected and respected

The problem of juvenile crime tends to be exacerbated by economic decline and focused especially in the poorer areas of big cities. Juvenile crime is primarily an urban problem. It also has a relationship with the consumer lifestyle portrayed by the mass media, which creates a desire for products and experiences that are materially inaccessible to whole sectors of the population unless they resort to illegal activities. Drug abuse is also a major factor driving juvenile crime, as addiction is virtually impossible to finance with the incomes available to adolescents. Adolescents from disadvantaged groups, including ethnic minorities and migrants, are disproportionately likely to offend.[21]

"I wish for peace and stability on the African continent."

Kingford, 19, Ghana

Most adolescents who come into conflict with the law are still children, and they need to receive special treatment from the criminal justice system that reflects their status. There are still too many countries where adolescents are simply absorbed into the adult justice system, both to be tried and to serve any eventual sentence. Adolescents who spend periods of pre-trial detention or serve prison sentences alongside adults are much less likely to be reintegrated into society when they are released and much more likely to revert to criminal behaviour.

While incarceration is clearly unavoidable in some circumstances, it is essential to explore alternatives to custodial

Migration and children: A cause for urgent attention

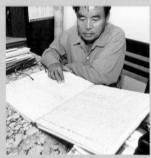

An official from the Ministry of Labour and Social Welfare in Thailand reviews a logbook of migrant workers and victims of trafficking who have been officially repatriated to the Lao People's Democratic Republic.

Today, it is estimated that approximately 214 million migrants live outside their countries of birth. This figure includes 33 million young children and adolescents under the age of 20 who have migrated either with their parents or unaccompanied. There are also many other children and adolescents who are directly or indirectly affected by migration, including those left in the country of origin when one or both of their parents emigrate.

Figures from the recently created United Nations Global Migration Database show that in industrialized countries, adolescents aged 10–19 account for around 53 per cent of international migrants under 20. Overall, however, developing countries tend to host a greater number of migrants under 20, of which around 68 per cent are adolescents aged 10–19.

There are wide geographical variations in migration trends for young children and adolescents. For instance, migrants under the age of 20 constitute the largest group of the total migrant population in Africa (28 per cent). They also make up a substantial percentage of migrants in Asia and Oceania (20 per cent), the Americas (11 per cent) and Europe (11 per cent).

A gender gap exists among the global migrant population under 20, with 94 migrant girls for every 100 migrant boys. This trend is in line with the global gender balance for that age cohort. In industrialized countries, however, migrant girls outnumber boys, with 100 girls for every 98 migrant boys under 20. This gap is sharply reversed in developing countries, with only 80 migrant girls under 20 for every 100 boys of the same age.

The risks of adolescent migration

Young children and adolescents – especially those who are undocumented or have been separated from their families – are particularly vulnerable to violations of human rights and protection abuses directly or indirectly related to migration and migration policies and regulation. The United Nations Special Rapporteur on the Human Rights of Migrants has underscored the exceptional vulnerability of children across the spectrum of migration. A fundamental concern is that young children and adolescents crossing borders may not be entitled to the same protection and rights as those who reside in a given country, leaving them at greater risk of invisibility, discrimination and exploitation. And while it is often reported that many migrants are not necessarily among the poorest in their countries of transit or destination, it is also true that they often disproportionately face discrimination and exclusion in their countries of origin, transit or destination – or all three.

The urgent need for a child and adolescent perspective in migration policies

A rights-based approach to migration is urgently required to reinforce the steady build-up of support and attention to migration issues at the international and national levels. This approach must begin by addressing the root causes of migration (e.g., poverty, inequality, discrimination, instability) in the country of origin, and it should incorporate policies specifically targeted for young children and adolescents, girls and young women, and vulnerable populations, including those left behind when family members migrate.

The absence of a child and adolescent perspective in migration-related detention, deportation and repatriation policies, and in fulfilling the economic, social and cultural rights of children is widely evident in both industrialized and developing countries. Urgent action is required to ensure that migration policies meet the principles of the Convention and other human rights treaties and that, in all cases, the best interests of the child are paramount.

Encouragingly, across the world, governments and their partners are increasingly working on research, policies and programmes aimed at promoting and protecting the rights of children and adolescents affected by migration. Though much more remains to be done, the examples that follow illustrate what can be achieved when political will is combined with adequate resources and sound strategies.

- In the **Philippines**, the Government has devised policies and institutions such as the Overseas Workers Welfare Administration, which manages a trust fund that supports health care, welfare assistance education and training programmes for migrant workers and families. The Philippines Overseas Employment Administration is also working to protect the rights of migrants and of families left behind.

- In **Mexico**, the National Family Development System (NFDS) and the National Migration Institute (NMI) jointly operate eight care units in northern border states to provide essential services, rest and communication with families for repatriated children. In conjunction with non-governmental organizations, the NFDS also provides a network of 27 transitory shelters to protect unaccompanied children and adolescents. A special corps of child protection officers, currently numbering over 300, has been established within the NMI since 2008; the corps has recorded higher rates of detection of and response to trafficking, sexual exploitation and violence and abuse against these children.

- In **Albania**, a programme launched by the Government and the UN, and supported by Spain's Millennium Development Goals Achievement Fund, aims to provide job opportunities and streamline national strategies for youth employment and migration. Through labour programmes targeting at-risk youth, this programme specifically aims to reach youth employees in two regions, Shkodra and Kukes, which are characterized by high levels of informal employment and youth migration. In addition, it seeks to foster ties between communities of origin and expatriate Albanians, using social media and web-based tools.

See References, page 78.

sentencing wherever possible, including counselling, probation and community service, as well as restorative justice that involves the child, family, community and victim and promotes restitution and reconciliation.[22] The ultimate aim must always be that of reintegration, of encouraging young people towards responsible citizenship.

Conflict and emergency settings

A lack of peace and security exacerbates the difficulties of growing into adulthood

Conflict is one situation of violence that has clear and unequivocal risks for all adolescents. Although they are not as vulnerable as young children to death and disease produced by conflict, this group is at greater risk in other ways. Adolescents may be targeted for recruitment by military groups, whether to carry weapons and participate in atrocities or to act in effect as sexual and other types of slaves. Although the activities may involve violence, adolescents may also become involved because of their growing interest in actively participating in politics.

In emergencies, adolescents, particularly girls, are often forced to discontinue their education, owing to disruption, economic considerations or because they have to care for younger siblings in the absence of parents. They may

Striving for equity:
A look at marginalized adolescents in Zambia

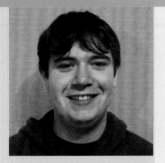

by Cian McLeod, 17, Ireland

"Girls who are disabled run a greater risk of physical and mental abuse."

Although I believe we are closer than ever to living in an equitable world, societies must still work towards changing social norms that allow discrimination, marginalization and exclusion. This is most apparent when we consider disabled children, girls' education and children living with HIV.

In November 2009, I had the opportunity to volunteer for a couple of weeks in a home for disabled children in Mongu, Zambia, and I gained a vivid insight into their lives. I was shocked by the marginalization of these children, as they are among the most cheerful and playful I have ever met. As in many other countries, disabled children in Zambia are sometimes sent away and even disowned. They may be left unattended and uncared for; they may also receive less food.

Disabled children are often excluded from school because the education system makes no allowance for them. In addition, their parents do not recognize their right to education or development. They are denied the chance to learn the skills they need to work and achieve independence as adults.

Gender inequality is evident as well. Girls who are disabled run a greater risk of physical and mental abuse. Girls are not valued, and neither is their education. I see the rise in HIV and AIDS as a direct result of this social outlook.

Education plays a vital role in the prevention of sexual transmitted infections. In order to halt the spread of

HIV, it is fundamental that all adolescents learn about prevention and treatment. Although school enrolment of girls has increased in developing countries, it is still not equal to that of boys. In Zambia, when a family member is HIV-positive, the family's financial resources shift from education to health. As girls are responsible for the traditionally female tasks – cooking, cleaning and nursing – they are expected to drop out of school to care for the sick.

Globally, nearly 5 million young people were living with HIV in 2008. In Zambia, if a girl or boy is thought to be infected with HIV, she or he is no longer sent to school. This lack of education leads to a vicious cycle of gender inequality, increased HIV infection and poverty. When girls and women are not given access to education, they cannot gain independence from men; when girls do not learn about HIV prevention, they are more likely to be exposed to the virus.

It is evident that we do not yet live in a fair and non-discriminatory world: The rights of marginalized children need to be better protected. It is the responsibility of adolescents to focus our endeavours towards creating a more equitable society in our lifetime.

Cian McLeod lives in Balbriggan, Ireland. He is involved in his community's sports development programme and peer mentoring. His experience volunteering in Mongu was with the Sporting Fingal Zambian Mission. Cian's goal is to work as an economist for developing countries. He would like to make the world a fairer place.

Releasing the potential of adolescents:
Education reform in the Middle East and North Africa region

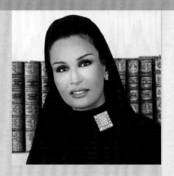

by Her Highness Sheikha Mozah bint Nasser Al Missned, UNESCO Special Envoy for Basic and Higher Education

"In order to release the potential of the next workforce – adolescents – we must ensure that their education properly prepares them for a career"

On 12 August 2010, the second United Nations International Year of Youth commenced. We stakeholders and advocates for children must therefore turn our attention to the problems adolescents face today. In the Middle East and North Africa region, these are particularly serious in the areas of education and future employment.

The region is also experiencing an unprecedented youth bulge. In the next 10 years, 65 per cent of the population will be 24 years old or younger. In addition to the demographic pressure, young people are finding it increasingly difficult to break into the labour market, especially with the larger number of new entrants every year. The region has a rapidly growing labour force, and both unemployment and underemployment are major concerns for young people trying to provide for themselves and their families. By the time a 13-year-old today turns 23, as many as 100 million jobs will be needed to accommodate these rising numbers. That means creating 6.5 million jobs per year.

While the Gulf countries have experienced a surge of wealth during recent decades, this has not been entirely beneficial for our young people. Many adolescents have grown accustomed to a materialistic lifestyle that distracts them from reaching their full potential. Likewise, the seduction of consumerism traps adolescents in an endless quest for possessions and encourages them to disregard their role as citizens responsible for community involvement and positive self-development. Moreover, the labour market cannot support the current youth bulge, impeding young people's ability to achieve financial independence. Unable to find work, they extend their studies, in turn delaying marriage and parenthood.

Acknowledging that our youth are consumers rather than producers is alarming, but it is not their fault alone. The education system in Arab countries is partly responsible for the soaring unemployment rate, because it focuses more on granting diplomas than on effectively training students in practical skills. It does not prepare young people for the global job market, as it neither encourages versatility nor enables them to apply a diverse set of abilities across a number of

disciplines. In today's rapidly changing technological world, young people need to learn critical thinking, writing skills and flexibility – areas virtually absent from our curricula at present. If we do not reform our current practice and aim to transform today's adolescents into creative, productive and diligent contributors, our economies will not be able to compete globally.

My work with the United Nations Alliance of Civilizations inspired me to launch Silatech, a regional youth initiative whose name derives from the Arabic term 'your connection'. Particularly active in the Gulf countries, the initiative aims to partner young people with leaders, corporations and organizations globally to promote opportunities for innovation and enterprise. In order to release the potential of the next workforce – adolescents – we must ensure that their education properly prepares them for a career. If we do not invest in this generation, I believe that the devastating cycle of unemployment will continue. Adolescents represent a tremendous asset for our future, and this historic opportunity to empower them and help them flourish must not be missed.

Her Highness Sheikha Mozah bint Nasser Al Missned serves as Chairperson of the Qatar Foundation for Education, Science and Community Development; Vice Chair of the Supreme Education Council; President of the Supreme Council for Family Affairs; and Chairperson of the Sidra Medical and Research Center project. She established the Silatech initiative to help generate new jobs and opportunities for young people in the Arab world.

be stranded in poverty by conflict or other emergencies, unable to pursue a livelihood, and they are often at greater risk of sexual violence and exploitation.[23] They may be lured or dragged into participation in criminal activities as a way of coping with the material and emotional uncertainties of their lives.[24]

The risks adolescents face, and the contributions they make in conflict and emergency settings, deserve great recognition

The past two decades has witnessed a growing recognition of the impact of armed conflict on children and youth, and a strengthening international response to the issue. The Convention on the Rights of the Child stipulates that children under age 15 should not take a direct part in hostilities and should be protected from the effects of armed conflict. This legal safeguard was then extended and reinforced in the Optional Protocol on the Involvement of Children in Armed Conflict, adopted by the UN General Assembly in 2000 and which entered into force in 2002. The Optional Protocol raised the minimum age for recruitment into military service to 18 and criminalized the recruitment of children under 18 by rebel groups.

The bar was raised even farther in 2007, when representatives of 59 countries committed themselves to ending the unlawful recruitment and use of children and adolescents in armed conflicts in what were called the Paris Commitments and Principles. As of the beginning of 2010, 84 countries had endorsed the Commitments.

Adolescents are not only victims and witnesses to conflict, however; given the chance, they can also be an integral part of its resolution and societal renewal. Ever since the first International Youth Year was designated in 1985 with a theme of 'Participation, Development and Peace', UN organizations have regularly attempted to stress the positive contribution adolescents and youth have made to resolving social problems and the even greater contribution they could make.

During the two-and-a-half decades that have ensued between the first and the current (August 2010–2011) UN International Year of Youth, the focus on involving adolescents and young people in conflict resolution and postconflict rebuilding has been greatly strengthened. There has also been increasing recognition of the importance of adolescent participation in emergency situations, as noted in chapter 2. Encouraging the participation of adolescents in all aspects of community life is not only the best way to realize their potential but also often the best means of ensuring their protection – though care clearly has to be taken when adolescents are politically outspoken in conflict and post-conflict situations.

Adolescent participation in challenging situations can be both a means and an end. It can allow young people to develop their problem-solving and negotiating skills while fostering a wider atmosphere of tolerance, democratic practice and non-violence. There is a virtuous circle within reach here: Just as adolescents are more likely to flourish and realize their potential in conditions of peace and security, so those conditions of peace and security are more likely to be attained if young people are encouraged to play a full part.

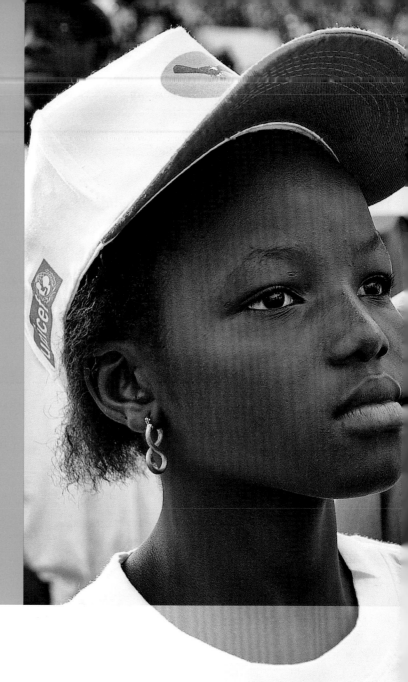

Attendance and completion of secondary school, access to quality health care, participation in decision-making and protection from violence, exploitation and abuse are fundamental to empowering adolescents to realize their full potential. *Adolescents from local schools attend Global Handwashing Day at Mobido Keita Stadium, Bamako, Mali.*

CHAPTER 4

Investing in Adolescents

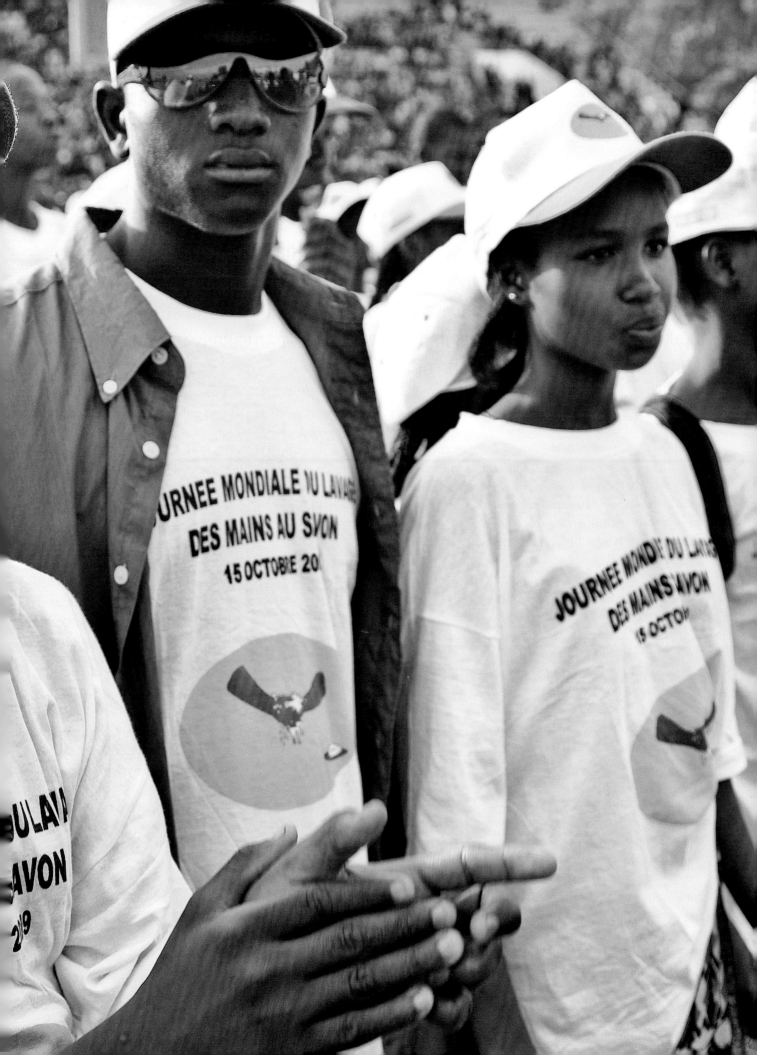

CHALLENGES AND

Over the course of the next five years, the world has an unprecedented opportunity to improve the lives of young children and adolescents by achieving the Millennium Development Goals (MDGs) with equity. Great strides have been made towards the goals in the past decade, particularly for those children currently still in the first decade of life.

The global under-five mortality rate, long considered a reliable gauge of child well-being, fell by 22 per cent between 2000 and 2009 – double the rate of decline achieved in the preceding decade. Immunization against major childhood diseases has risen in all regions. Primary education has seen a strong boost in enrolment and attendance, which in turn has served to narrow the gender divide as girls steadily gain greater access to basic schooling.

With these successes comes a responsibility to ensure that children who have survived the first five years of life and gone on to attend and complete primary school are given continued support in the second decade of life. As this report has shown, once children have navigated their way successfully through infancy and childhood, a new set of challenges awaits.

Lack of educational and employment opportunities, accidents and injuries, early sex, HIV and AIDS, mental health issues, child labour, adolescent marriage and teenage pregnancy are just some of the risks that can prevent adolescents from realizing their capacities as they transition to adulthood. Global challenges, including climate change, economic uncertainty, globalization, demographic shifts and humanitarian crises, present an uncertain backdrop for adolescents during the pivotal decade of their lives.

> "I wish governments would invest more in our safety and education to strengthen our values and knowledge."
>
> Santiago, 15, Venezuela

Support for these young people, most of whom are still children under the Convention on the Rights of the Child, must not stop at the end of their first decade of life. A good start in life is necessary but not sufficient to break the bonds of poverty and inequity: To make a lasting difference, for both individuals and societies, support in early and middle childhood must be complemented by investment in adolescent education, health care, protection and participation – particularly for the poorest and most marginalized. Families, communities, national governments, donors, development agencies and all other stakeholders must join together with young people as they prepare for their future.

Attendance and completion of secondary school, access to quality health care, participation in decision-making, and protection from violence, exploitation and abuse are fundamental to empowering adolescents to realize their potential. Evidence shows that the realization of these rights increases the likelihood that adolescents will become economically independent, make informed decisions about sex, participate in community and civic affairs and be better equipped to obtain productive employment that will help end the cycle of poverty. As adults, they will also be better prepared to handle the global challenges facing their generation.

This report has identified five key areas in which partners can come together and invest in adolescents. These are

OPPORTUNITIES

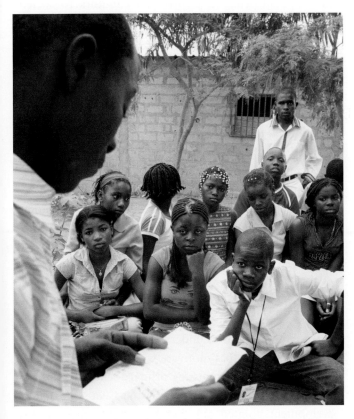

Contribution to family decisions and volunteering in the community are all part of a young person's rights and responsibilities. *An adolescent boy gives a presentation on HIV and AIDS during a Sunday school class in Luanda Province, Angola.*

data collection and analysis, education and training, participation, establishing a supportive environment for adolescent rights and addressing poverty and inequities. The proposals cited are not new, but they require a fresh look and an intensification of efforts if we are to move towards a 'tipping point' that can make a significant difference in the lives of adolescents and their communities.

There is no need to wait for the global economy to fully recover to take action. The solutions in question, from education to improved data collection, have been tried and proven to work. Evidence exists on the merits of investing in adolescents and young people. Particularly in the developing world, where the majority of adolescents live, such investment has the poten-

tial to rapidly accelerate progress in reducing poverty over the coming decades and to set economies on the path to more equitable, sustained growth.

Improve data collection and analysis

Start with data collection and analysis. Major gaps in data on adolescents pose one of the biggest challenges to promoting their rights. While this report has examined a rich vein of factual information on late adolescence, the knowledge base remains limited.

Data on early adolescents aged 10–14 is relatively scarce, thus denying us the knowledge of the most important and crucial period of adolescence. In addition, our understanding of pre-adolescence – middle childhood, ranging from ages 5–9 – is even more restricted, with fewer international indicators disaggregated for this age than for early childhood (0–4) or adolescence.

Recent initiatives by the United Nations and others have expanded our understanding of such vital issues as violence, sexual abuse and reproductive health in adolescence – but not all countries are covered. Additionally, there are a considerable number of areas, such as adolescent mental health, disability and quality indicators for secondary education, where data in most developing countries are simply unavailable in sufficient quantities. And in other areas, notably adolescent participation, the attempt to determine a set of core indicators to measure both inputs and outcomes continues.

It is not just more data that is needed; a deeper level of disaggregation and causal analysis is also imperative. The available data suggest that poverty is a major factor preventing adolescents from fully participating in education, and that it sustains conditions that heighten their risk of protection abuses. Few countries, however, have key indicators broken down by geographic location or wealth quintiles. Internationally accepted indicators disaggregated by age, disability, sex, ethnicity, caste and religion are urgently required as a foundation for programmes and policies and as a measure of progress.

Population-based household surveys such as Demographic and Health Surveys and Multiple Indicator Cluster Surveys are increasingly providing some of these indicators, but these tools require further use and investment. Developing the capacity of national statistical systems to focus more keenly on adolescents will ensure better understanding of whether and how their rights are being fulfilled.

Indicators should be chosen that identify gaps and track progress in services specific to adolescents. National and international partners should coordinate and collaborate on statistical information to help foster comprehensive global knowledge about, and understanding of, adolescents and the challenges they face.

The Committee on the Rights of the Child not only urges governments to provide accurate data on children and adolescents, but also emphasizes that it should be inclusive. In General Comment No. 4, it is stated that "where appropriate, adolescents should participate in the analysis to ensure that the information is understood and utilized in an adolescent-sensitive way."

An excellent example of youth participation in data collection is an innovative study of sexual exploitation of young people in six countries of Eastern Europe. The project involved 60 young people as researchers responsible for gathering baseline data on the extent of sexual abuse, awareness of it and available support services. The young researchers participated in developing the methodology, created appropriate survey materials, conducted research and analysed data to produce recommendations for future action; they also subsequently helped produce training and advocacy materials and devise strategies to take a stand against the sexual abuse of minors.

More than 5,700 responses allowed for a robust analysis of the situation and enabled the project to conclude with meaningful recommendations for action to address sexual exploitation. Interestingly, some partner organizations questioned the study, arguing that young people lacked the competence and expertise to take responsibility for research in such a sensitive and complex field. To test their concerns, a pilot project was arranged in which a professional researcher and the young researchers interviewed a sample of respondents in turn. The adolescents, who were interviewing their own generation, were found to have elicited more comprehensive responses.[1]

Invest in education and training

Developing adolescents' capacities and values through education can enable an entire generation to become economically independent, positive contributors to society. Investing in education and training for adolescents and young people is perhaps the single most promising action to end extreme poverty during this decade.

Secondary education has a significant impact on individual earnings and overall economic growth. An increasingly technological labour market demands greater skills and advanced education to scale up productivity and spur capital investment. An analysis of 100 countries found a significant positive correlation between the average years of adult male secondary school attainment and economic growth between 1960 and 1995. Years of primary school, on the other hand, did not appear to have an influence on positive economic outcomes.[2]

Investing in secondary education can accelerate progress towards achieving several of the MDGs. For example, greater availability of secondary education will create realistic opportunities that motivate students to complete primary school, thereby boosting primary school completion rates (MDG 2).[3] A 2004 paper by the Center for Global Development pointed out that no country had achieved more than a 90 per cent net primary school enrolment rate without also having at least 35 per cent net enrolment in secondary school.[4]

Secondary education can also have a strong impact on promoting gender equality (MDG 3) and improving maternal health (MDG 5). Data for 24 sub-Saharan African countries show that adolescent girls with secondary education are six times less likely to be married than girls with little or no education. They are also three times less likely to get pregnant than their peers with only primary education.[5] In developing countries, women who have completed secondary education or higher are more likely to have a skilled attendant present at delivery than their counterparts, thereby improving their children's chances of survival.[6]

Investing in secondary education will require at least three key actions. The first is to extend compulsory schooling into the secondary level. Some countries already do this. A recent example is Brazil, whose Congress passed legislation in 2009 that augmented spending on education and increased compulsory school attendance from 9 to 14 years.[7] In Yemen, education from grades 1 through 9 has been free and compulsory since the early 1990s. Enrolment in these grades increased from 2.3 million in 1999 to 3.2 million in 2005.[8]

The second key action is to abolish school fees for both primary and secondary education. Eliminating such charges has proved to be an effective strategy for fostering equitable enrolment in primary school. Especially as children get older, the rising costs of their education force many parents to cut their academic life short. Not only does this limit their opportunities for the future, it also places adolescents at risk of other negative outcomes, such as child labour and child marriage.

Significant progress is being made in abolishing school fees. In many countries, primary school has been free for quite a while. Over the past decade, several sub-Saharan African countries have abolished school fees, including Cameroon, Kenya, Lesotho, Malawi, Uganda, the United Republic of Tanzania and Zambia. As result, many of these countries have seen dramatic increases in school attendance.

Unfortunately, increased attendance can create its own complications, as the sudden surge of students may lead to overcrowding and poor quality education. Governments must therefore be prepared to meet the increased demand by building more schools, hiring more teachers and ensuring that quality standards are maintained.[9]

Collaborative initiatives such as the School Fee Abolition Initiative (SFAI), launched in 2005 by UNICEF and the World Bank, work with national governments to promote

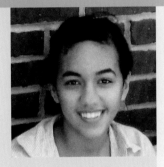

Preparing adolescents for adulthood and citizenship

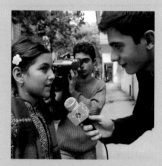

A young girl is interviewed by 16-year-old journalists from the Young People's Media Network, which promotes youth participation in media training and the establishment of youth networks, Tbilisi, Georgia.

An active role for adolescents in decision-making in families, communities and societies

As they mature and develop, adolescents and young people seek to more actively shape their environment, their society and the world they live in and will inherit. Preparing adolescents for adulthood, and particularly for their citizenship responsibilities, is the key task for families, communities and governments during this stage of their development. For adolescents to be active and empowered citizens, they must be aware of their rights and have opportunities for civic engagement through a variety of institutions that encourage basic civic values such as fairness, mutual respect and understanding, justice, tolerance and accountability for one's actions.

The Convention on the Rights of the Child broke new ground by establishing children's right to be heard (Article 12), giving children and adolescents the right to express their views freely on all matters affecting them – especially within the family, school and community – and to have those opinions duly taken into account. This and the other 'participation rights' enumerated in the Convention enable adolescents to exercise progressively more control over decisions that concern them, in line with their evolving capacities. Participation thus stands alongside the principles of universality, the best interests of the child, and child survival and development as one of the cornerstones of the Convention.

In addition to being a fundamental right, participation stimulates the full development of the child's personality and capacities. Young people learn best when they have real choices and are actively involved in dealing with their circumstances. Participation boosts confidence, builds skills and empowers children to protect their own rights. It allows adolescents to step out of the passive roles to which they were relegated as young children and gives them opportunities to create knowledge rather than merely receive it. It empowers adolescents to plan and implement their own projects, to lead and, accordingly, to be accountable for their actions. Mounting evidence shows that active adolescents have fewer problems than their peers, are more skilled and tend to develop a greater sense of social responsibility. Involvement in social organizations also opens the door to economic opportunities, making it especially valuable for adolescents from previously excluded groups.

Encouraging participation not only empowers adolescents, it also has numerous benefits for the societies in which they live. Investment in well-informed and empowered citizens can lead to healthier populations, stronger economic growth and more cohesive communities. When young people are involved in broader peer and community initiatives, they bring into play fresh perspectives and a strong sense of commitment that can result in innovative solutions, especially in the midst of complex crises. Youth engagement can enhance collective action, increasing pressure on governments to provide good public services and driving social, economic and political change.

Finally, evidence shows that participation is one of the best ways of informing children of their rights, especially their right to protection from violence, harm and abuse. This knowledge, in turn, is crucial to ensuring that these rights are respected. Enabling adolescents to access a broad spectrum of information – on topics such as family planning, accident prevention and substance abuse – is a very cost-effective way for states to promote health and development.

Despite the benefits of enabling children to exercise their participation rights, and despite the formal commitment of governments to do so, the principle is not yet being implemented effectively or consistently. Many long-standing practices and attitudes, as well as political and economic barriers, continue to impede adolescents' right to be heard – especially for those who may have difficulties expressing themselves, including adolescents with disabilities and minority, indigenous and migrant children.

Engagement in youth service and public policy initiatives

Over the past two decades, and particularly during the past 10 years, many countries have adopted innovative and successful initiatives to encourage adolescent and youth participation. Several have gone on to form youth councils or parliaments to foster dialogue about relevant issues while offering youth leaders a formal, consultative relationship with the government. A survey of 22 youth councils in industrialized and developing countries reveals that the top three priorities for most such bodies are increased youth participation, international cooperation and greater engagement in the direction of youth policy.

While national youth councils do not have the power to dictate a country's youth policy, they can successfully influence decision-making. In Lithuania, for instance, young people form half of the Council of Youth Affairs, which formally advises the Department of Youth Affairs as it prepares and implements national youth policies. In South Africa, adolescents contributed to a 'Children's Charter of South Africa' and provided substantial inputs to the drafting of the 2005 Children's Act, which includes child participation as one of its founding principles.

Children should be encouraged to create their own, child-led organizations, through which they can carve out a space for meaningful participation and representation. An excellent example of such an organization is the African Movement of Working Children and Youth (AMWCY), which in 2008 had associations in 196 cities and villages in 22 countries of sub-Saharan Africa, with a membership of over 260,000 working girls and boys. Strengthened by the active participation of children who have experience of the issues it seeks to address, AMWCY is uniquely able to reach out to the most marginalized children, including child migrants, for whom it offers a variety of services and support.

The growing number of organizations created and led by young people serves as a testament to young people's activism and also to the fact that existing adult-led organizations fall short in addressing their needs. Networking among youth-led organizations offers excellent opportunities for sharing best practices and creating a shared platform for advocacy.

Adolescent involvement in political action has also received a boost from new communications technologies, which have great potential to broaden and lend momentum and geographical breadth to child-led activism. Over time, more children will have access to information, leading to heightened awareness of their own rights and linking new members to existing networks and associations that represent their views. Enabling all children to voice their opinions via a common platform could potentially level inequalities and overcome discrimination, especially for adolescents with disabilities, girls and those living in rural areas where youth associations may not exist. For example, in 2005 UNICEF created a Rural Voices of Youth (RVOY) platform, which connects 'offline' young people with their 'online' peers, giving them the opportunity to engage in dialogue on child rights and participation issues.

Used appropriately, the Internet, social networking and related technologies can be powerful tools that enable adolescents to speak out on matters that are important to them. Rather than seeking formal representative participation in local government, the youth of this century are increasingly turning to online or interactive activism, creating relevant and agile networks on the Web. The old model of 'dutiful citizenship', in which people respond to mass media and are mobilized by government or civil society initiatives, is being replaced by a form of 'self-actualizing citizenship'. Politicians, policymakers and educators should resist the temptation to dismiss young people as uninterested or apathetic and instead focus on tapping into the power of new and different forms of engagement that are expressed in a different 'language'.

Myriad legal, political, economic, social and cultural barriers impede adolescents' participation in making decisions that affect their lives. Dismantling these barriers is a challenge that requires a willingness to re-examine assumptions about adolescents' potential and to create environments in which they can truly thrive, building their capacities in the process.

See References, page 78.

free education. SFAI researches and analyses past country experiences and uses that knowledge to guide and support countries in their efforts to remove school fees.[10] Families and communities must also have a voice and urge their governments to abolish fees.

The third key action is to promote equitable access to post-primary education. Extending education to those currently excluded will be a particular challenge in the current decade; if it can be achieved, however, it has the potential to break the intergenerational cycle of adolescent poverty.

Attendance and completion of secondary school is still largely beyond the reach of the poorest and most marginalized groups and communities in many countries. Girls, adolescents with disabilities and those from minority groups are especially disadvantaged. While most countries have reached gender parity in primary school, fewer have approached this goal for secondary education. The 2010 *United Nations Millennium Development Goals Report* looked at secondary-school-aged girls in 42 countries and found that twice as many girls from the poorest 60 percent of households were out of school, compared with girls from the wealthiest 40 per cent of households (50 per cent compared with 24 per cent). The disparities were similar for boys of secondary school age. Extending quality compulsory education and abolishing school fees will help reduce these gender gaps.

Additional efforts to reach indigenous, disabled and other marginalized children must also be made. Recent reforms in Bolivia, for example, aim to reach minorities and indigenous groups through intercultural and bilingual education. In South Africa, including disabled children in mainstream schooling – rather than sending them to special schools – has led to increased school enrolment of disabled children and support for specialized teaching practices.[11]

Another group needing special support are teenage mothers who are forced to leave school. In Namibia, 1 in 7 young women aged 15–19 have already begun childbearing. Young motherhood is more common in rural areas than in urban areas, and young women with no education are more than 10 times more likely to have started childbearing by the age of 19 than those who have completed secondary school (58 per cent versus 6 per cent).[12] Although primary school enrolment is over 90 per cent, the prevalence of girls among those who make the transition to secondary school is still very low, and many drop out due to teenage pregnancy. In 2008, the Ministry of Education, in collaboration with UNICEF, addressed this issue by developing a new, flexible policy regarding student pregnancy that, with input from the student, her family and the school, works to create a more supportive environment to enable the young mother to return to school with a suitable care plan in place.[13]

Finally, governments and other stakeholders must take into account that one type of education does not fit all. Other post-secondary options, such as job training programmes, may be more appealing to families who might otherwise take their children out of school because of economic burdens.

Adolescents who have been out of school for several years may need specialized programmes to fit their educational needs. Following the conflict in Sri Lanka in 2009, UNICEF worked with the Government to develop a curriculum to reintegrate children and adolescents who had been out of school for at least six months. The curriculum included a psychosocial component that helped young people cope with the stresses of the conflict.[14]

Institutionalize mechanisms for youth participation

Active participation of adolescents in family and civic life fosters positive citizenship as they mature into adults. Furthermore, adolescents' contributions enrich and inform policies that benefit society as a whole. Adults at all levels of community and political life must challenge processes and systems that exclude youth involvement.

The personal benefits of participation for adolescents are immense. Building decision-making abilities in young people empowers them when it comes to making decisions about their own health and well-being. Adolescents who participate actively in civic life are more likely to avoid risky activities such as drug use or criminal activity, to make informed decisions about sex, to take ownership over their legal rights and to navigate their way through the array of challenges they encounter on their journey to adulthood. When they become adults, this empowerment will inform the decisions they make on behalf of their own children.

National youth councils, community service initiatives, digital communication and other forms of adolescent participation mentioned in this report are all effective means of educating youth about their rights while empowering them as decision-makers. These efforts should not, however, overshadow the meaningful contributions that young people can make in their daily lives. Contributing to family decisions, joining school governments, volunteering in the community and meeting with local representatives are all part of a young person's rights and responsibilities.

Determining roles in the partnership between adults and adolescents has always been challenging, and it can become even more so as both parties work to understand what

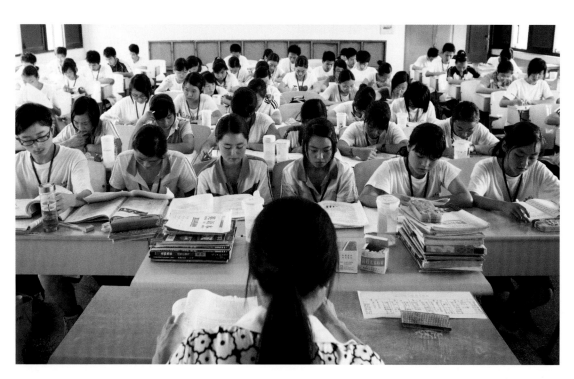

Investing in secondary education has a significant impact on overall economic growth and can accelerate progress towards achieving several of the MDGs. *Adolescents, orphaned or separated from their families by earthquake, study for their university entrance exams at Sichuan University in Chengdu, China.*

Doing our part:
Mass media's responsibility to adolescents

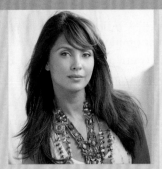

by Lara Dutta, Goodwill Ambassador of the United Nations Population Fund

"Such support and protection can moderate children's exposure to inappropriate content and prevent them from being taken advantage of by opportunistic adults."

'Infotainment' is a buzzword of our times. Information combined with entertainment floods adolescent minds, and there are few ways to filter it before it gets absorbed. Violence, sex, social prejudice and offensive language are all products of the mass media these days. To what extent can we guide youth to recognize what is true or valuable in what they see and read, while protecting them from objectionable images and ideas?

While estimates vary by region and culture, studies show that the average child in the developed world watches TV or a computer screen for about four to six hours per day. The entertainment industry and the Internet offer a seemingly endless array of activities. With the globe at their fingertips, teenagers easily forget about the real world around them and spend their leisure time watching movies, playing video games and participating in online chat rooms and forums.

Schools and colleges have recognized the potential of electronic media and made curricula more interactive. Education today is no longer restricted to textbooks and classrooms; children are encouraged to surf the net, use digital media in their presentations and expand their computer knowledge. Schools and parents are also aware of the worrying trend of 'cyber-bullying', whereby a child is tormented or threatened through interactive and digital technologies such as instant messages, email and mobile phones. The limitless nature of new technology can be harmful to vulnerable youth.

Parents and children often clash over using the Internet, watching TV or movies and listening to music. Parents want to protect their children from negative influences and may feel they know what is best for them, while adolescents struggle for independence. Family decisions and open lines of communication between parents, teachers and children can ensure that young people are given the proper guidance as they engage in this vast network of information and experience. Such support and protection can moderate children's exposure to inappropriate content and prevent them from being taken advantage of by opportunistic adults.

The power of the media over adolescents can be neither ignored nor denied. It has given the stars of films,

music and sports a disproportionate influence on the lives of adolescents, who admire these figures and often emulate them. A film or musical artist with mass appeal and the ability to reach out should therefore aim to offer entertainment that is also educational – without being preachy or boring. For every three or four 'light' movies churned out by the Mumbai film industry, for example, one movie that conveys a special message can do a world of good. We have seen this with films like *Taare Zameen Par*, the story of an 8-year-old boy who feels depressed and humiliated as he struggles in school until a new art teacher determines that he is dyslexic, helps him improve his learning skills and changes his life for the better.

A movie or song can inspire a generation to think in global, humanitarian ways. The single 'We Are the World', for example, was recorded by USA for Africa in the 1980s to benefit famine relief in Ethiopia. Twenty-five years after its release, the title was re-recorded in February 2010 following Haiti's devastating 7.0 magnitude earthquake. Dozens of artists came together to perform the legendary piece, with the aim of raising money to help the Haitian people. The entertainment industry and the Internet can be powerful partners in involving young people in helping regions deal with disasters and addressing social ills such as gender discrimination and the spread of HIV.

Being an adolescent is hard. I know; I've been there. It is a life stage during which one is still growing and becoming self-aware. Adolescents search for inspiration, acceptance and guidance as they blossom into adulthood. Celebrities with the power to affect their impressionable minds therefore have a moral responsibility to impart positive messages. I am committed to using any influence I may have to do just that as a Goodwill Ambassador of the United Nations Population Fund (UNFPA). In the words of USA for Africa's famous song, "We are the ones who make a brighter day so let's start giving."

Lara Dutta was appointed as a UNFPA Goodwill Ambassador in 2001. She was crowned Miss Universe in May 2000 in Cyprus. Formerly Miss India, Ms. Dutta was a print and fashion model. She has since joined the Indian film industry as an actress. She has a degree in economics with a minor in communications.

exactly 'youth participation' looks like. A recent report in the *Journal of Community Psychology* sheds light on this issue, explaining that youth organizing gives a new role to adults. "Rather than leading, adults need to be in the background, monitoring, mentoring, facilitating, but not being in charge. Young people want support from adults in the form of dialogue, coaching, and providing connections to sources of institutional, community, and political power."[15]

The Committee on the Rights of the Child has encouraged governments to put in place legal and policy frameworks and mechanisms to ensure the systematic participation of children and young people at all levels of society. A good example is the recent development of a National Strategy on Child Participation by the Government of Mongolia. Formulation of the strategy involved extensive consultations with adolescents and youth at the local, provincial and national levels.

The positive experience of active youth engagement in this process has given greater impetus to child and youth participation in national and local decision-making forums.

Young people must also be given a voice in deciding how best to allocate resources. This can be done through the formation of youth groups, forums or other channels through which youth can express their opinions. Some countries are even taking steps to include youth as partners in the development of Poverty Reduction Strategy Papers.[16]

UNICEF Brazil, for example, has encouraged adolescents to become partners in social budgeting initiatives. Adolescents received training to help them identify areas of public policy relevant to them, undertake research, estimate the benefits of additional expenditures on social spending and become effective advocates.

Map Kibera and Regynnah's empowerment

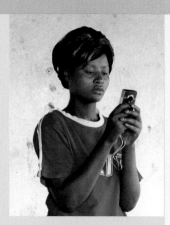

by Regynnah Awino and Map Kibera

Map Kibera – a partnership between local youth, non-governmental organizations and several United Nations agencies including UNICEF – is based in Kibera in Nairobi, Kenya. It engages young people, particularly young women and girls, in the participatory digital mapping of risks and vulnerabilities in their community, which is Africa's largest slum. Through this process, young people gain new awareness about their surroundings, empowering them to amplify their voices on critical issues. The project is helping identify safe and unsafe physical spaces, as well as raising awareness and offering advocacy opportunities around the issues of HIV and AIDS and other vulnerabilities.

Map Kibera involves five steps:

- *Stakeholder meetings*: Implementers consider issues of gender-based violence, HIV and AIDS or related topics to identify the most appropriate map data to collect.
- *Map data collection:* Thirteen young mappers from the community use global positioning system (GPS) devices and open source software to create a map of safe and dangerous areas; then the data is uploaded to OpenStreetMap.

- *Community consultations*: Using printed maps, tracing paper and coloured pens, the mappers conduct discussions with girls and young women about safety and vulnerability, leading to better situational awareness for both girls and planners.
- *Narrative media:* Young people from the community use videos, photos and audio to create short narratives about the issues they face, which are then interwoven into the map narrative.
- *Advocacy:* Quantitative and qualitative data are used for advocacy with local governments, community leaders and other decision-makers to obtain better services and protection for young people.

Results from the mapping process will be used to identify physical and psychological areas of risk or vulnerability and patterns of risk perception. The information will be publicly owned and available, helping keep grass-roots advocates and policy planners more accountable to young people in the community.

Regynnah, one of the mappers, provides below an account of her involvement in the project.

Many governments have also developed or updated national youth policies to better address the diverse needs of adolescents and youth. The development of the national youth policy in South Africa – in which a participatory approach involving adolescents and young adults as key contributors produced a comprehensive, rights-based national youth framework – is often seen as a model. While most national youth policies have tried to cater to the needs and concerns of youth in an age range extending to 24 years and sometimes beyond, it is also important to focus on adolescents, who require special support, protection and preparation for their transition to adulthood.

A supportive environment

Conventions, legislation, policies and programmes for adolescent rights require a supportive environment to uphold them. Creating an environment that is conducive to positive adolescent development entails addressing the values, attitudes and behaviours of the institutions in the adolescent's domain – family, peers, schools and services – as well as the broader context of norms established within communities, the media, legislation, policies and budgets.

A national government may build secondary schools and expand compulsory education, but it must also address the underlying factors of poverty and inequity that lead many parents to take their children out of school. Donors who make significant contributions to HIV and AIDS prevention and treatment initiatives need to recognize that the availability of condoms, testing sites and vaccines must be complemented with efforts to remove stigmas and change gender constructs that serve to sustain the spread of the epidemic. Systemic changes are required on all levels to create an environment where children have the greatest chance of thriving.

Regynnah's story

I am Regynnah Awino, a 22-year-old from Kibera. My father died when I was a little child, leaving my mother to raise a family of six. Three of my sisters died. Growing up as a young girl in Kibera was a challenge. I did my fourth form in 2007, and since then I have not been able to pursue further education because my family cannot afford the fees. My mother is a businesswoman, and the little money she gets goes to sustain us. I always had aspirations to become a journalist.

Until November 2009, when Map Kibera came about, I used to stay at home doing casual jobs to help out. Now I am one of a group of 13 who have been trained to use GPS devices and upload data to the Internet. Mapping has been educational, fun and challenging. In the field I learned many things, though the work could also be a challenge due to unfavourable weather conditions or a poor response from interviewees. Map Kibera has really helped my people know what we have in our community and how to make use of and improve what is available. We were able to collect information on all the schools, toilets, shops, kiosks, heath centres and street lights, producing a complete and detailed map.

We spend a week on every mapping theme and then another week creating awareness and helping other people better understand mapping's benefits and impact. For example, one of the most sensitive themes is girls' security. At meetings with a community girls' group called Binti Pamoka (Daughters United), which helps young girls deal with gender-based violence, I helped lead a discussion of what we found on the map, as well as the places they felt were safe or dangerous. Through this we gained not only local knowledge, but also excitement about the project, because we found that the community could respond positively.

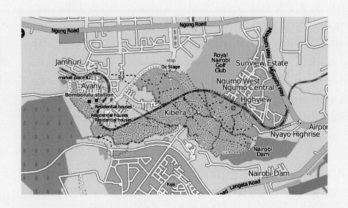

To me, this is a lifetime achievement. So many people are impressed with what the group is doing, and I think it will continue to build maps for the community in the future.

The training and the whole process of mapping have changed me. For example, I used to be very shy and afraid of speaking in public, but now I feel much more confident and well informed. Mapping Kibera also allows me to meet people from all walks of life – different people every day. I believe that if by the grace of God I am able to fulfil my dreams, I will not leave Kibera but will stay and make it a better place to live.

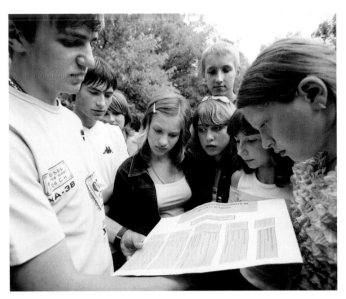

Active participation of adolescents in family and civic life fosters positive citizenship as they mature into adults. *A boy shares a poster about the effects of iodine deficiency disorders with a group of adolescents as part of a peer-to-peer education programme, Ukraine.*

Building a protective environment requires breaking the silence around taboo topics such as sexual exploitation and abuse. It involves promoting open discussion by both media and society and ensuring that adolescents have access to hotlines, social workers, shelters and youth clubs so they can talk about these topics and seek respite from violence, exploitation, abuse and discrimination that occur within the family or community.

In Brazil, adolescent-created media have created forums for adolescents to discuss such sensitive issues as teenage pregnancy with peers and adults. Where the majority of young mothers are neither studying nor working, illustrated stories and multi-media digital products were used to initiate debate on adolescent motherhood. The stories, written by adolescents themselves, served to inspire discussions aimed at dispelling both the 'romantic' perception of pregnancy and the 'guilty' vision of pregnancy that burden adolescent girls with condemning attitudes.

Promoting open, fluid and honest communication supports adolescents in their interaction with parents and families, communities and policymakers, and helps adults and communities positively appreciate their contributions. Community-based activities can promote inter-generational dialogue that may propel societal change.

In São Paulo, Brazil, squares, alleys, cinemas, cafes, cultural centres and theatres have been transformed into learning spaces as part of Aprendiz, the 'Neighborhood as School' project. Children and adolescents participate in a variety of activities – such as IT courses, mosaics, theatre, guitar lessons, skateboarding, and English lessons – that build skills and enhance opportunities for physical and creative expression. The key to the project's success lies in the partnerships that have been developed among schools, families, public authorities, entrepreneurs, associations, craftspeople, non-governmental organizations and volunteers.[17]

Media-based and technology-based communications are popular tools for adolescents to have their voices heard and to play a powerful role in forming, influencing and changing public perceptions and opinions.

In 2004, UNICEF India supported a Child Reporters Initiative in a district in the state of Orissa. This programme, which began with 100 adolescent reporters aged 10–18, has turned into a movement in 14 states, with child reporters now numbering in the thousands. The target is to have 10 child reporters for each of the *gram panchayats*. Aspiring child reporters first participated in workshops to become sensitized on child rights and to learn to express, observe, analyse and freely write about their experiences and observations.

Addressing poverty and inequity

Poverty is one of the biggest threats to adolescent rights. It catapults young people prematurely into adulthood by pulling them out of school, pushing them into the labour market or forcing them to marry young. The World Bank estimates that approximately 73 per cent of the population in South Asia and sub-Saharan Africa live on under US$2 per day. These are also the two regions with the fastest-growing adolescent populations.

Article 19 of the Convention on the Rights of the Child commits governments to the "establishment of social programmes to provide necessary support for the child and for those who have the care of the child." Governments are responsible for providing safety nets such as cash transfers and other social protection programmes that alleviate the financial burden of parents in the poorest households. The international community should continue to advocate for social protection initiatives and research their effectiveness.

One such example is Ethiopia's Productive Safety Net Programme, which provides employment and social protection for communities made vulnerable by external shocks such as drought. Evaluations of the initiative have found that around 15 per cent of the cash transfers are used for education, and parents report keeping their children in school longer as a result. A programme component dedicated to building classrooms ensures that increased school attendance does not result in overcrowding.[18]

Similarly, Liberia's Economic Empowerment of Adolescent Girls and Young Women (EPAG) Project, a collaborative effort between the Ministry of Gender and Development, the World Bank, the Nike Foundation and the Government of Denmark, provides skills training for wage employment, combined with job placement assis-

tance; at the same time it facilitates business development services and links to microcredit for young women entrepreneurs.[19]

Inequity is also a major barrier to the fulfillment of adolescent rights outlined in the Convention on the Rights of the Child and the Convention on the Elimination of All Forms of Discrimination against Women. The importance of equal access to education was discussed earlier, but equal rights to health, employment, juvenile justice, religion, culture and identity are also imperative to the positive development of young people.

Adolescents today are healthier, better protected, better educated and more connected than ever. However, millions

The Campus Initiative
Advocating for children's rights at colleges and universities

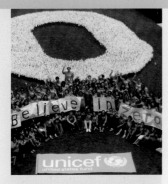

Students at the UNICEF Campus Initiative Summit in June 2010. More than 140 students gathered on the lawn at Columbia University to stake 24,000 flags in the shape of a zero as a symbolic representation of the daily number of preventable child deaths, and their commitment to help make that number zero.

On more than 100 college campuses across the United States, students are choosing to play a powerful role in helping the world's children survive. The Campus Initiative, run by the US Fund for UNICEF, is a rapidly growing grass-roots movement of dynamic college students who champion the organization's mission. The goal of the program, which began in 1988, is to build global citizens who will generate funding, attention and political will to help combat preventable child deaths.

Education, advocacy and fund-raising are at the heart of the UNICEF Campus Initiative's work. Students initiate and conduct a wide range of activities that include advocating for child survival by contacting elected officials, writing campus newspaper editorials about UNICEF's work and partnering with local children's organizations for service projects. During the 2009–2010 academic year, 2,033 active members – defined as those attending at least 50 per cent of planned campus activities – undertook 358 events between August and December 2009.

The US National Committee and a student-led Campus Initiative National Council provide support for campus clubs across the country. This team of staff and volunteers also sets the agenda by creating national goals and plans, and it implements the Campus Initiative Summit each year. The nationwide gathering enables club members and campus leaders

to learn from each other and share best practices. The summit also provides leadership opportunities as well as skill-building and knowledge-building workshops, and it motivates campus members to stay engaged with UNICEF.

Keeping pace with the advancing digital age is pivotal for the Campus Initiative, as members of younger generations become more and more technologically savvy. To connect with individuals aged 19–24, we must provide them with the organizing tools they have come to expect in other areas of their online experience. Advocacy expertise and mobilization is another area of growth for the Campus Initiative. Students have shown time and time again that they will use their political muscle when they are motivated and supported.

A lifetime of service and commitment to children can be fostered among all of levels of supporters, but especially among college students. Adolescents and young people can and should be an integral part of the solution to ending the preventable deaths of children, alleviating child poverty, fighting child exploitation and forced labour, combating HIV and AIDS, ensuring access to quality education and providing opportunities for the world's children.

See References, page 78.

Adolescent girls:
The best investment you can make

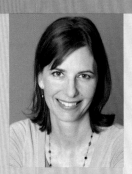

*by Maria Eitel,
President of the
Nike Foundation*

There are more than 515 million adolescent girls living in the developing world today. These girls have the potential to accelerate growth and progress in every sector, to break the cycle of intergenerational poverty and to advance whole economies. And yet girls are often overlooked. Adolescent girls are more likely to be pulled out of school, married off and infected with HIV. They also face the reality that a leading cause of death for a girl 15 to 19 years old is related to pregnancy and childbirth. Families who have nothing else may resort to treating their daughters as commodities, to be married off or sold. Despite such adversities, adolescent girls are the most powerful force for transformative change.

Yes, girls often face immense barriers, but they also hold unique promise. That is the other side of the story – the Girl Effect. This is the story of girls who are counted, invested in and included in society. When a girl in the developing world receives seven or more years of education, she marries four years later. An extra year of primary school boosts girls' eventual wages by 10 to 20 per cent. Studies in 2003 showed that when women and girls earn income, they reinvest 90 per cent of it into their families, as compared to the 30 to 40 per cent that men and boys contribute. Research has also shown that higher levels of schooling among mothers correlate with better infant and child health. Yes, this is the Girl Effect, and we have only begun to see its myriad effects.

It is truly remarkable how investing in one girl can generate ripples of change that benefit her family, her village and her country. Girls all over the world are putting the Girl Effect into motion every day despite the countless obstacles in their lives. Sanchita, a 17-year-old from Bangladesh, is one of these girls. Born into poverty, Sanchita had no money for school, clothes or food. Thanks to BRAC, she received a small loan to buy a cow. She sold the cow's milk and used the money to pay for her own schooling and that of her brother. BRAC also helped her learn skills that have enabled her to grow her own vegetables and continue to earn an income for her family and herself. Stories like Sanchita's serve as beacons of hope – and as tangible proof that investments in girls can result in significant economic and social change. The Girl Effect is real, and its impact is both extensive and profound.

I have seen this change take hold in Bangladesh, Brazil, Burundi, Kenya, Uganda, the United Republic of Tanzania and countless other countries. Girls around the world are putting the Girl Effect into motion when they are given the tools to do so. At this very moment, girl entrepreneurs in India are drafting their business plans, girls in Bangladesh are studying to be nurses so they can meet the health needs of those who have been largely ignored, and girls in Uganda and the United Republic of Tanzania are receiving life-skills training and gaining access to microfinance, benefiting from safe spaces where they are allowed to dream big and to translate these dreams into reality.

But there is still much work to be done. In order to know what is happening to girls, and to track their progress or lack thereof, we urgently need data disaggregated by sex and age. We need to show the value in girls and convince governments, villages, corporations and families that investing in adolescent girls is a smart endeavour. We must bring girls into the center of our discussions, acknowledge them as a unique population and address their particular needs.

Unleashing the potential of adolescent girls begins with our doing the following:
1. Stop using girls as the infrastructure of poverty.
2. Don't assume you have girls covered in your programmes. Specifically address them.
3. Count girls – look for them in your numbers.
4. You don't need to change your strategy, just include girls in what you already do.
5. Enforce policies that are already in place.
6. Men and boys can be champions for girls.
7. Don't treat girls as the issue of the day.

This approach will yield numerous benefits for decades to come. If we wholeheartedly invest in girls, we will see stronger communities and families, sustainable economies, lower rates of maternal mortality and morbidity, lower rates of HIV and AIDS, less poverty, more innovation, reduced rates of joblessness and more equitable prosperity. The Girl Effect is real, and it is powerful – but we won't fully realize its ripple effect until we start taking it seriously and expanding its scope.

Maria Eitel is the founding President and CEO of the Nike Foundation, where she works to promote the Girl Effect – the powerful social and economic change that ensues when girls have opportunities. Prior to her work with the Foundation, Ms. Eitel served as the first Vice President of Corporate Responsibility at NIKE, Inc. Before that, she served at the White House, the Microsoft Corporation, the Corporation for Public Broadcasting and MCI Communications Corporation.

Working together for adolescent girls: The United Nations Adolescent Girls Task Force

In 2007, a number of United Nations agencies* founded the United Nations Adolescent Girls Task Force. With support from the UN Foundation, the Task Force aims to strengthen interagency collaboration at both the global and country levels; facilitate the development of effective programmes to address the rights and needs of adolescent girls; support the drive to achieve the MDGs; and eliminate all forms of violence and discrimination against girls and young women.

In March 2010, the Task Force launched a Joint Statement for Accelerated Efforts to Advance the Rights of Adolescent Girls signed by the heads of the six agencies. The agencies committed to increasing support to govern- ments and civil societies over the next five years to advance policies and programmes to empower the hardest-to-reach adolescent girls.

The Joint Statement spells out the mandate and the responsibilities of the UN country teams in protecting the rights of the marginalized adolescent girl. It commits agencies to mobilizing the financial and technical resources to work together to identify five strategic priorities for fulfilling the rights of adolescent girls. These priorities include:

- Educating adolescent girls.
- Improving the health of adolescent girls.
- Keeping adolescent girls free from violence, abuse and exploitation.
- Promoting leaders among adolescent girls.
- Counting adolescent girls to advance their well-being and realize their human rights.

See References, page 78.

* Participating agencies include International Labour Organization, United Nations Children's Fund, United Nations Educational, Scientific and Cultural Organization, United Nations Population Fund, United Nations Entity for Gender Equality and Empowerment of Women, and World Health Organization.

have been left behind. Policies and programmes aimed at achieving the MDGs too often ignore the situation of the poorest and most marginalized adolescents and youth, even those in middle-income and industrialized countries. Fulfilling their rights to education, health and recreation; to an environment without violence; and to having their voic- es heard in decision-making processes are all conditions for achieving social equality, pro-poor economic growth and expanded citizenship.

Moreover, an equity approach to adolescent development highlights the urgent need to identify the most marginalized and vulnerable adolescents in every society, to design and develop relevant and innovative approaches to reach and engage them, and to ensure that investments are targeted to give them equal access and opportunities for growth and development.

In an effort to move towards greater equity in health, national governments are taking action, with international support, to abolish user fees for critical health services. Countries that have done so include Burundi, Ghana, Kenya, Lesotho, Liberia, the Niger, Senegal and Zambia. Donor countries such as France and the United Kingdom offer incentives to eliminate fees by providing additional aid to countries that remove them. Development agencies such as the World Health Organization and the World Bank have also taken strong positions against user fees in health care.[20] When partners come together in this way, significant advances in human rights can be achieved.

Working together for adolescents

In 2010–2011, the world celebrates the International Year of Youth (IYY). Since the first IYY 25 years ago, the world has come a long way in recognizing and advancing the rights of young people. Governments adopted the Convention on the Rights of the Child (1989), two optional protocols protect- ing children from armed conflict and sexual exploitation (2000), the International Labour Organization Convention on the Worst Forms of Child Labour (1999) and the Millennium Development Goals (2000).

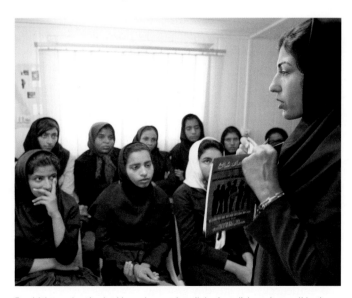

Equal rights to education, health, employment, juvenile justice, religion, culture and identity are all imperative to the positive development of young people. *A peer education trainer discusses a film,* Born with AIDS, *at the Adolescent-Friendly Services Centre at Bandar Abbas Health Complex, Islamic Republic of Iran.*

From victims to activists:
Children and the effects of climate change in Pakistan

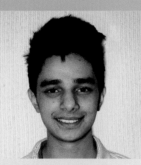

by Syed Aown Shahzad,
16, Pakistan

"As adolescents, we face a common opponent: greenhouse gases."

Adolescents in Pakistan – where we account for 40.5 million out of a population of over 176 million people – are keenly aware that we are inheriting a planet suffering from climate change. Like other developing countries that will be hit hardest by the effects of global warming, Pakistan has contributed minimally to global emissions but still has to deal with the dreadful impacts of storm surges, natural disasters and heavy rains. Rising sea levels and dramatic changes in weather patterns have already caused flooding and drought, limiting food harvests and access to fresh water and affecting industrial production. We need to take all remedial measures to avoid becoming 'environmental refugees'.

Climate change, in Pakistan and worldwide, is especially hard on children, who are more vulnerable than adults to disease, malnutrition and exploitation. Rising temperatures and extreme climate events contribute to the spread of diseases such as malaria, diarrhoea and pneumonia. These are some of the main causes of death for Pakistani children under 5 years old. With drought, agriculture – 24 per cent of our gross domestic product – suffers as the crop yield is reduced and supplies are depleted.

Recent events have provided dramatic evidence of the catastrophic impact on Pakistan of changing weather patterns. Unprecedented heavy rains gave way in July 2010 to devastating floods. The initial death toll was approximately 1,600 people, but many more are unaccounted for. An estimated 20 million men, women and children have been affected by the floods, and huge numbers are stranded, waiting for help. Most escaped from their homes with nothing but what they were wearing. Compounding the health risks resulting from the flooding and the lack of food, water and shelter, the country is beleaguered by the economic catastrophe resulting from the destruction of its agricultural backbone. Millions of hectares of crops have been soaked or washed away, and livestock have been destroyed.

This drowning nation now faces a further disaster: The floods are threatening to decimate Pakistan's youth. One of the biggest threats is the outbreak of water-borne diseases such as cholera and diarrhoea. As in most natural catastrophes, children are also at a high risk of separation from their families and exposure to the dangers of child labour, abuse and exploitation. More than 5,500 schools have been ruined or wiped out. We cannot stand by and watch this generation disappear. As global citizens, we must help them survive this shattering event and emerge as role models of courage, endurance and determination.

It is time to take action – not only to deal with this immediate tragedy, but also to address the issue of global warming. As adolescents, we face a common opponent: greenhouse gases. In order to prevail, we must come together to help others, employ alternative energy sources and create laws to protect our planet and its people.

Syed Aown Shahzad is a youth activist and a native of Lahore, Pakistan. He was part of the youth delegations at the 2009 Summit on Climate Change and the 20th anniversary of the Convention on the Rights of the Child, and he continues to spread awareness about global issues such as climate change and children's rights in Pakistan and beyond.

As noted throughout this report, the results have been encouraging. Health and education levels have improved, particularly for young children. Protection is higher on the international agenda. Participation initiatives are being rolled out in industrialized and developing countries alike with increasing intensity. And the body of knowledge on adolescent development and participation – in terms of data and analysis, best practices and lessons learned, and understanding of disparities and bottlenecks – is steadily growing.

A collaborative effort must be made to continue building on this progress, so that investments made now will reap rewards not only for the children of today, but for their children as well. As this report points out in Chapter 2, the number of adolescents is expected to increase, especially in poor countries. Many key development agents have already joined in a global consensus on the importance of investing in adolescence and youth. These stakeholders, at all levels, must now pull together to support young people in developing the skills and capacities they need to pull themselves out of poverty. Only then will we ensure that adolescence truly becomes an age of opportunity for all.

Violent conflict and the vulnerability of adolescents

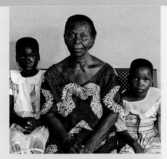

A grandmother cares for her grandchildren following the death of their parents from AIDS.

"Post-conflict programmes for youth have focused on improving services and providing opportunities for them to return to school."

Since civil war broke out in 2002, Côte d'Ivoire has faced grave obstacles in its political, social and economic development. Although a fragile compromise was reached between the Government and the New Force rebel movement in 2007, elections planned for November 2009 were postponed indefinitely, and United Nations and French troops remain in the country to maintain security. The United Nations Office for the Coordination of Humanitarian Affairs reports that the country entered the post-conflict phase for the first time in 2009, with thousands of internally displaced persons returning voluntarily to their places of origin. Still, the peace process is gradual and requires national and global commitment.

The conflict resulted in horrific gender-based violence and widespread military conscription, while also disrupting education and destroying medical services. The health of civilians, especially children and women, has been directly compromised, as illustrated by the resurgence of polio in 2008 and the interruption in reproductive and maternal and child health care generally and in treatment services for those living with HIV and AIDS in particular.

In such a situation adolescents, who made up 23 per cent of the total population of Côte d'Ivoire in 2009, have been and remain uniquely vulnerable. In addition to military conscription, sexual slavery and forced migration, adolescent girls and boys suffer in other ways that are direct and indirect results of the civil war. Boys, for example, are subject to involvement in the worst forms of child labour on cocoa plantations, which are one of the country's most important sources of revenue; between 1994 and 2003, Côte d'Ivoire accounted for 38 per cent of global cocoa bean production. While children have long worked on these farms, and while data on the prevalence of child labour in the country are difficult to obtain, conflicts over land for farming were in part a catalyst for the war and have intensified the scramble to find workers for an industry that is crucial for redevelopment. It is estimated that the majority of child labourers on these

farms are under 14 years old and come from specific Ivorian ethnic groups or are migrants from Burkina Faso. The most vulnerable are those dislocated by the war and lacking ties to farmers or local communities.

Adolescent girls are also suffering from the effects of the war. In some regions of the country – particularly in the west, where violence was most intense – rape and other unspeakable acts, including forced incest and cannibalism, have left not only permanent physical impairment but also psychological and emotional scars that will take a long time to heal.

Post-conflict programmes for youth have focused on improving services and providing opportunities for youth to return to school and to protect themselves and their communities in a fragile environment. UNICEF, for example, is supporting more than 40 School Girl Mothers' Clubs (CMEFs) to help adolescent girls stay in school and complete their education. A National Action Plan for the implementation of United Nations Security Council Resolution 1325 on women, peace and security has also been put in place, and its first priority is the protection of women and girls from sexual violence.

One area of success in post-conflict rehabilitation has been heightened awareness of HIV prevention, which is particularly important because Côte d'Ivoire had the highest prevalence in West Africa in 2008. A partnership between CARE and Population Services International has targeted soldiers, many of whom long believed they were too powerful to contract the disease. However, more work remains to be done, particularly for girls, who lag behind boys in comprehensive knowledge of HIV and condom use. In 2008, just 18 per cent of girls aged 15 to 24 had comprehensive knowledge of HIV, compared to 28 per cent of their male counterparts, while the prevalence of HIV among girls was three times higher (2.4 per cent) than among boys (0.8 per cent).

See References, page 78.

References

CHAPTER 1

1. United Nations, Department of Economic and Social Affairs, Population Division, *World Population Prospects: The 2008 revision*, <www.esa.un.org/unpd/wpp2008/index.htm>, accessed October 2010; and UNICEF global databases, accessed October 2010.

2. United Nations Children's Fund, *Progress for Children: Achieving the MDGs with equity*, no. 9, UNICEF, New York, 2010; and Statistical Tables 1–10, pp. 88–129.

3. Figures provided by UNICEF Brazil, October 2010.

4. Statistical Table 5, p. 104

5. Derived from United Nations Children's Fund, *Children and AIDS: Fifth Stocktaking Report*, 2010, UNICEF, New York, December 2010, p. 17; and Joint United Nations Programme on HIV/AIDS, *Global Report: UNAIDS report on the Global AIDS epidemic*, 2010, UNAIDS, Geneva, p. 184.

6. Statistical Table 9, p. 120.

7. Statistical Table 5, p. 104.

8. International Labour Office, *Global Employment Trends for Youth August 2010: Special issue on the impact of the global economic crisis on youth,* International Labour Organization, Geneva, 2010, pp. 3–6.

9. Ibid.

10. World Bank, *World Development Report 2006: Equity and development*, World Bank, Washington, D.C. 2005.

11. United Nations Children's Fund, *Progress for Children: A report card on child protection*, no. 8, UNICEF, New York, 2009, pp. 46–47; and Statistical Table 9, p. 120.

12. United Nations Children's Fund, *Tracking Progress on Child and Maternal Nutrition: A survival and development priority*, UNICEF, New York, November 2009, pp. 12–14.

13. World Health Organization, Joint United Nations Program on HIV/AIDS and United Nations Population Fund, *Seen but Not Heard: Very young adolescents aged 10–14 years*, UNAIDS, Geneva, 2004, pp. 5–7.

14. Ibid., p. 7.

15. The Civil Code of the Islamic Republic of Iran, p. 118; Ministry of Gender Equality and Child, Draft Child Care and Protection Bill, Summary, Ministry of Gender Equality and Child, Government of the Republic of Namibia, Windhoek, 2009.

16. Johnson, Carolyn C., et al., 'Co–Use of Alcohol and Tobacco Among Ninth Graders in Louisiana', *Preventing Chronic Diseases*, Practice and Policy, vol. 6, no.3, July 2009.

17. Pakpahan Medina Yus, Daniel Suryadarma and Asep Suryahadi, 'Destined for Destitution: intergenerational poverty persistence in Indonesia', Working Paper no. 134, Chronic Poverty Research Centre, SMERU Research Institute, Jakarta, January 2009.

18. Diallo, Yacouba, et al., *Global Child Labour Developments: Measuring trends from 2004 to 2008*, International Labour Organization, Geneva, 2010.

19. Statistical Table 9, p. 120.

20. UNICEF's mandate, based on the Convention on the Rights of the Child, defines 'children' as persons between 0 and 18 years of age. 'Adolescents' are defined by UNICEF and partners (UNFPA, WHO, UNAIDS) as persons between 10 and 19 years.

The United Nations General Assembly defines 'youth' as persons between 15 and 24 years of age, and 'young people' as those between 10 and 24 years of age. These definitions were adopted during the International Year of Youth in 1985 and have been generally used by United Nations agencies and other partners. In general, the overlapping use of these definitions is recognized, with 'adolescents' and 'youth' often used interchangeably with 'young people'.

In addition to these agreed definitions by the United Nations and its agencies, each national government has its own definition and age threshold for children, adolescents, young people and youth.

CHAPTER 1 PANELS

Haiti: Building back better together with young people

United Nations Children's Fund, 'Children of Haiti: Milestones and looking forward to six months', UNICEF, New York, July 2010, pp. 2, 4–5; United Nations Children's Fund, *The State of the World's Children Special Edition: Celebrating 20 Years of the Convention on the Rights of the Child*, UNICEF, New York, 2009, p. 25; United Nations Children's Fund, *The State of Latin American and Caribbean Children 2008*, UNICEF, New York, 2008, pp. 4, 16; Hudson, Lynne, et al., 'Picking Up the Pieces: Women's health needs assessment, Fond Parisien Region, Haiti, January–February 2010', Circle of Health Initiative, Bolton, Mass., 2010, pp. 9–11; Pan American Health Organization, 'Earthquake in Haiti: PAHO/WHO situation report on health activities post earthquake', PAHO, Washington, D.C., May 2010, pp. 2, 7; Government of the Republic of Haiti, 'Action Plan for National Recovery and Development of Haiti: Immediate key initiatives for the future', Port-au-Prince, March 2010, pp. 36–38; Iezzoni, Lisa I., and Laurence J. Ronan, 'Disability Legacy of the Haitian Earthquake', *Annals of Internal Medicine*, vol. 152, no. 12, 15 June 2010, pp. 812–814; UNICEF global databases, <www.childinfo.org>, accessed September 2010.

Early and late adolescence

Johnson, Sara B., et al., 'Adolescent Maturity and the Brain: The promise and pitfalls of neuroscience research in adolescent health policy', *Journal of Adolescent Health*, vol. 45, no. 3, September 2009, pp. 216–221; United Nations Joint Programme on HIV/AIDS, *Seen But Not Heard: Very young adolescents aged 10–14 years*, UNAIDS, Geneva, 2004, pp. 7, 24; United Nations Children's Fund, *Adolescence: A time that matters*, UNICEF, New York, 2002, p. 7; United Nations Children's Fund, 'Adolescent Development: Perspectives and frameworks – A summary of adolescent needs, an analysis of the various programme approaches and general recommendations for adolescent programming', Learning Series No. 1, UNICEF, New York, May 2006, p. 3.

Jordan: Ensuring productive work for youth

United Nations Children's Fund, *The State of the World's Children Special Edition: Celebrating 20 years of the Convention on the Rights of the Child – Statistical tables*, UNICEF, New York, 2009, p. 33; United Nations Children's Fund, *UNICEF Jordan Annual Report 2009*, p. 5; UNICEF global databases, <www.childinfo.org>, accessed September 2010; European Training Foundation, *Unemployment in Jordan*, ETF, Torino, 2005, p. 9; The Hashemite Kingdom of Jordan, The National Social and Economic Development Plan (2004–2006), Ministry of Planning and International Cooperation, p. 7.

CHAPTER 2

1. Peden, Margie, et al., eds., *World Report on Child Injury Prevention*, World Health Organization and United Nations Children's Fund, Geneva, 2008, p. 2.

2. Ibid., p. 5.

3. Sleet, David A., et al., 'A review of unintentional injuries in adolescents', *Annual Review of Public Health*, vol. 31, 2010, p. 195.

4. World Health Organization, *Adolescent Friendly Health Services*, WHO, Geneva, 2001, p. 15. Ibid., p .13.

5. Ibid., p. 14.

6. UNICEF Innocenti Research Centre, *Child Poverty in Perspective: An overview of child well-being in rich countries*, Report Card 7, UNICEF IRC, Florence, 2007, p. 31.

7. United Nations Children's Fund, *Progress for Children: Achieving the MDGs with equity*, no. 9, UNICEF, New York, 2010.

8. UNICEF global databases, accessed September 2010. More detailed information on methodology and data sources is available at <www.childinfo.org>.

9. UNICEF global databases, accessed September 2010. More detailed information on methodology and data sources is available at <www.childinfo.org>; and Statistical Table 9.

10. UNICEF global databases, accessed September 2010. More detailed information on methodology and data sources is available at <www.childinfo.org>; and Statistical Table 9.

11. UNICEF global databases, accessed September 2010. More detailed information on methodology and data sources is available at <www.childinfo.org>.

12. *Child poverty in perspective*, p. 28.

13. UNICEF global databases, accessed September 2010. More detailed information on methodology and data sources is available at <www.childinfo.org>.

14. UNICEF global databases, accessed September 2010. More detailed information on methodology and data sources is available at <www.childinfo.org>.

15. UNICEF global databases, accessed September 2010. More detailed information on methodology and data sources is available at <www.childinfo.org>.

16. Conde-Agudelo, A., J. M. Belizán and C. Lammers, 'Maternal-Perinatal Morbidity and Mortality Associated with Adolescent Pregnancy in Latin America: Cross-sectional study', *American Journal of Obstetrics and Gynecology*, vol. 192, no. 2, February 2005, pp. 342–349.

17. Goicolea, Isabel, et al., 'Risk Factors for Pregnancy among Adolescent Girls in Ecuador's Amazon Basin: A case-control study', *Revista Panamericana de Salud Public*, vol. 26, no. 3, September 2009, pp. 221–228.

18. World Health Organization, *Unsafe Abortion: Global and regional estimates of the incidence of unsafe abortions and associated mortality*, 5th ed., WHO, Geneva, 2003.

19. Grimes, David A., et al., 'Unsafe Abortion: The preventable epidemic', Journal paper, Sexual and Reproductive Health no. 4, World Health Organization, Geneva, 2005.

20. World Health Organization, *Adolescent Friendly Health Services: An agenda for change*, WHO, Geneva, 2002, p. 13.

21. United Nations Children's Fund, United Nations Joint Programme on HIV/AIDS, World Health Organization and United Nations Population Fund, *Children and AIDS: Fifth Stocktaking Report*, UNICEF, New York, December 2010, p. 41.

22. Ibid., p. 45.

23. Ibid., pp. 43–45.

24. UNICEF global databases, accessed September 2010. More detailed information on methodology and data sources is available at <www.childinfo.org>.

25. UNICEF global databases, accessed September 2010. More detailed information on methodology and data sources is available at <www.childinfo.org>.

26. United Nations, Convention on the Rights of Persons with Disabilities and Optional Protocol, <www.un.org/disabilities/documents/convention/convoptprot-e.pdf>, accessed 22 November 2010.

27. Statistical Table 6, p. 108.

28. United Nations Educational, Scientific and Cultural Organization Institute of Statistics, *Out-of-School Adolescents*, UIS, Montreal, 2010, p. 10.

29. Ibid.

30. United Nations Educational, Scientific and Cultural Organization, *Education for All Global Monitoring Report 2010: Reaching the marginalized*, UNESCO, Paris, 2010, p. 74.

31. Ibid.

32. Ibid.

33. Ibid., p. 75.

34. UNICEF global databases, accessed September 2010. More detailed information on methodology and data sources is available at <www.childinfo.org>.

35. United Nations Children's Fund, *Beijing+15: Bringing girls into focus*, UNICEF, New York, 2010.

36 Nickerson, Amanda B., and Richard J. Nagle, 'The Influence of Parent and Peer Attachments on Life Satisfaction in Middle Childhood and Early Adolescence', *Social Indicators Research*, vol. 66, no. 1–2, April 2004, p. 49.

37 United Nations, Keeping the Promise: A forward-looking review to promote an agreed action agenda to achieve the Millennium Development Goals by 2015 – Report of the Secretary-General, A/64/665, 12 February 2010, pp. 10, 14.

38 Ibid., p. 14.

39 *EFA Global Monitoring Report 2010*, pp. 76–93.

40 United Nations Educational, Scientific and Cultural Organization, *Another Way to Learn: Case studies*, UNESCO, Paris, 2007, pp. 6–9.

41 UNICEF global databases, accessed September 2010. More detailed information on methodology and data sources is available at <www.childinfo.org>.

42 UNICEF global databases, accessed September 2010. More detailed information on methodology and data sources is available at <www.childinfo.org>.

43 Statistical Table 9, p. 120.

44 UNICEF global databases, accessed September 2010. More detailed information on methodology and data sources is available at <www.childinfo.org>.

45 UNICEF global databases, accessed September 2010. More detailed information on methodology and data sources is available at <www.childinfo.org>; and Statistical Table 9, p. 120.

46 UNICEF global databases, accessed September 2010. More detailed information on methodology and data sources is available at <www.childinfo.org>.

47 UNICEF global databases, accessed September 2010. More detailed information on methodology and data sources is available at <www.childinfo.org>.

48 United Nations Children's Fund, *Progress for Children: A report card on child protection*, no. 8, UNICEF, New York, 2009, p. 15.

49 International Labour Office, The End of Child Labour: Within reach – Global report on the follow-up to the ILO Declaration on Fundamental Principles and Rights at Work, International Labour Conference 95th Session, Report I(B), ILO, Geneva, 2006.

50 International Labour Organization, *Good Practices and Lessons Learned on Child and Adolescent Domestic Labour in Central America and the Dominican Republic: A gender perspective*, ILO, San Jose, 2005, p. 10.

51 *Progress for Children 8*, pp. 17, 20.

52 Levine, Ruth et al., *Girls Count: A global investment and action agenda*, Center for Global Development, Washington D.C., 2009, p. 61.

53 Ibid.

54 Ibid.

55 Ibid.

56 Ibid.

57 Ibid.

58 Ibid.

59 Pulerwitz, Julie, et al., 'Promoting More Gender Equitable Norms and Behaviors among Young Men as an HIV Prevention Strategy', Population Council, Washington, D.C., 2009, p. 51; and Levine, op. cit., p. 61.

CHAPTER 2 PANELS

Demographic trends for adolescents: Ten key facts
United Nations, Department of Economic and Social Affairs, Population Division, World Population Prospects: The 2008 Revision, <www.esa.un.org/unpd/wpp2008/index.htm>, accessed October 2010; and UNICEF global databases, accessed October 2010.

India: Risks and opportunities for the world's largest national cohort of adolescents
Parasuraman, Sulabha, et al., *A Profile of Youth in India*, National Family Health Survey (NFHS-3) India 2005–2006, International Institute for Population Sciences, Mumbai, and ICF Macro, Calverton, Md., 2009; United Nations Development Programme, *Human Development Report 2009: Overcoming barriers – Human mobility and development*, UNDP, New York, 2009, p. 183; Child Development and Nutrition Programme, United Nations Children's Fund India, 'Unlocking the Indian Enigma: Breaking the inter-generational cycle of under-nutrition through a focus on adolescent girls', Paper

presented at the UNICEF-New School Graduate Program in International Affairs conference 'Adolescent Girls: Cornerstone of society – Building evidence and policies for inclusive societies', New York, 26–28 April 2010, p. 9; Ministry of Women and Child Development, Government of India, *Handbook on the Prohibition of Child Marriage Act, 2006*, Government of India, Ministry of Women and Child Development, Delhi, 2006.

Adolescent mental health: An urgent challenge for investigation and investment
World Health Organization and World Organization of Family Doctors, *Integrating Mental Health into Primary Care: A global perspective*, WHO and Wonca, Geneva and London, 2008; World Health Organization, *Adolescent Mental Health in Resource-Constrained Settings: A review of the evidence, nature, prevalence and determinants of common mental health problems and their management in primary health care*, WHO, Geneva, 2010 (in press); World Health Organization, 'Strengthening the Health Sector Response to Adolescent Health and Development', WHO, Geneva, 2009, <www.who.int/child-adolescent-health>, accessed 18 November 2010; World Health Organization, *mhGAP: Mental Health Gap Action Programme – Scaling up care for mental, neurological and substance use disorders*, WHO, Geneva, 2008; World Health Organization, *Mental Health Policy and Service Guidance Package: Child and adolescent mental health policies and plans*, WHO, Geneva, 2005; World Health Organization, *The World Health Report 2001: Mental health – New understanding, new hope*, WHO, Geneva, 2001; Patel, Vikram, et al., 'Mental Health of Young People: A global public-health challenge', *The Lancet*, vol. 369, no. 9569, 14 April 2007, pp. 1302–1313; Patricia J. Mrazek and Robert J. Haggerty, eds., *Reducing Risks for Mental Disorders: Frontiers for preventive intervention research*, National Academies Press, Washington, D.C., 1994.

Inequality in childhood and adolescence in rich countries – Innocenti Report Card 9: The children left behind
UNICEF Innocenti Research Centre, *The Children Left Behind: A league table of inequality in child well-being in the world's rich countries*, Report Card 9, UNICEF IRC, Florence, December 2010.

Ethiopia: Gender, poverty and the challenge for adolescents
United Nations Children's Fund, *Annual Report for Ethiopia 2009*, pp. 8–10; United Nations Children's Fund, *State of the World's Children 2009: Maternal and newborn health – Statistical tables*, UNICEF, New York, 2009, pp. 8, 28; World Health Organization, 'Adolescent Pregnancy: A culturally complex issue', *Bulletin of the World Health Organization*, vol. 87, no. 6, June 2009, pp. 405–484, <www.who.int/bulletin/volumes/87/6/09-020609/en/>, accessed 22 November 2010; Ethiopian Society of Population Studies, 'Levels, Trends and Determinants of Lifetime and Desired Fertility in Ethiopia: Findings from EDHS 2005', Ethiopian Society of Population Studies, Addis Ababa, October 2008, p. 8; Annabel Erulkar and Tekle-ab Mekbib, 'Reaching Vulnerable Youth in Ethiopia', *Promoting Healthy, Safe and Productive Transitions to Adulthood*, Brief no. 6, Population Council, New York, August 2007, pp. 1–3; United Nations Children's Fund, 'Ethiopia: Adolescence', <www.unicef.org/ethiopia/children_395.html>, accessed 22 November 2010; Annabel Erulkar, Tekle-Ab Mekbib, Negussie Smith and Tsehai Gulema, 'Differential Use of Adolescent Reproductive Health Programs in Addis Ababa, Ethiopia', *Journal of Adolescent Health*, vol. 38, 2006, pp. 256–258; Annabel Erulkar and Eunice Muthengi, 'Evaluation or Berhane Hewan: A program to delay child marriage in rural Ethiopia', *International Perspectives on Sexual and Reproductive Health*, vol. 35, no. 1, March 2009, pp. 7, 12; Craig Hadley, David Lindstrom, Fasil Tessema and Tefara Belachew, 'Gender Bias in the Food Insecurity Experience of Ethiopian Adolescents', *Social Science and Medicine*, vol. 66, no. 2, January 2008, pp. 427–438, 435.

Mexico: Protecting unaccompanied migrant adolescents
United Nations Children's Fund, *The State of the World's Children: Special edition – Celebrating 20 years of the Convention on the Rights of the Child*, UNICEF, New

York, 2009, p. 66; The Economist Intelligence Unit, *Mexico Country Profile: Main report 2008*, EIU, London, 2008, pp. 15–16; United Nations Children's Fund, 'Examples of Good Practices in Implementation of the International Framework for the Protection of the Rights of the Child in the Context of Migration: A draft report', UNICEF, New York, 2008, p. 36.

CHAPTER 3

1 United Nations Children's Fund, *Climate Change and Children: A human security challenge*, Policy Review Paper, UNICEF Innocenti Research Centre, Florence, 2008, pp. 9–12.

2 Ibid., pp. 3, 4.

3 United Nations Framework Convention on Climate Change, *Growing Together in a Changing Climate: The United Nations, young people and climate change*, United Nations, New York, 2009, p. 1.

4 United Nations Environment Programme, 'TUNZA 2009 Youth Conferences: What we want from Copenhagen', *TUNZA: The UNEP magazine for youth*, vol. 7, no. 3, 2009.

5 Kelsey-Fry, Jamie, and Anita Dhillon, *The Rax Active Citizenship Toolkit: GCSE Citizenship Studies – Skills and processes*, New Internationalist, Oxford, 2010, p. 75.

6 Institute of Development Studies, 'Children in a Changing Environment: Lessons from research and practice – Rights, needs and capacities of children in a changing climate' and 'Children in a Changing Environment: Lessons from research and practice – Climate change, child rights and intergenerational justice', *IDS in Focus Policy Briefing*, nos. 13.1 and 13.2, November 2009.

7 Institute of Development Studies, 'Children in a Changing Environment: Lessons from research and practice – Rights, needs and capacities of children in a changing climate', *IDS in Focus Policy Briefing*, no. 13.1, November 2009.

8 International Labour Organization, *Global Employment Trends for Youth 2010*, ILO, Geneva, 2010, pp. 3–6.

9 World Bank, *World Development Report 2007: Development and the next generation*, World Bank, Washington, D.C., 2006, p. 3.

10 United Nations, *World Youth Report 2005: Young people today and in 2015*, Department of Economic and Social Affairs, United Nations, New York, 2005, pp. 17, 46.

11 World Bank, *World Development Report 2007: Development and the next generation*, World Bank, Washington, D.C., 2006, pp. 4–5.

12 Barrientos, Armando, *Social Protection and Poverty*, United Nations Research Institute for Social Development, Geneva, 2010, p. 10.

13 Department for International Development, United Kingdom; HelpAge International; Hope & Homes for Children; Institute of Development Studies; International Labour Organization; Overseas Development Institute; Save the Children UK; United Nations Children's Fund; United Nations Development Programme and the World Bank, 'Advancing Child-Sensitive Social Protection', June 2009, p. 1.

14 United Nations Development Programme, *Youth and Violent Conflict: Society and development in crisis?*, UNDP, New York, 2006.

15 United Nations General Assembly, United Nations Guidelines for the Prevention of Juvenile Delinquency (The Riyadh Guidelines), adopted by the General Assembly 14 December 1990, A/RES/45/112, available at: <www.un.org/documents/ga/res/45/a45r112.htm>, accessed 12 September 2010.

16 United Nations, *World Youth Report 2003: The global situation of young people*, Department of Economic and Social Affairs, United Nations, New York, 2004, pp. 189–190.

17 United Nations Children's Fund, *Progress for Children: A report card on child protection*, no. 8, UNICEF, New York, 2009, p. 20.

18 United Nations Children's Fund, *The Impact of Small Arms on Children and Adolescents in Central America and the Caribbean: A case study of El Salvador, Guatemala, Jamaica and Trinidad and Tobago*, UNICEF, New York, 2007, p. 5.

[19] United Nations Children's Fund, *Child Protection Information Sheets*, UNICEF, New York, 2006, p. 19.

[20] Defence for Children International. *No Kids Behind Bars: A global campaign on justice for children in conflict with the law*, DCI, 2005, pp. 2–4.

[21] United Nations, *World Youth Report 2003. The global situation of young people*, Department of Economic and Social Affairs, United Nations, New York, 2004, pp. 190–192, 194–195.

[22] United Nations Children's Fund, *Child Protection Information Sheets*, UNICEF, New York, 2006, p. 19.

[23] United Nations Children's Fund, *Adolescent Programming Experiences during Conflict and Post-conflict: Case studies*, UNICEF, New York, 2004, p. 6.

[24] Women's Commission for Refugee Women and Children, *Untapped Potential: Adolescents affected by armed conflict – A review of programs and policies*, Women's Commission for Refugee Women and Children, New York, 2000, p. 5.

CHAPTER 3 PANELS

Ukraine: Establishing a protective environment for vulnerable children
United Nations Children's Fund, *The State of the World's Children: Celebrating 20 Years of the Convention on the Rights of the Child – Statistical tables*, UNICEF, New York, 2009, pp. 19, 27; Joint United Nations Programme on HIV/AIDS and World Health Organization, *2009 AIDS Epidemic Update*, UNAIDS and WHO, Geneva, 2009, p. 48; Teltschik, Anja, *Children and Young People Living or Working on the Streets: The missing face of the HIV epidemic in Ukraine*, United Nations Children's Fund and AIDS Foundation East-West, Kyiv, 2006, pp. 27–29.

The Philippines: Strengthening the participation rights of adolescents
United Nations Development Programme, 'Philippine Commitment to the Millennium Development Goals', <www.undp.org.ph/?link=mdg_ph>, accessed 23 August 2010; United Nations Children's Fund, *The State of the World's Children Special Edition: Celebrating 20 Years of the Convention on the Rights of the Child – Statistical tables*, UNICEF, New York, 2009, p. 26; Huasman, Ricardo, Laura D. Tyson and Saadia Zahidi, eds., *The Global Gender Gap Report 2007*, World Economic Forum, Geneva, 2007, p. 7; Economist Intelligence Unit, *Country Profile Philippines: Main report*, 2008, EIU, London, 2008, p. 3; Philippine Institute for Development Studies, 'Global Study on Child Poverty and Disparities: The case of the Philippines', Discussion Paper Series No. 2009–27, September 2009; UNICEF Innocenti Research Centre, *Law Reform and Implementation of the Convention on the Rights of the Child*, Florence, 2007, p. 24; United Nations Children's Fund, *Young People's Civic Engagement in East Asia and the Pacific: A regional study conducted by Innovations in Civic Participation*, UNICEF East Asia and Pacific Regional Office, Bangkok, 2008, p. 47.

Migration and children: A cause for urgent attention
United Nations, Department of Economic and Social Affairs, Population Division, *Population Facts*, no. 2010/6, November 2010, p. 2; United Nations Children's Fund, 'Examples of Good Practices in the Implementation of the International Framework for the Protection of the Rights of the Child in the Context of Migration', Draft report, UNICEF, New York, 18 June 2010, p.1; Abramovich, Victor, Pablo Ceriani Cernades and Alejandro Morlachetti, 'Migration, Children and Human Rights: Challenges and opportunities', Draft working paper, United Nations Children's Fund, New York, November 2010, pp. 1–12; United Nations Children's Fund, 'Children, Adolescents and Migration: Filling the evidence gap', UNICEF, October 2009.

CHAPTER 4

[1] Warburton, J., et al., *A Right to Happiness: Positive prevention and intervention strategies with children abused through sexual exploitation*, Regional Seminars Action Research Youth Projects in the CIS and Baltics, BICE, Geneva, 2001.

[2] World Bank, *Expanding Opportunities and Building Competencies for Young People: A new agenda for secondary education*, The International Bank for Reconstruction and Development/The World Bank, Washington, D.C., 2005, pp. 17, 18.

[3] Ibid., p. 21.

[4] Clemens, Michael, 'The Long Walk to School: International education goals in historical perspective', Working Paper 37, Center for Global Development, Washington, D.C., 2004, cited in *Expanding Opportunities and Building Competencies*, p. 21.

[5] Levine, Ruth, et al., *Girls Count: A global investment and action agenda*, Center for Global Development, Washington, D.C., 2008, p. 48.

[6] United Nations, *The Millennium Development Goals Report 2007*, UN, New York, 2007, p. 17.

[7] Poirier, Marie-Pierre, 'Brazil Ranks amongst Countries Taking Responsibility for Longer Mandatory Education', *Panorama*, no. 96, 11 November 2009.

[8] United Nations Educational, Scientific and Cultural Organization, *Education for All Global Monitoring Report 2010: Reaching the marginalized*, UNESCO and Oxford University Press, Paris, 2010, p. 65.

[9] Huebler, Friedrich, 'Child Labour and School Attendance: Evidence from MICS and DHS surveys', Seminar on Child Labour, Education and Youth Employment, Understanding Children's Work Project, Madrid, 11–12 September 2008, pp. 17–18.

[10] United Nations Girls' Education Initiative, 'Global Section: The School Fee Abolition Initiative (SFAI)', <www.ungei.org/infobycountry/247_712.html>, accessed 12 November 2010.

[11] *Education for All Global Monitoring Report 2010*, pp. 12, 202.

[12] Ministry of Health and Social Services and Macro International, Inc., *Namibia: Demographic and Health Survey 2006–07*, MoHSS and Macro International, Inc., Windhoek, Namibia, and Calverton, Md., 2008.

[13] Murtaza, Rushnan, 'Visibility of Girls in the Education Sector Policy in Namibia', UNICEF Namibia, Windhoek, 2009.

[14] Mead, Francis, 'New Syllabus Helps Conflict-Affected Children Get Back to School in Sri Lanka', Back on Track, 5 November 2007, <www.educationandtransition.org/resources/stories/new-syllabus-helps-conflict-affected-children-get-back-to-school-in-sri-lanka/>, accessed 12 November 2010.

[15] Watts, Roderick J., and Constance Flanagan, 'Pushing the Envelope on Youth Civic Engagement: A developmental and liberation psychology perspective', *Journal of Community Psychology*, vol. 35, no. 6, 2007, p. 782.

[16] United Nations Children's Fund, Adolescent Development and Participation Unit, 'Youth Participation in Poverty Reduction Strategies and National Development Plans: A desk study', ADAP Learning Series No. 4, UNICEF, New York, March 2009.

[17] UNICEF, *What Works: Promoting adolescent development in Latin America and Caribbean*, UNICEF, Panama City, 2010.

[18] *Education for All Global Monitoring Report 2010*, p. 208.

[19] Republic of Liberia, Ministry of Gender and Development, 'Economic Empowerment of Adolescent Girls and Young Women (EPAG) Project, http://www.supportliberia.com/assets/108/EPAG_one-pager_1_.pdf>.

[20] *Education for All Global Monitoring Report 2010*, p. 48.

CHAPTER 4 PANELS

Preparing adolescents for adulthood and citizenship
United Nations Children's Fund, *Promoting Adolescent Development in Latin America and the Caribbean*, UNICEF, Panama City, 2009 p. 22; United Nations Children's Fund, *The State of the World's Children Special Edition: Celebrating 20 Years of the Convention on the Rights of the Child*, UNICEF, New York, 2010, p. 30; United Nations Children's Fund, *Voices of Hope: Adolescents and the tsunami*, UNICEF, New York, 2005; Pittman, Karen Johnson, et al., *Preventing Problems, Promoting Development, Encouraging Engagement: Competing priorities or inseparable goals?*, Forum for Youth Investment, Washington, D.C., 2003, reprint 2005; TakingITGlobal, *National Youth Councils: Their creation, evolution, purpose and governance*, Ontario, April 2006, pp. 7, 41, 43; Bennett, W. Lance, 'Changing Citizenship in the Digital Age', in *Civic Life Online: Learning how digital media can engage youth*, edited by W. Lance Bennett, MIT Press, Cambridge, Mass., 2008, pp. 1–24.

United States: The Campus Initiative – Advocating for children's rights at colleges and universities.
Information provided by the US Fund for UNICEF.

Working together for adolescent girls: The United Nations Adolescent Girls Task Force
International Labour Organization, United Nations Educational, Scientific and Cultural Organization, United Nations Population Fund, United Nations Children's Fund, United Nations Development Fund for Women and World Health Organization. 'Accelerating Efforts to Advance the Rights of Adolescent Girls: A Joint UN Statement, March 2010.

Côte d'Ivoire: Violent conflict and the vulnerability of adolescents
United Nations Office for the Coordination of Humanitarian Affairs, 'Côte d'Ivoire', <http://ochaonline.un.org/OCHAHome/WhereWeWork/Cocircted8217Ivoire/tabid/6410/language/en-US/Default.aspx>, accessed 19 November 2010; Betsi, N. A., et al., 'Effect of an Armed Conflict on Human Resources and Health Systems in Côte d'Ivoire', *AIDS Care*, vol. 18, no. 4, May 2006, pp. 360–363; Human Rights Watch, *"My Heart is Cut": Sexual violence by rebels and pro-government forces in Côte d'Ivoire*, vol. 19, no. 11(a), Human Rights Watch, New York, August 2007, pp. 86–91; Bøås, Morten, and Anne Huser, 'Child Labour and Cocoa Production in West Africa: The case of Côte d'Ivoire and Ghana', Report 522, Fafo Institute for Applied International Studies, Research Program on Trafficking and Child Labour, Oslo, 2006, p. 8; Yapo, Serge Armand, 'Improving Human Security in Post-Conflict Cote d'Ivoire: A local governance approach', United Nations Development Programme, Oslo Governance Center, 2007, pp. 21, 23, 27; Ministry of the Family, Women and Social Affairs/Gender Equity and Promotion Directorate, 'National Action Plan for the Implementation of Resolution 1325 of the Security Council (2008–2012): Background document', Abidjan, <www.un.org/womenwatch/feature/wps/nap1325_cote_d_ivoire.pdf>, accessed 19 November 2010; Joint United Nations Programme on HIV/AIDS and World Health Organization, 'Sub-Saharan Africa', *AIDS Epidemic Update 2009*, UNAIDS and WHO, Geneva, November 2009, pp. 21–36.

STATISTICAL TABLES

Economic and social statistics on the countries and territories of the world, with particular reference to children's well-being.

OVERVIEW

This reference guide presents the most recent key statistics on child survival, development and protection for the world's countries, territories and regions in a single volume. For the first time this year, two new tables have been included:

- Table 11: Adolescents
- Table 12: Equity

The Adolescents table provides data relevant to this specific age group. The indicators include: proportion of the total population that are 10–19 years old; current marital status of girls aged 15–19; percentage of girls aged 20–24 who gave birth before age 18; adolescent fertility; attitudes towards domestic violence of girls and boys aged 15–19; secondary education; and HIV/AIDS knowledge of adolescents.

The Equity table provides data on disparities by household wealth for four indicators – birth registration, skilled attendant at delivery, underweight prevalence and immunization – as well as disparity data by area of residence (urban and rural) for use of improved sanitation facilities.

The statistical tables presented in this volume help to meet the demand for timely, reliable, comparable and comprehensive data on the state of the world's children. They also support UNICEF's focus on progress and results on internationally agreed goals and compacts on children's rights and development. UNICEF is the lead agency responsible for global monitoring of the Millennium Declaration child-related goals as well as Millennium Development Goals and indicators; the organization is also a key partner in the United Nations' work on monitoring these targets and indicators.

All of the numbers presented in this reference guide are available online at <www.unicef.org/publications> and <www.unicef.org/sowc2011>. The data will also be available via the UNICEF global statistical databases at <www.childinfo.org>. Please refer to these websites for the latest versions of the statistical tables and for any updates or corrigenda subsequent to printing.

General note on the data

The data presented in the following statistical tables are derived from the UNICEF global databases, which include only internationally comparable and statistically sound data; these data are accompanied by definitions, sources and explanations of symbols. In addition, data from other United Nations organizations have been used. The report draws on inter-agency estimates and nationally representative household surveys such as Multiple Indicator Cluster Surveys (MICS) and Demographic and Health Surveys (DHS). Data presented in this year's statistical tables generally reflect information available as of July 2010.

More detailed information on methodology and data sources is available at <www.childinfo.org>.

Several of the indicators, such as the data for life expectancy, total fertility rates and crude birth and death rates, are part of the regular work on estimates and projections undertaken by the United Nations Population Division. These and other internationally produced estimates are revised periodically, which explains why some data will differ from those published in earlier UNICEF publications.

This report includes the latest estimates and projections from World Population Prospects: The 2008 revision (United Nations Department of Economic and Social Affairs, Population Division). Data quality is likely to be adversely affected for countries that have recently suffered human-caused or natural disasters. This is particularly true where basic country infrastructure has been fragmented or where major population movements have occurred.

Child mortality estimates

Each year, in its flagship publication The State of the World's Children, UNICEF reports a series of mortality estimates for children – including the annual infant mortality rate, the under-five mortality rate and the number of under-five deaths – for at least two reference years. These figures represent the best estimates available at the time the report goes to print. The estimates are based on the work of the Inter-agency Group for Child Mortality Estimation (IGME), which includes UNICEF, the World Health Organization (WHO), the United Nations Population Division and the World Bank.

IGME updates these mortality estimates each year, undertaking a detailed review of all newly available data points. This exercise often results in adjustments to previously reported estimates; as a result, estimates published in consecutive editions of The State of the World's Children may not be comparable and **should not be used for analysing mortality trends over time.** Comparable under-five mortality estimates for the period 1970–2009 are presented below, according to UNICEF Regional and Country Classifications.

Under-five mortality rate (per 1,000 live births)

Region	1970	1975	1980	1985	1990	1995	2000	2005	2007	2008	2009
Africa	223	201	186	172	165	161	147	131	125	121	118
Sub-Saharan Africa	226	204	193	185	180	175	160	143	136	133	129
Eastern and Southern Africa	210	185	177	168	166	158	141	124	116	112	108
West and Central Africa	258	227	213	205	199	195	181	163	156	153	150
Middle East and North Africa	192	161	131	97	77	66	56	47	44	43	41
Asia	150	129	115	98	87	83	70	59	54	52	50
South Asia	194	175	158	141	125	112	97	81	76	73	71
East Asia and Pacific	121	94	73	59	53	49	40	31	28	27	26
Latin America and Caribbean	121	103	83	66	52	43	33	27	24	23	23
CEE/CIS	89	81	70	59	51	49	37	27	24	23	21
Industrialized countries	24	19	15	12	10	8	7	6	6	6	6
Developing countries	157	139	125	109	99	95	84	74	70	68	66
Least developed countries	239	223	205	187	178	164	146	131	126	123	121
World	**138**	**123**	**112**	**97**	**89**	**86**	**77**	**67**	**63**	**62**	**60**

Under-five deaths (millions)

Region	1970	1975	1980	1985	1990	1995	2000	2005	2007	2008	2009
Africa	3.6	3.6	3.8	4.0	4.2	4.4	4.4	4.2	4.2	4.1	4.1
Sub-Saharan Africa	2.9	3.0	3.3	3.6	3.9	4.2	4.2	4.1	4.1	4.0	4.0
Eastern and Southern Africa	1.3	1.3	1.4	1.5	1.7	1.7	1.7	1.6	1.6	1.5	1.5
West and Central Africa	1.6	1.6	1.8	1.9	2.1	2.3	2.4	2.4	2.4	2.3	2.3
Middle East and North Africa	1.3	1.2	1.1	0.9	0.8	0.6	0.5	0.4	0.4	0.4	0.4
Asia	10.4	8.8	7.5	7.2	6.8	5.9	4.9	4.0	3.7	3.6	3.4
South Asia	5.3	5.2	5.2	4.9	4.6	4.3	3.6	3.1	2.9	2.7	2.6
East Asia and Pacific	5.0	3.5	2.3	2.2	2.2	1.6	1.3	0.9	0.9	0.8	0.8
Latin America and Caribbean	1.2	1.1	0.9	0.8	0.6	0.5	0.4	0.3	0.3	0.3	0.2
CEE/CIS	0.6	0.6	0.5	0.5	0.4	0.3	0.2	0.2	0.1	0.1	0.1
Industrialized countries	0.3	0.2	0.2	0.1	0.1	0.1	0.1	0.1	0.1	0.1	0.1
Developing countries	15.9	14.3	13.0	12.6	12.2	11.2	10.0	8.9	8.4	8.2	8.0
Least developed countries	3.3	3.5	3.6	3.6	3.7	3.8	3.6	3.5	3.4	3.4	3.3
World	**16.3**	**14.8**	**13.4**	**12.9**	**12.4**	**11.4**	**10.2**	**9.0**	**8.5**	**8.3**	**8.1**

Country-specific mortality indicators for 1970–2009, based on the most recent IGME estimates, are presented in Table 10 (for the years 1970, 1990, 2000 and 2009) and are also available at <www.childinfo.org> and <www.childmortality. org>, the IGME website.

Multiple Indicator Cluster Surveys: For more than a decade, UNICEF has supported countries in collecting statistically sound and internationally comparable data through MICS. Since 1995, nearly 200 surveys have been conducted in approximately 100 countries and territories. The third round of MICS was conducted in more than 50 countries during 2005–2006, allowing for a new and more comprehensive assessment of the situation of children and women globally. The fourth round of surveys is now under way and will run until 2011. The UNICEF-supported MICS are among the largest sources of data for monitoring progress towards internationally agreed development goals for children, including the Millennium Development Goals (MDGs). Many of the MICS indicators have been incorporated into the statistical tables appearing in this report. More information on these data is available at <www.childinfo.org>.

Regional Classification: In the 2009 edition of *The State of the World's Children,* UNICEF added two new regional groupings: Africa and Asia. In addition, the number of countries classified in the sub-Saharan Africa region increased with the inclusion of Djibouti and the Sudan. As a result, regional estimates for sub-Saharan Africa published in previous issues of *The State of the World's Children* may not be comparable with those published in this issue. All other regions remain unchanged.

For details of the countries included in all UNICEF regions, please refer to the UNICEF Regional Classification, page 124.

Revisions to Statistical Tables

Table 1. Basic Indicators:
Neonatal mortality rates: The neonatal mortality rates presented in this report were produced by WHO and are consistent with the under-five mortality rates. Both indicators are for the year 2009.

Table 2. Nutrition:
Underweight, stunting and wasting: Prevalence of underweight, stunting and wasting among children under 5 years of age is estimated by comparing actual measurements with an international standard reference population. In April 2006, WHO released the WHO Child Growth Standards to replace the widely used National Center for Health Statistics/World Health Organization (NCHS/WHO) reference population, which was based on a limited sample of children from the United States. The new standards are the result of an intensive study project involving more than 8,000 children from Brazil, Ghana, India, Norway, Oman and the United States.

Overcoming the technical and biological drawbacks of the old reference population, the new standards confirm that children born anywhere in the world and given the optimum start in life have the potential to develop to within the same range of height and weight. Differences in children's growth to age 5 are more influenced by nutrition, feeding practices, environment and health care than genetics or ethnicity.

In this report, all of the child anthropometry indicators are reported according to the WHO Child Growth Standards. An additional column displays underweight prevalence (moderate and severe) based on the NCHS/WHO standard. Owing to the differences between the old reference population and the new standards, prevalence estimates of child anthropometry indicators published in consecutive editions of *The State of the World's Children* may not be fully comparable.

Vitamin A supplementation: Only full coverage (two doses) of vitamin A supplementation is presented in this report, emphasizing the importance for children of receiving two annual doses of vitamin A, spaced 4–6 months apart. In the absence of a direct method to measure this indicator, full coverage is reported as the lower coverage estimate from rounds 1 and 2 in a given year.

Table 3. Health:
Water and Sanitation: The drinking water and sanitation coverage estimates in this report come from the WHO/UNICEF Joint Monitoring Programme for Water Supply and Sanitation (JMP). These are the official United Nations estimates for measuring progress towards the MDG target for drinking water and sanitation, and they are based on a standard classification of what constitutes coverage. JMP estimates coverage using a linear regression line that is fitted to coverage data from all available household sample surveys and censuses. Full details of the JMP methodology and country estimates can be found at <www.childinfo.org> and <www.wssinfo.org>.

Table 4. HIV and AIDS:
In 2010, the Joint United Nations Programme on HIV/AIDS (UNAIDS) released new global HIV and AIDS estimates for 2009 that reflect more reliable data available from population-based surveys, expanded national sentinel surveillance systems and programme service statistics in a number of countries. As a result, UNAIDS has retrospectively generated new estimates for HIV prevalence, the number of people living with HIV and the number of children whose parents have died due to all causes or AIDS for past years based on the refined methodology.

Figures published in this report are not comparable to previous estimates and therefore do not reflect trends over time. UNAIDS has published comparable estimates by applying the new methods to earlier HIV and AIDS estimates; these data can be accessed at <www.unaids.org>. In addition to presenting the HIV prevalence among young males and females aged 15–24, this year's table presents the total HIV prevalence among young people aged 15–24.

Table 5. Education:
Survival rate to the last grade of primary school: The survival rate to Grade 5 (percentage of primary school entrants reaching Grade 5) was replaced in 2008 by the survival rate to the last grade of primary school (percentage of children entering the first grade of primary school who are expected to reach the last grade). The survival rate to the last grade became an official indicator for MDG 2 (Universal Primary Education) in January 2008.

Table 6. Demographic Indicators:
Population annual growth rate and average annual growth rate of urban population: These indicators have been further disaggregated to include data for 1990–2000.

Table 7. Economic Indicators:
Proportion of the population living below US$1.25 per day: In 2008, the World Bank announced a new poverty line that is based on revised estimates of purchasing power parity (PPP) price levels around the world. Table 7 reflects this updated poverty line and reports on the proportion of the population living below US$1.25 per day at 2005 prices, adjusted for PPP. The new poverty threshold reflects revisions to PPP exchange rates based on the results of the 2005 International Comparison Program. The revisions reveal that the cost of living is higher across the developing world than previously estimated. As a result of these revisions, poverty rates for individual countries cannot be compared with poverty rates reported in previous editions. More detailed information on the definition, methodology and sources is available at <www.worldbank.org>.

Table 8. Women:
Delivery care coverage: For the first time, the table includes Caesarean section (C-section) as part of the indicator on delivery care coverage. C-section is an essential part of comprehensive emergency obstetric care.

Maternal mortality ratio (adjusted): The table presents the new 'adjusted' maternal mortality ratios for the year 2008. The new 'adjusted' maternal mortality estimates were produced by the Maternal Mortality Estimation Inter-agency Group (MMEIG), which is composed of WHO, UNICEF, the United Nations Population Fund (UNFPA) and the World Bank, together with independent technical experts. The inter-agency group has used a dual approach in deriving estimates of maternal mortality, which involves making adjustments to existing estimates of maternal mortality from civil registration systems to correct for misclassification and under-reporting, and generating model-based estimates for countries that do not have reliable national-level estimates of maternal mortality from civil registration systems.

These 'adjusted' estimates should not be compared to previous inter-agency estimates, as the methodological approach is not the same. A full report with complete country estimates and detailed methodological information, as well as statistical tables including new country and regional maternal mortality ratios for the years 1990, 1995, 2000, 2005 and 2008, can be found at <www.childinfo.org/maternal_mortality.html>.

Table 9. Child Protection:
Previous estimates used in UNICEF publications and in MICS country reports were calculated using household weights that did not take into account the last stage selection of children for the administration of the child discipline module in MICS surveys. (A random selection of one child aged 2–14 is undertaken for the administration of the child discipline module.) In January 2010, it was decided that more accurate estimates are produced by using a household weight that takes the last-stage selection into account. MICS 3 data were recalculated using the new approach. The *State of the World's Children 2011* and all future UNICEF publications will use these modified estimates.

Child disability: The table in the current edition does not report on child disability because new, comparable data are unavailable for a significant number of countries.

Explanation of symbols

Because the aim of these statistical tables is to provide a broad picture of the situation of children and women worldwide, detailed data qualifications and footnotes are seen as more appropriate for inclusion elsewhere.

Sources and years for specific data points included in the statistical tables are available at <www.childinfo.org>.

Symbols specific to a particular table are included in the table footnotes. The following symbols are common across all tables:

– Data are not available.

x Data refer to years or periods other than those specified in the column heading, differ from the standard definition or refer to only part of a country. Such data are not included in the calculation of regional and global averages.

y Data refer to years or periods other than those specified in the column heading, differ from the standard definition or refer to only part of a country. Such data are included in the calculation of regional and global averages.

* Data refer to the most recent year available during the period specified in the column heading.

§ Includes territories within each category or regional group. Countries and territories in each country category or regional group are listed on page 124.

Under-five mortality rankings

The following list ranks countries and territories in descending order of their estimated 2009 under-five mortality rate (U5MR), a critical indicator of the well-being of children. Countries and territories are listed alphabetically in the tables on the following pages.

	Under-5 mortality rate (2009) Value	Rank		Under-5 mortality rate (2009) Value	Rank		Under-5 mortality rate (2009) Value	Rank
Chad	209	1	Micronesia (Federated States of)	39	66	Bahrain	12	130
Afghanistan	199	2	Morocco	38	68	Belarus	12	130
Democratic Republic of the Congo	199	2	Kyrgyzstan	37	69	Lebanon	12	130
Guinea-Bissau	193	4	Solomon Islands	36	70	Oman	12	130
Sierra Leone	192	5	Uzbekistan	36	70	Romania	12	130
Mali	191	6	Guyana	35	72	Russian Federation	12	130
Somalia	180	7	Marshall Islands	35	72	Saint Vincent and the Grenadines	12	130
Central African Republic	171	8	Trinidad and Tobago	35	72	Seychelles	12	130
Burkina Faso	166	9	Tuvalu	35	72	Barbados	11	140
Burundi	166	9	Azerbaijan	34	76	Costa Rica	11	140
Angola	161	11	Democratic People's			Qatar	11	140
Niger	160	12	Republic of Korea	33	77	The former Yugoslav Republic		
Cameroon	154	13	Philippines	33	77	of Macedonia	11	140
Equatorial Guinea	145	14	Algeria	32	79	Bulgaria	10	144
Guinea	142	15	Dominican Republic	32	79	Dominica	10	144
Mozambique	142	15	Iran (Islamic Republic of)	31	81	Kuwait	10	144
Zambia	141	17	Jamaica	31	81	Chile	9	147
Nigeria	138	18	Honduras	30	83	Montenegro	9	147
Congo	128	19	Occupied Palestinian Territory	30	83	Latvia	8	149
Uganda	128	19	Georgia	29	85	United States	8	149
Côte d'Ivoire	119	21	Kazakhstan	29	85	Brunei Darussalam	7	151
Benin	118	22	Mongolia	29	85	Malta	7	151
Mauritania	117	23	Cape Verde	28	88	Poland	7	151
Liberia	112	24	Nicaragua	26	89	Serbia	7	151
Rwanda	111	25	Suriname	26	89	Slovakia	7	151
Malawi	110	26	Jordan	25	91	United Arab Emirates	7	151
Sudan	108	27	Samoa	25	91	Canada	6	157
United Republic of Tanzania	108	27	Ecuador	24	93	Cuba	6	157
Comoros	104	29	Viet Nam	24	93	Estonia	6	157
Ethiopia	104	29	Panama	23	95	Hungary	6	157
Gambia	103	31	Paraguay	23	95	Lithuania	6	157
Togo	98	32	Armenia	22	97	Malaysia	6	157
Djibouti	94	33	Brazil	21	98	New Zealand	6	157
Senegal	93	34	Egypt	21	98	United Kingdom	6	157
Zimbabwe	90	35	Peru	21	98	Australia	5	165
Cambodia	88	36	Saudi Arabia	21	98	Belgium	5	165
Haiti	87	37	Tunisia	21	98	Croatia	5	165
Pakistan	87	37	Saint Lucia	20	103	Republic of Korea	5	165
Kenya	84	39	Turkey	20	103	Andorra	4	169
Lesotho	84	39	China	19	105	Austria	4	169
Bhutan	79	41	Colombia	19	105	Cyprus	4	169
Sao Tome and Principe	78	42	Libyan Arab Jamahiriya	19	105	Czech Republic	4	169
Swaziland	73	43	Tonga	19	105	Denmark	4	169
Myanmar	71	44	Belize	18	109	France	4	169
Gabon	69	45	Fiji	18	109	Germany	4	169
Ghana	69	45	Venezuela (Bolivarian Republic of)	18	109	Ireland	4	169
Papua New Guinea	68	47	El Salvador	17	112	Israel	4	169
India	66	48	Mauritius	17	112	Italy	4	169
Yemen	66	48	Mexico	17	112	Monaco	4	169
South Africa	62	50	Republic of Moldova	17	112	Netherlands	4	169
Tajikistan	61	51	Syrian Arab Republic	16	116	Portugal	4	169
Lao People's Democratic Republic	59	52	Vanuatu	16	116	Spain	4	169
Madagascar	58	53	Albania	15	118	Switzerland	4	169
Botswana	57	54	Cook Islands	15	118	Finland	3	184
Timor-Leste	56	55	Grenada	15	118	Greece	3	184
Eritrea	55	56	Palau	15	118	Iceland	3	184
Bangladesh	52	57	Saint Kitts and Nevis	15	118	Japan	3	184
Bolivia (Plurinational State of)	51	58	Sri Lanka	15	118	Luxembourg	3	184
Namibia	48	59	Ukraine	15	118	Norway	3	184
Nepal	48	59	Argentina	14	125	Singapore	3	184
Kiribati	46	61	Bosnia and Herzegovina	14	125	Slovenia	3	184
Turkmenistan	45	62	Thailand	14	125	Sweden	3	184
Iraq	44	63	Maldives	13	128	Liechtenstein	2	193
Nauru	44	63	Uruguay	13	128	San Marino	2	193
Guatemala	40	65	Antigua and Barbuda	12	130	Holy See	–	
Indonesia	39	66	Bahamas	12	130	Niue	–	

TABLE 1. BASIC INDICATORS

Countries and territories	Under-5 mortality rank	Under-5 mortality rate 1990	Under-5 mortality rate 2009	Infant mortality rate (under 1) 1990	Infant mortality rate (under 1) 2009	Neonatal mortality rate 2009	Total population (thousands) 2009	Annual no. of births (thousands) 2009	Annual no. of under-5 deaths (thousands) 2009	GNI per capita (US$) 2009	Life expectancy at birth (years) 2009	Total adult literacy rate (%) 2005–2008*	Primary school net enrolment/attendance (%) 2005–2009*	% share of household income 2000–2009* lowest 40%	% share of household income 2000–2009* highest 20%
Afghanistan	2	250	199	167	134	52	28150	1302	237	370 x	44	–	61	–	–
Albania	118	51	15	41	14	4	3155	47	1	3950	77	99	91 x	20	41
Algeria	79	61	32	51	29	17	34895	723	23	4420	73	73	95	18 x	42 x
Andorra	169	9	4	7	3	1	86	1	0	41130	–	–	80	–	–
Angola	11	258	161	153	98	42	18498	784	116	3490	48	70	58 x, s	8	62
Antigua and Barbuda	130	–	12	–	11	6	88	1	0	12130	–	99	88	–	–
Argentina	125	28	14	25	13	8	40276	691	10	7600	76	98	99	12	53
Armenia	97	56	22	48	20	13	3083	48	1	3100	74	100	99 s	22	39
Australia	165	9	5	8	4	3	21293	270	1	43770	82	–	97	18 x	41 x
Austria	169	9	4	8	3	2	8364	76	0	46850	80	–	97 x	22	38
Azerbaijan	76	98	34	78	30	15	8832	169	6	4840	71	100	73 s	30	30
Bahamas	130	25	12	17	9	6	342	6	0	21390 x	74	–	91	–	–
Bahrain	130	16	12	14	10	6	791	14	0	25420 x	76	91	98	–	–
Bangladesh	57	148	52	102	41	30	162221	3401	171	590	67	55	85	22	41
Barbados	140	18	11	15	10	7	256	3	0	d	78	–	–	–	–
Belarus	130	24	12	20	11	5	9634	96	1	5540	69	100	94	22	38
Belgium	165	10	5	9	4	2	10647	120	1	45310	80	–	98	21	41
Belize	109	43	18	35	16	8	307	7	0	3740 x	77	–	98	–	–
Benin	22	184	118	111	75	32	8935	349	39	750	62	41	67 s	18	46
Bhutan	41	148	79	91	52	33	697	15	1	2020	66	53	87	14	53
Bolivia (Plurinational State of)	58	122	51	84	40	22	9863	262	13	1630	66	91	94	9	61
Bosnia and Herzegovina	125	23	14	21	13	10	3767	34	1	4700	75	98	98 s	18	43
Botswana	54	60	57	46	43	22	1950	48	3	6260	55	83	87	9 x	65 x
Brazil	98	56	21	46	17	12	193734	3026	61	8070	73	90	94	10	59
Brunei Darussalam	151	11	7	9	5	3	400	8	0	d	77	95	93	–	–
Bulgaria	144	18	10	14	8	5	7545	73	1	5770	74	98	96	22	38
Burkina Faso	9	201	166	110	91	36	15757	738	121	510	53	29	46 s	18	47
Burundi	9	189	166	114	101	42	8303	283	46	150	51	66	71 s	21	43
Cambodia	36	117	88	85	68	30	14805	367	32	650	62	78	89	16	52
Cameroon	13	148	154	91	95	36	19522	711	108	1170	51	76	88	15	51
Canada	157	8	6	7	5	4	33573	358	2	42170	81	–	99 x	20	40
Cape Verde	88	63	28	49	23	12	506	12	0	3010	72	84	84	13	56
Central African Republic	8	175	171	115	112	45	4422	154	26	450	47	55	59 s	15	49
Chad	1	201	209	120	124	45	11206	508	100	620	49	33	36 x, s	17	47
Chile	147	22	9	18	7	5	16970	252	2	9460	79	99	94	12	57
China	105	46	19	37	17	11	1345751	18294	347	3620	73	94	100	16	48
Colombia	105	35	19	28	16	12	45660	917	17	4950	73	93	90	8	62
Comoros	29	128	104	90	75	37	676	22	2	870	66	74	31 x, s	8	68
Congo	19	104	128	67	81	36	3683	126	16	1830	54	–	86 s	13	53
Cook Islands	118	18	15	16	13	8	20	0	0	–	–	–	85 x	–	–
Costa Rica	140	18	11	16	10	6	4579	76	1	6260	79	96	92	13	55
Côte d'Ivoire	21	152	119	105	83	40	21075	729	83	1060	58	55	62 s	14	54
Croatia	165	13	5	11	5	3	4416	42	0	13810	76	99	90	22	38
Cuba	157	14	6	10	4	3	11204	116	1	c	79	100	99	–	–
Cyprus	169	10	4	9	3	2	871	10	0	26940 x	80	98	99	–	–
Czech Republic	169	12	4	10	3	2	10369	111	0	17310	77	–	90	25 x	36 x
Democratic People's Republic of Korea	77	45	33	23	26	18	23906	327	11	a	68	100	–	–	–
Democratic Republic of the Congo	2	199	199	126	126	52	66020	2930	558	160	48	67	61 s	15	51
Denmark	169	9	4	8	3	2	5470	62	0	58930	79	–	96	23 x	36 x
Djibouti	33	123	94	95	75	35	864	24	2	1280	56	–	66 s	17	47
Dominica	144	18	10	15	8	6	67	1	0	4900	–	–	72	–	–
Dominican Republic	79	62	32	48	27	17	10090	224	7	4530	73	88	89 s	13	54
Ecuador	93	53	24	41	20	11	13625	279	7	3940	75	84	97	11	59
Egypt	98	90	21	66	18	11	82999	2029	42	2070	70	66	94	22	41
El Salvador	112	62	17	48	15	7	6163	125	2	3370	72	84	94	13	52
Equatorial Guinea	14	198	145	120	88	39	676	26	4	12420	51	93	66 x	–	–
Eritrea	56	150	55	92	39	17	5073	185	10	300 x	60	65	39	–	–
Estonia	157	17	6	13	4	3	1340	16	0	14060	73	100	94	18	43
Ethiopia	29	210	104	124	67	36	82825	3132	315	330	56	36	45 s	23	39
Fiji	109	22	18	19	15	9	849	18	0	3950	69	–	89	–	–
Finland	184	7	3	6	3	2	5326	59	0	45680	80	–	96	24	37

	Under-5 mortality rank	Under-5 mortality rate		Infant mortality rate (under 1)		Neonatal mortality rate 2009	Total population (thousands) 2009	Annual no. of births (thousands) 2009	Annual no. of under-5 deaths (thousands) 2009	GNI per capita (US$) 2009	Life expectancy at birth (years) 2009	Total adult literacy rate (%) 2005–2008*	Primary school net enrolment/attendance (%) 2005 2009*	% share of household income 2000–2009*	
		1990	2009	1990	2009									lowest 40%	highest 20%
France	169	9	4	7	3	2	62343	745	3	43990	81	–	98	20 x	40 x
Gabon	45	93	69	68	52	25	1475	40	3	7370	61	87	94 x, s	16	48
Gambia	31	153	103	104	78	32	1705	62	6	440	56	45	61 s	13	53
Georgia	85	47	29	41	26	20	4260	52	2	2530	72	100	99	16	47
Germany	169	9	4	7	4	2	82167	659	3	42560	80	–	98	22	37
Ghana	45	120	69	76	47	27	23837	766	50	700	57	66	77	15	48
Greece	184	11	3	9	3	2	11161	106	0	28630	80	97	99	19	41
Grenada	118	40	15	33	13	8	104	2	0	5580	76	–	93	–	–
Guatemala	65	76	40	57	33	12	14027	456	18	2630	71	74	95	11	58
Guinea	15	231	142	137	88	41	10069	397	54	370	58	38	51 s	15	50
Guinea-Bissau	4	240	193	142	115	46	1611	66	12	510	48	51	52 x	19	43
Guyana	72	61	35	47	29	22	762	13	0	1450 x	67	–	95	–	–
Haiti	37	152	87	105	64	27	10033	274	24	a	61	–	50 s	8	63
Holy See	–	–	–	–	–	–	1	–	–	–	–	–	–	–	–
Honduras	83	55	30	43	25	14	7466	202	6	1820	72	84	79 s	9	58
Hungary	157	17	6	15	5	4	9993	99	1	12980	74	99	90	22	39
Iceland	184	7	3	6	2	1	323	5	0	43220	82	–	98	–	–
India	48	118	66	84	50	34	1198003	26787	1726	1170	64	63	83 s	19	45
Indonesia	66	86	39	56	30	19	229965	4174	163	2230	71	92	85 s	18	46
Iran (Islamic Republic of)	81	73	31	55	26	17	74196	1390	43	4530	72	82	100 x	17	45
Iraq	63	53	44	42	35	23	30747	949	41	2210	68	78	87	–	–
Ireland	169	9	4	8	4	2	4515	70	0	44310	80	–	97	20	42
Israel	169	11	4	10	3	2	7170	140	1	25740	81	–	97	16	45
Italy	169	10	4	8	3	2	59870	543	2	35080	81	99	99	18	42
Jamaica	81	33	31	28	26	12	2719	52	2	5020	72	86	97 s	14	51
Japan	184	6	3	5	2	1	127156	1014	3	37870	83	–	100	25 x	36 x
Jordan	91	39	25	32	22	15	6316	158	4	3740	73	92	99 s	18	45
Kazakhstan	85	60	29	51	26	15	15637	308	9	6740	65	100	98 s	21	40
Kenya	39	99	84	64	55	27	39802	1530	124	770	55	87	74 s	13	53
Kiribati	61	89	46	65	37	19	98	2	0	1890	–	–	97 x	–	–
Kuwait	144	17	10	14	8	5	2985	52	1	43930 x	78	94	88	–	–
Kyrgyzstan	69	75	37	63	32	17	5482	122	5	870	68	99	92 s	21	43
Lao People's Democratic Republic	52	157	59	108	46	22	6320	172	10	880	65	73	82	21	41
Latvia	149	16	8	12	7	5	2249	23	0	12390	73	100	97 x	18	43
Lebanon	130	40	12	33	11	7	4224	66	1	7970	72	90	90	–	–
Lesotho	39	93	84	74	61	34	2067	59	5	1020	46	90	85 s	10	56
Liberia	24	247	112	165	80	37	3955	149	16	160	59	88	40 s	18	45
Libyan Arab Jamahiriya	105	36	19	32	17	11	6420	148	3	12020	74	58	–	–	–
Liechtenstein	193	10	2	9	2	–	36	0	0	113210 x	–	–	90	–	–
Lithuania	157	15	6	12	5	3	3287	32	0	11410	72	100	92	18	43
Luxembourg	184	9	3	8	2	1	486	6	0	74430	80	–	96	–	–
Madagascar	53	167	58	102	41	21	19625	695	38	420 x	61	71	76 x, s	16	53
Malawi	26	218	110	129	69	30	15263	608	64	280	54	73	91	18	46
Malaysia	157	18	6	16	6	3	27468	550	3	7230	75	92	96	17	44
Maldives	128	113	13	80	11	8	309	6	0	3870	72	98	96	17	44
Mali	6	250	191	139	101	50	13010	551	101	680	49	26	44 s	17	46
Malta	151	11	7	10	6	2	409	4	0	16690 x	80	92	91	–	–
Marshall Islands	72	49	35	39	29	15	62	1	0	3060	–	–	66	–	–
Mauritania	23	129	117	81	74	41	3291	109	12	960	57	57	57 s	17	46
Mauritius	112	24	17	21	15	10	1288	18	0	7240	72	88	94	–	–
Mexico	112	45	17	36	15	7	109610	2021	34	8960	76	93	98	12	56
Micronesia (Federated States of)	66	58	39	45	32	16	111	3	0	2220	69	–	92 x	7	64
Monaco	169	8	4	7	3	2	33	0	0	203900 x	–	–	–	–	–
Mongolia	85	101	29	73	24	11	2671	50	1	1630	67	97	97 s	18	44
Montenegro	147	17	9	15	8	6	624	8	0	6550	74	–	97 s	18	44
Morocco	68	89	38	69	33	20	31993	651	25	2790	72	56	89	17	48
Mozambique	15	232	142	155	96	41	22894	877	121	440	48	54	80	15	53
Myanmar	44	118	71	84	54	33	50020	1016	70	a	62	92	84 x, s	–	–
Namibia	59	73	48	49	34	19	2171	59	3	4310	62	88	89	4 x	78 x
Nauru	63	–	44	–	36	25	10	0	0	–	–	–	72	–	–
Nepal	59	142	48	99	39	27	29331	730	34	440	67	58	84 s	15	54

TABLE 1. BASIC INDICATORS

	Under-5 mortality rank	Under-5 mortality rate 1990	Under-5 mortality rate 2009	Infant mortality rate (under 1) 1990	Infant mortality rate (under 1) 2009	Neonatal mortality rate 2009	Total population (thousands) 2009	Annual no. of births (thousands) 2009	Annual no. of under-5 deaths (thousands) 2009	GNI per capita (US$) 2009	Life expectancy at birth (years) 2009	Total adult literacy rate (%) 2005–2008*	Primary school net enrolment/ attendance (%) 2005–2009*	% share of household income 2000–2009* lowest 40%	% share of household income 2000–2009* highest 20%
Netherlands	169	8	4	7	4	3	16592	183	1	49350	80	–	99	21 x	39 x
New Zealand	157	11	6	9	5	3	4266	59	0	26830 x	80	–	99	18 x	44 x
Nicaragua	89	68	26	52	22	12	5743	140	4	1010	73	78	92	12	57
Niger	12	305	160	144	76	35	15290	815	122	340	52	29	38 s	16	50
Nigeria	18	212	138	126	86	39	154729	6081	794	1140	48	60	61	15	49
Niue	–	–	–	–	8	1	0	–	–	–	–	–	99 x	–	–
Norway	184	9	3	7	3	2	4812	58	0	86440	81	–	99	24	37
Occupied Palestinian Territory	83	43	30	35	25	–	4277	150	4	b	74	94	75	–	–
Oman	130	48	12	37	9	6	2845	62	1	17890 x	76	87	68	–	–
Pakistan	37	130	87	101	71	42	180808	5403	460	1020	67	54	71 s	22	41
Palau	118	21	15	18	13	7	20	0	0	8940	–	–	96 x	–	–
Panama	95	31	23	25	16	10	3454	70	2	6740	76	94	98	9	58
Papua New Guinea	47	91	68	67	52	26	6732	208	14	1180	61	60	–	12 x	56 x
Paraguay	95	42	23	34	19	12	6349	154	3	2280	72	95	90	11	57
Peru	98	78	21	62	19	11	29165	605	13	4160	73	90	94	11	55
Philippines	77	59	33	41	26	15	91983	2245	75	1790	72	94	92	15	50
Poland	151	17	7	15	6	4	38074	375	3	12260	76	100	96	19	42
Portugal	169	15	4	12	3	2	10707	103	0	20940	79	95	99	17 x	46 x
Qatar	140	19	11	17	10	5	1409	16	0	d	76	93	94 x	–	52
Republic of Korea	165	9	5	8	5	2	48333	450	2	19830	80	–	99	21 x	37 x
Republic of Moldova	112	37	17	30	15	8	3604	45	1	1590	69	98	88	18	45
Romania	130	32	12	25	10	6	21275	212	3	8330	73	98	90	21	40
Russian Federation	130	27	12	23	11	6	140874	1559	19	9370	67	100	–	15	50
Rwanda	25	171	111	103	70	33	9998	413	42	460	51	70	86 s	14	53
Saint Kitts and Nevis	118	26	15	22	13	10	52	0	0	10150	–	–	93	–	–
Saint Lucia	103	20	20	16	19	11	172	3	0	5190	74	–	91	–	–
Saint Vincent and the Grenadines	130	24	12	19	11	8	109	2	0	5130	72	–	95	–	–
Samoa	91	50	25	40	21	12	179	4	0	2840	72	99	93	–	–
San Marino	193	15	2	14	1	1	31	0	0	50670 x	–	–	–	–	–
Sao Tome and Principe	42	95	78	62	52	27	163	5	0	1140	66	88	96	14	56
Saudi Arabia	98	43	21	35	18	12	25721	593	12	17700 x	73	86	85	–	–
Senegal	34	151	93	73	51	31	12534	476	43	1040	56	42	58 s	17	46
Serbia	151	29	7	25	6	4	9850	114	1	5990	74	98	95	23	37
Seychelles	130	15	12	13	11	7	84	3	0	8480	–	92	99 x	9	70
Sierra Leone	5	285	192	166	123	49	5696	227	43	340	48	40	69 s	16	49
Singapore	184	8	3	6	2	1	4737	37	0	37220	81	95	–	14 x	49 x
Slovakia	151	15	7	13	6	4	5406	56	0	16130	75	–	–	24 x	35 x
Slovenia	184	10	3	9	2	2	2020	20	0	23520	79	100	97	21	39
Solomon Islands	70	38	36	31	30	15	523	16	1	910	67	77 x	67	–	–
Somalia	7	180	180	109	109	52	9133	402	69	a	50	–	23 s	–	–
South Africa	50	62	62	48	43	19	50110	1085	66	5770	52	89	87	9	63
Spain	169	9	4	8	4	2	44904	499	2	31870	81	98	100	19	42
Sri Lanka	118	28	15	23	13	9	20238	364	5	1990	74	91	99	17	48
Sudan	27	124	108	78	69	36	42272	1300	139	1230	58	69	54 s	–	–
Suriname	89	51	26	44	24	11	520	10	0	4760 x	69	91	90	–	–
Swaziland	43	92	73	67	52	20	1185	35	3	2350	46	87	83	12	56
Sweden	184	7	3	6	2	2	9249	108	0	48930	81	–	95	23	37
Switzerland	169	8	4	7	4	3	7568	73	0	56370 x	82	–	94	20	41
Syrian Arab Republic	116	36	16	30	14	8	21906	596	10	2410	74	84	95 x	–	–
Tajikistan	51	117	61	91	52	24	6952	195	12	700	67	100	97	20	42
Thailand	125	32	14	27	12	8	67764	977	13	3760	69	94	98 s	16	49
The former Yugoslav Republic of Macedonia	140	36	11	32	10	6	2042	22	0	4400	74	97	95 s	15	49
Timor-Leste	55	184	56	138	48	27	1134	46	3	2460 x	62	–	76	21	41
Togo	32	150	98	89	64	32	6619	215	20	440	63	65	79 s	16	47
Tonga	105	23	19	19	17	9	104	3	0	3260	72	99	99	–	–
Trinidad and Tobago	72	34	35	30	31	23	1339	20	1	16560	70	99	98 s	16 x	46 x
Tunisia	98	50	21	40	18	12	10272	165	3	3720	74	78	98	16	47
Turkey	103	84	20	69	19	12	74816	1346	28	8730	72	89	95	16	47
Turkmenistan	62	99	45	81	42	19	5110	111	5	3420	65	100	99 s	16 x	47 x
Tuvalu	72	53	35	42	29	15	10	0	0	–	–	–	100 x	–	–
Uganda	19	184	128	111	79	30	32710	1502	184	460	53	75	82 s	16	49

	Under-5 mortality rank	Under-5 mortality rate		Infant mortality rate (under 1)		Neonatal mortality rate 2009	Total population (thousands) 2009	Annual no. of births (thousands) 2009	Annual no. of under-5 deaths (thousands) 2009	GNI per capita (US$) 2009	Life expectancy at birth (years) 2009	Total adult literacy rate (%) 2005 2008*	Primary school net enrolment/ attendance (%) 2005–2009*	% share of household income 2000–2009*	
		1990	2009	1990	2009									lowest 40%	highest 20%
Ukraine	118	21	15	18	13	7	45708	468	7	2800	68	100	97 s	23	37
United Arab Emirates	151	17	7	15	7	4	4599	63	0	d	78	90	92	–	–
United Kingdom	157	10	6	8	5	3	61565	749	4	41520	80	–	100	18 x	44 x
United Republic of Tanzania	27	162	108	99	68	33	43739	1812	188	500	56	73	73 s	19	42
United States	149	11	8	9	7	4	314659	4413	35	47240	79	–	92	16	46
Uruguay	128	24	13	21	11	7	3361	50	1	9400	76	98	98	13	52
Uzbekistan	70	74	36	61	32	17	27488	558	20	1100	68	99	100 s	19	44
Vanuatu	116	40	16	33	14	8	240	7	0	2620	70	81	81 s	–	–
Venezuela (Bolivarian Republic of)	109	32	18	27	15	10	28583	600	10	10200	74	95	90	14	49
Viet Nam	93	55	24	39	20	12	88069	1485	35	1010	75	93	94 x	18	45
Yemen	48	125	66	88	51	29	23580	861	56	1060	63	61	73	18	45
Zambia	17	179	141	108	86	35	12935	549	74	970	46	71	80 s	11	55
Zimbabwe	35	81	90	54	56	29	12523	379	33	a	46	91	90	13 x	56

SUMMARY INDICATORS

		Under-5 mortality rate		Infant mortality rate		Neonatal	Total population	Annual births	Under-5 deaths	GNI per capita	Life expectancy	Adult literacy	Primary enrolment	lowest 40%	highest 20%
Africa#		165	118	102	75	34	1008354	35762	4072	1500	56	63	69	14	52
Sub-Saharan Africa#		180	129	109	81	37	841775	32044	3976	1147	53	63	65	13	55
Eastern and Southern Africa		166	108	103	69	32	392853	14480	1504	1496	53	68	71	11	59
West and Central Africa		199	150	118	92	40	405786	16241	2331	841	51	57	62	15	49
Middle East and North Africa		77	41	57	32	19	413313	10012	410	3029	70	74	83	18	45
Asia#		87	50	63	39	25	3632042	68469	3417	2550	69	80	88	17	47
South Asia		125	71	89	55	35	1619757	38008	2635	1092	64	62	82	20	45
East Asia and Pacific		53	26	40	21	14	2012285	30460	782	3748	73	93	96	16	48
Latin America and Caribbean		52	23	41	19	11	576790	10661	239	7195	74	92	93	11	57
CEE/CIS		51	21	42	19	11	404153	5629	120	6854	69	97	95	17	46
Industrialized countries§		10	6	8	5	3	988390	11221	66	40463	80	–	96	18	43
Developing countries§		99	66	68	47	26	5580485	122921	7988	2988	67	79	83	15	50
Least developed countries§		178	121	112	78	37	835486	28641	3330	638	57	60	67	17	48
World		89	60	62	42	24	6813327	136712	8087	8686	69	81	85	17	45

\# For a complete list of countries and territories in the regions and subregions, see page 124.

§ Includes territories within each country category or regional group. Countries and territories in each country category or regional group are listed on page 124.

DEFINITIONS OF THE INDICATORS

Under-five mortality rate – Probability of dying between birth and exactly 5 years of age, expressed per 1,000 live births.

Infant mortality rate – Probability of dying between birth and exactly 1 year of age, expressed per 1,000 live births.

Neonatal mortality rate – Probability of dying during the first 28 completed days of life, expressed per 1,000 live births.

GNI per capita – Gross national income (GNI) is the sum of value added by all resident producers, plus any product taxes (less subsidies) not included in the valuation of output, plus net receipts of primary income (compensation of employees and property income) from abroad. GNI per capita is gross national income divided by midyear population. GNI per capita in US dollars is converted using the World Bank Atlas method.

Life expectancy at birth – Number of years newborn children would live if subject to the mortality risks prevailing for the cross section of population at the time of their birth.

Adult literacy rate – Number of literate persons aged 15 and above, expressed as a percentage of the total population in that age group.

Primary school net enrolment/attendance ratios – Number of children enrolled in or attending primary school, expressed as a percentage of the total number of children of primary school age. The indicator is either the primary school net enrolment ratio or the primary school net attendance ratio. In general, if both indicators are available, the primary school net enrolment ratio is preferred unless the data for primary school attendance is considered to be of superior quality. Definitions for both the primary school net enrolment ratio and the primary school net attendance ratio are given on page 27.

Income share – Percentage of income received by the 20 per cent of households with the highest income and by the 40 per cent of households with the lowest income.

MAIN DATA SOURCES

Under-five and infant mortality rates – Inter-agency Group for Child Mortality Estimation (UNICEF, World Health Organization, United Nations Population Division and the World Bank).

Neonatal mortality rate – World Health Organization, using civil registrations, surveillance systems and household surveys.

Total population – United Nations Population Division.

Births – United Nations Population Division.

Under-five deaths – UNICEF.

GNI per capita – World Bank.

Life expectancy – United Nations Population Division.

Adult literacy – UNESCO Institute for Statistics (UIS).

School enrolment/attendance – UIS, Multiple Indicator Cluster Surveys (MICS) and Demographic and Health Surveys (DHS).

Household income – World Bank.

NOTES

a: low income ($995 or less).
b: lower-middle income ($996 to $3,945).
c: upper-middle income ($3,946 to $12,195).
d: high income ($12,196 or more).

– Data not available.

x Data refer to years or periods other than those specified in the column heading, differ from the standard definition or refer to only part of a country. Such data are not included in the calculation of regional and global averages.

s National household survey data.

* Data refer to the most recent year available during the period specified in the column heading.

TABLE 2. NUTRITION

Countries and territories	% of infants with low birthweight 2005–2009*	Early initiation of breastfeeding (%) 2005–2009*	% of children (2005–2009*) who are: exclusively breastfed (<6 months)	breastfed with complementary food (6–9 months)	still breastfeeding (20–23 months)	underweight (NCHS/WHO) moderate & severe	underweight (WHO) moderate & severe	underweight (WHO) severe	wasting (WHO) moderate & severe	stunting (WHO) moderate & severe	Vitamin A supplementation coverage rate (6–59 months) 2009 Full coverage△ (%)	% of households consuming iodized salt 2003–2009*
Afghanistan	–	–	–	29 x	54 x	39 y	33 y	12 y	9 y	59 y	95	28 y
Albania	7	43	39	54	31	6	5	2	9	19	–	76
Algeria	6	50	7	39	22	4	3	1	4	15	–	61
Andorra	–	–	–	–	–	–	–	–	–	–	–	–
Angola	12 x	55	11 x	77 x	37 x	–	16 y	7 y	8 y	29 y	28	45
Antigua and Barbuda	5	–	–	–	–	–	–	–	–	–	–	–
Argentina	7	–	–	–	28	4 y	2 y	0 y	1 y	8 y	–	90 x
Armenia	7	28	33	57	15	4	4	1	5	18	–	97
Australia	7 x	–	–	–	–	–	–	–	–	–	–	–
Austria	7 x	–	–	–	–	–	–	–	–	–	–	–
Azerbaijan	10	32	12	44	16	10	8	2	7	25	79 w	54
Bahamas	11	–	–	–	–	–	–	–	–	–	–	–
Bahrain	8 x	–	34 x	65 x	41 x	9 x	–	–	–	–	–	–
Bangladesh	22	43	43	74	91	46	41	12	17	43	91	84 y
Barbados	14	–	–	–	–	–	–	–	–	–	–	–
Belarus	4	21	9	38	4	1	1	1	2	4	–	55 y
Belgium	8 x	–	–	–	–	–	–	–	–	–	–	–
Belize	14	51	10	–	27	6	4	1	2	22	–	90 x
Benin	15	32	–	76	92 y	23	18	5	8	43	56	67
Bhutan	9	–	–	–	–	19 x	14 x	3 x	3 x	48 x	–	96 x
Bolivia (Plurinational State of)	6	61	60	81	40	6	4	1	1	27	45	89 y
Bosnia and Herzegovina	5	57	18	29	10	2	1	0	4	10	–	62 y
Botswana	13	20	20	46	6	14	–	–	–	–	89	66 x
Brazil	8	43	40	70	25 y	–	2	–	2	7	–	96 y
Brunei Darussalam	10 x	–	–	–	–	–	–	–	–	–	–	–
Bulgaria	9	–	–	–	–	–	–	–	–	–	–	100
Burkina Faso	16	20	16	–	–	31	26	7	11	35	100	34
Burundi	11	–	45	88	–	35	–	–	–	–	90	98 y
Cambodia	9	35	66	89	47	–	29	9	9	40	98	73 y
Cameroon	11	20	21	64	21	19	16	5	7	36	–	49 y
Canada	6 x	–	–	–	–	–	–	–	–	–	–	–
Cape Verde	6	73	60	80	13	9 y	–	–	–	–	–	0 x
Central African Republic	13	39	23	55	47	29	24	8	12	43	87	62
Chad	22 x	34 x	2 x	77 x	65 x	37	–	–	–	–	71	56
Chile	6	–	–	–	–	1 y	–	–	–	–	–	100 x
China	3	41	28	43	–	7	6	–	–	15	–	96 x
Colombia	6	49	47	65	32	7 y	5 y	2 y	2 y	15 y	–	92 x
Comoros	25 x	25 x	21 x	34 x	45 x	25	–	–	–	–	40	82 x
Congo	13	39	19	78	21	14	11	3	8	30	8	82
Cook Islands	3 x	–	19 x	–	–	10 x	–	–	–	–	–	–
Costa Rica	7	–	15	–	49	5 x	–	–	–	–	–	92 x
Côte d'Ivoire	17	25	4	54	37	20	16	5	8	40	88	84 x
Croatia	5	–	23 x	–	–	1 x	–	–	–	–	–	90 x
Cuba	5	70	26	47	16	4	–	–	–	–	–	88
Cyprus	–	–	–	–	–	–	–	–	–	–	–	–
Czech Republic	7 x	–	–	–	–	–	–	–	–	–	–	–
Democratic People's Republic of Korea	7 x	–	65 x	31 x	37 x	23 y	18 y	7 y	9 y	45 y	99	40 y
Democratic Republic of the Congo	10	48	36	82	64	31	25	8	10	46	89	79
Denmark	5 x	–	–	–	–	–	–	–	–	–	–	–
Djibouti	10	55	1	23	18	33 y	31 y	9 y	17 y	33 y	94	0
Dominica	10	–	–	–	–	–	–	–	–	–	–	–
Dominican Republic	11	74	9	62	21	4	7	2	3	18	–	19
Ecuador	10	–	40 x	77 x	23 x	9	6	–	–	–	–	99 x
Egypt	13	56	53	66	35 y	8	6	1	7	29	–	79
El Salvador	7 x	33	31	72	54	9 y	6 y	1 y	1 y	19 y	–	62 x
Equatorial Guinea	13 x	–	24 x	–	–	19 x	16 x	5 x	9 x	43 x	–	33 x
Eritrea	14 x	78	52 x	43 x	62 x	40 x	35 x	13 x	15 x	44 x	44	68 x
Estonia	4 x	–	–	–	–	–	–	–	–	–	–	–
Ethiopia	20	69	49	54	88 y	38	33	11	12	51	84	20
Fiji	10 x	57 x	40 x	–	–	–	–	–	–	–	–	31 x
Finland	4 x	–	–	–	–	–	–	–	–	–	–	–

| | % of infants with low birthweight 2005–2009* | Early initiation of breastfeeding (%) 2005–2009* | % of children (2005–2009*) who are: | | | % of under-fives (2003–2009*) suffering from: | | | | | Vitamin A supplementation coverage rate (6–59 months) 2009 | % of households consuming iodized salt 2003–2009* |
			exclusively breastfed (<6 months)	breastfed with complementary food (6–9 months)	still breastfeeding (20–23 months)	underweight (NCHS/WHO) moderate & severe	underweight (WHO) moderate & severe	underweight (WHO) severe	wasting (WHO) moderate & severe	stunting (WHO) moderate & severe	Full coverage△ (%)	
France	7 x	–	–	–	–	–	–	–	–	–	–	–
Gabon	14 x	71 x	6 x	62 x	9 x	12 x	8 x	2 x	4 x	25 x	0	36 x
Gambia	20	48	41	44	53	20	16	4	7	28	–	7
Georgia	5	65	–	43	17	–	1	1	2	11	–	100
Germany	7 x	–	–	–	–	–	–	–	–	–	–	–
Ghana	13	52	63	75	44	17	14	3	9	28	90	32
Greece	8 x	–	–	–	–	–	–	–	–	–	–	–
Grenada	9	–	39 x	–	–	–	–	–	–	–	–	–
Guatemala	12 x	60 x	50	71	46	19	–	–	–	–	43	76
Guinea	12	35	48	32	–	26	21	7	8	40	–	41
Guinea-Bissau	24	23	16	35	61	19	15	4	8	47	80	1
Guyana	19	43	33	59	49	–	11	2	5	18	–	–
Haiti	25	44	41	87	35	22	18	6	10	29	–	3
Holy See	–	–	–	–	–	–	–	–	–	–	–	–
Honduras	10	79	30	69	48	11	8	1	1	29	–	80 x
Hungary	9 x	–	–	–	–	–	–	–	–	–	–	–
Iceland	4 x	–	–	–	–	–	–	–	–	–	–	–
India	28	41	46	57	77	48	43	16	20	48	66	51
Indonesia	9	44	32	75	50	–	18	5	14	37	84	62 y
Iran (Islamic Republic of)	7	56	23	68	58	5	–	–	–	–	–	99 y
Iraq	15	31	25	51	36	8	6	2	6	26	–	28
Ireland	6 x	–	–	–	–	–	–	–	–	–	–	–
Israel	8 x	–	–	–	–	–	–	–	–	–	–	–
Italy	6 x	–	–	–	–	–	–	–	–	–	–	–
Jamaica	12	62	15	36	24	–	2	–	2	4	–	100 x
Japan	8 x	–	–	–	–	–	–	–	–	–	–	–
Jordan	13	39	22	66	11	–	2	0	2	8	–	88 x
Kazakhstan	6	64	17	39	16	4	4	1	5	17	–	92
Kenya	8	58	32	83	54	20	16	4	7	35	51	98
Kiribati	5 x	–	80 x	–	–	13 x	–	–	–	–	–	–
Kuwait	7 x	–	12 x	26 x	9 x	10 x	–	–	–	–	–	–
Kyrgyzstan	5	65	32	49	26	3	2	0	3	18	99	76
Lao People's Democratic Republic	11	30	26	70	48	37	31	9	7	48	88	84 y
Latvia	5 x	–	–	–	–	–	–	–	–	–	–	–
Lebanon	6 x	–	27 x	35 x	11 x	4	–	–	–	–	–	92
Lesotho	13 x	63 x	54	58	35	–	13	2	4	39	–	91
Liberia	14	67	29	62	47	24	19	6	8	39	92	–
Libyan Arab Jamahiriya	7 x	–	–	–	23 x	5 x	4 x	–	4 x	21 x	–	90 x
Liechtenstein	–	–	–	–	–	–	–	–	–	–	–	–
Lithuania	4 x	–	–	–	–	–	–	–	–	–	–	–
Luxembourg	8 x	–	–	–	–	–	–	–	–	–	–	–
Madagascar	16	72	51	89	61	–	–	–	–	50	95	53
Malawi	13	58	57	89	72	21	15	3	4	53	95	50
Malaysia	11	–	29 x	–	12 x	8	–	–	–	–	–	–
Maldives	22 x	–	10 x	85 x	–	30 x	26 x	7 x	13 x	32 x	52	44 x
Mali	19	46	38	30	56	32	27	10	15	38	100	79
Malta	6 x	–	–	–	–	–	–	–	–	–	–	–
Marshall Islands	18	73	31	77	53	–	–	–	–	–	–	–
Mauritania	34	64	35	62	47	20 y	14 y	2 y	6 y	23 y	89	23
Mauritius	14 x	–	21 x	–	–	15 x	–	–	–	–	–	0 x
Mexico	8	–	20 x	–	25 x	5	3	–	2	16	–	91
Micronesia (Federated States of)	18 x	–	60 x	–	–	15 x	–	–	–	–	–	–
Monaco	–	–	–	–	–	–	–	–	–	–	–	–
Mongolia	5	81	57	57	65	6	5	1	3	27	–	83 y
Montenegro	4	25	19	35	13	3	2	1	4	7	–	71 x
Morocco	15 x	52 x	31 x	66 x	15 x	10	9	2	10	23	–	21
Mozambique	15	63	37	84	54	18	18	5	4	44	97	25
Myanmar	15 x	–	15 x	66 x	67 x	32	30	9	11	41	95	93
Namibia	16	71	24	72	28	21	17	4	8	29	–	63 x
Nauru	27	76	67	65	65 y	–	5	1	1	24	–	–
Nepal	21	35	53	75	95	45	39	11	13	49	95	63 x
Netherlands	–	–	–	–	–	–	–	–	–	–	–	–
New Zealand	6 x	–	–	–	–	–	–	–	–	–	–	83 x

TABLE 2. NUTRITION

Countries and territories	% of infants with low birthweight 2005–2009*	Early initiation of breastfeeding (%) 2005–2009*	% of children (2005–2009*) who are: exclusively breastfed (<6 months)	breastfed with complementary food (6–9 months)	still breastfeeding (20–23 months)	% of under-fives (2003–2009*) suffering from: underweight (NCHS/WHO) moderate & severe	underweight (WHO) moderate & severe	severe	wasting (WHO) moderate & severe	stunting (WHO) moderate & severe	Vitamin A supplementation coverage rate (6–59 months) 2009 Full coverage△ (%)	% of households consuming iodized salt 2003–2009*
Nicaragua	8	54	31	76	43	7	6	1	1	22	6	97
Niger	27	40	10	52	–	41 y	34 y	11 y	12 y	46 y	95	46
Nigeria	12	38	13	75	32	29	24	9	11	43	78	97
Niue	0 x	–	–	–	–	–	–	–	–	–	–	–
Norway	5 x	–	–	–	–	–	–	–	–	–	–	–
Occupied Palestinian Territory	7	–	27	–	–	3	–	–	–	–	–	86
Oman	9	85	–	91 x	73 x	18 x	11 x	2 x	7 x	13 x	–	69 x
Pakistan	32	29	37	36	55	38 x	31 x	13 x	14 x	42 x	91	17 x
Palau	9 x	–	59 x	–	–	–	–	–	–	–	–	–
Panama	10 x	–	25 x	38 x	21 x	–	4 y	–	1 y	19 y	–	95 x
Papua New Guinea	10	–	56	76	72	26 y	18 y	5 y	5 y	43 y	12	92
Paraguay	9 x	21 x	22 x	60 x	–	4	3	–	1	18	–	94 y
Peru	8	53	70	81	51	6	4	1	1	24	–	91
Philippines	21	54	34	58	34	26	22	–	7	32	91	45
Poland	6 x	–	–	–	–	–	–	–	–	–	–	–
Portugal	8 x	–	–	–	–	–	–	–	–	–	–	–
Qatar	10 x	–	12 x	48 x	21 x	6 x	–	–	–	–	–	–
Republic of Korea	4 x	–	–	–	–	–	–	–	–	–	–	–
Republic of Moldova	6	65	46	18	2	4	3	1	5	10	–	60
Romania	8 x	–	16 x	41 x	–	3 x	4 x	1 x	4 x	13 x	–	74
Russian Federation	6	–	–	–	–	3 x	–	–	–	–	–	35 y
Rwanda	6	68	88	69	77	23	18	4	5	51	94	88
Saint Kitts and Nevis	11	–	56 x	–	–	–	–	–	–	–	–	100 x
Saint Lucia	11	–	–	–	–	–	–	–	–	–	–	–
Saint Vincent and the Grenadines	8	–	–	–	–	–	–	–	–	–	–	–
Samoa	4 x	–	–	–	–	–	–	–	–	–	–	–
San Marino	–	–	–	–	–	–	–	–	–	–	–	–
Sao Tome and Principe	8	35	51	77	20	–	13	3	11	29	37	37
Saudi Arabia	11 x	–	31 x	60 x	30 x	14 x	–	–	–	–	–	–
Senegal	19	23	34	61	42	17	14	4	9	19	97	41
Serbia	6	17	15	39	8	2	1	0	4	7	–	32
Seychelles	–	–	–	–	–	–	–	–	–	–	–	–
Sierra Leone	14	51	11	73	50	25	21	7	10	36	99	58
Singapore	8 x	–	–	–	–	3 x	3 x	0 x	4 x	4 x	–	–
Slovakia	7 x	–	–	–	–	–	–	–	–	–	–	–
Slovenia	–	–	–	–	–	–	–	–	–	–	–	–
Solomon Islands	13	75	74	81	67	–	12	2	4	33	–	–
Somalia	–	26	9	15	35	36	32	12	13	42	62	1
South Africa	15 x	61 x	8 x	49 x	31 x	12	–	–	–	–	–	62 x
Spain	6 x	–	–	–	–	–	–	–	–	–	–	–
Sri Lanka	17	80	76	87	84	27	21	4	15	17	–	92 y
Sudan	31 x	–	34	56	35	31	27	10	16	40	84	11
Suriname	13 x	34	2	34	15	10	7	1	5	11	–	–
Swaziland	9	44	33	–	23 y	10	7	1	1	40	27	80
Sweden	4 x	–	–	–	–	–	–	–	–	–	–	–
Switzerland	6 x	–	–	–	–	–	–	–	–	–	–	–
Syrian Arab Republic	9	32	29	37	16	10	9	2	10	28	–	79
Tajikistan	10	57 y	25	15	34	18	15	6	7	39	87	62
Thailand	9	50	5	43	19	9	7	1	5	16	–	47
The former Yugoslav Republic of Macedonia	6	–	37 x	8 x	10 x	2	2	0	3	11	–	94 x
Timor-Leste	12 x	–	52	80	33	–	49	15	25	54	45	60
Togo	12	53	48	70 y	–	21	21	3	6	27	100	25
Tonga	3 x	–	62 x	–	–	–	–	–	–	–	–	–
Trinidad and Tobago	19	41	13	43	22	6 x	–	–	–	–	–	28
Tunisia	5	87	6	61	15	3	–	–	–	–	–	97 x
Turkey	11	39	42	68	22	3	2	0	1	12	–	69
Turkmenistan	4	60	11	54	37	11	8	2	7	19	–	87
Tuvalu	5 x	–	35	40	51 y	–	2	0	3	10	–	–
Uganda	14	42	60	80	54	20	16	4	6	38	64	96
Ukraine	4	41	18	55	6	1 x	–	–	–	–	–	18
United Arab Emirates	15 x	–	34 x	52 x	29 x	14 x	–	–	–	–	–	–
United Kingdom	8 x	–	–	–	–	–	–	–	–	–	–	–

	% of infants with low birthweight 2005 2009*	Early initiation of breastfeeding (%) 2005 2009*	% of children (2005–2009*) who are: exclusively breastfed (<6 months)	breastfed with complementary food (6–9 months)	still breastfeeding (20–23 months)	% of under-fives (2003–2009*) suffering from: underweight (NCHS/WHO) moderate & severe	underweight (WHO) moderate & severe	underweight (WHO) severe	wasting (WHO) moderate & severe	stunting (WHO) moderate & severe	Vitamin A supplementation coverage rate (6–59 months) 2009 Full coverage△ (%)	% of households consuming iodized salt 2003–2009*
United Republic of Tanzania	10	67	41 x	91 x	55 x	22	17	4	4	44	94	43
United States	8 x	–	–	–	–	2 x	1 x	0 x	0 x	3 x	–	–
Uruguay	8	60	57	35	28	5 x	5 x	2 x	2 x	15 x	–	–
Uzbekistan	5	67	26	45	38	5	4	1	4	19	65	53
Vanuatu	10	72	40	62	32	16	–	–	–	–	–	23
Venezuela (Bolivarian Republic of)	8	–	7 x	50 x	31 x	5	–	–	–	–	–	90 x
Viet Nam	5	58	17	70	23	20	–	–	–	–	99 w	93
Yemen	32 x	30	12 x	76 x	–	46	43	19	15	58	–	30
Zambia	11	57	61	93	42	19	15	3	5	45	91	77 x
Zimbabwe	11	69	26	89	21	16 y	12 y	2 y	2 y	35 y	77	91 y

SUMMARY INDICATORS

Africa#	13	49	34	69	49	24	20	6	9	40	81	62
Sub-Saharan Africa#	14	49	33	70	51	27	22	7	9	42	81	61
Eastern and Southern Africa	14	61	47	72	64	25	21	6	7	44	77	53
West and Central Africa	13	39	23	70	43	28	23	8	10	40	84	74
Middle East and North Africa	10	47	32	57	35	14	14	5	10	31	–	60
Asia#	18	41	38	54	68	31	27	13	17	35	76 **	73
South Asia	27	39	45	56	75	47	42	15	19	48	73	55
East Asia and Pacific	6	44	28	52	–	11	11	–	–	22	88 **	87
Latin America and Caribbean	8	49	43	70	32	7	4	–	2	14	–	89
CEE/CIS	7	47	29	52	21	5	4	1	3	16	–	51
Industrialized countries§	–	–	–	–	–	–	–	–	–	–	–	–
Developing countries§	15	44	36	59	56	26	22	9	12	34	77 **	72
Least developed countries§	16	50	42	69	68	33	28	9	11	44	87	57
World	15	44	36	59	56	26	22	9	12	34	77 **	71

For a complete list of countries and territories in the regions and subregions, see page 124.
§ Includes territories within each country category or regional group. Countries and territories in each country category or regional group are listed on page 124.

DEFINITIONS OF THE INDICATORS

Low birthweight – Percentage of infants weighing less than 2,500 grams at birth.

Early initiation of breastfeeding – Percentage of infants who are put to the breast within one hour of birth.

Underweight (NCHS/WHO) – Moderate and severe: Percentage of children aged 0–59 months who are below minus two standard deviations from median weight for age of the NCHS/WHO reference population.

Underweight (WHO) – Moderate and severe: Percentage of children aged 0–59 months who are below minus two standard deviations from median weight for age of the World Health Organization (WHO) Child Growth Standards; Severe: Percentage of children aged 0–59 months who are below minus three standard deviations from median weight for age of the WHO Child Growth Standards.

Wasting (WHO) – Moderate and severe: Percentage of children aged 0–59 months who are below minus two standard deviations from median weight for height of the WHO Child Growth Standards.

Stunting (WHO) – Moderate and severe: Percentage of children aged 0–59 months who are below minus two standard deviations from median height for age of the WHO Child Growth Standards.

Vitamin A supplementation (full coverage) – The estimated percentage of children aged 6–59 months reached with 2 doses of vitamin A supplements.

Iodized salt consumption – Percentage of households consuming adequately iodized salt (15 parts per million or more).

MAIN DATA SOURCES

Low birthweight – Demographic and Health Surveys (DHS), Multiple Indicator Cluster Surveys (MICS), other national household surveys, data from routine reporting systems, UNICEF and WHO.

Breastfeeding – DHS, MICS, other national household surveys and UNICEF.

Underweight, wasting and stunting – DHS, MICS, other national household surveys, WHO and UNICEF.

Vitamin A – UNICEF.

Salt iodization – DHS, MICS, other national household surveys and UNICEF.

NOTES
- – Data not available.
- w Identifies countries with national vitamin A supplementation programmes targeted towards a reduced age range. Coverage figure is reported as targeted.
- x Data refer to years or periods other than those specified in the column heading, differ from the standard definition or refer to only part of a country. Such data are not included in the calculation of regional and global averages.
- y Data refer to years or periods other than those specified in the column heading, differ from the standard definition or refer to only part of a country. Such data are included in the calculation of regional and global averages.
- △ Full coverage with vitamin A supplements is reported as the lower percentage of 2 annual coverage points (i.e., lower point between round 1 (January–June) and round 2 (July–December) of 2008).
- * Data refer to the most recent year available during the period specified in the column heading.
- ** Excludes China.

TABLE 3. HEALTH

Countries and territories	% of population using improved drinking-water sources 2008			% of population using improved sanitation facilities 2008			% of routine EPI vaccines financed by government 2009	Immunization 2009 — 1-year-old children immunized against:							% newborns protected against tetanus	% under-fives with suspected pneumonia taken to an appropriate health-care provider	% under-fives with suspected pneumonia receiving antibiotics	% under-fives with diarrhoea receiving oral rehydration and continued feeding	Malaria 2006–2009*		
	total	urban	rural	total	urban	rural	total	TB	DPT	DPT	Polio	Measles	HepB	Hib					% households owning at least one ITN	% under-fives sleeping under ITNs	% under-fives with fever receiving anti-malarial drugs
								BCG	DPT1β	DPT3β	polio3	measles	HepB3	Hib3		2005–2009*		2005–2009*			
Afghanistan	48	78	39	37	60	30	2	82	94	83	83	76	83	83	89	–	–	–	–	–	–
Albania	97	96	98	98	98	98	100	97	99	98	98	97	98	98	87	70	38	63	–	–	–
Algeria	83	85	79	95	98	88	100	99	97	93	92	88	91	93	71	53	59	24	–	–	–
Andorra	100	100	100	100	100	100	100	–	98	99	99	98	96	97	–	–	–	–	–	–	–
Angola	50	60	38	57	86	18	100	83	93	73	73	77	73	73	88	–	–	–	28	18	29
Antigua and Barbuda	–	95	–	–	98	–	100	–	99	99	98	99	98	99	–	–	–	–	–	–	–
Argentina	97	98	80	90	91	77	–	99	95	94	95	99	90	90	–	–	–	–	–	–	–
Armenia	96	98	93	90	95	80	60	99	97	93	94	96	93	–	–	36	11	59	–	–	–
Australia	100	100	100	100	100	100	100	–	97	92	92	94	92	92	–	–	–	–	–	–	–
Austria	100	100	100	100	100	100	–	–	97	83	83	83	83	83	–	–	–	–	–	–	–
Azerbaijan	80	88	71	81	85	77	100	81	79	73	79	67	46	–	–	36 x	–	31	–	1 x	1 x
Bahamas	–	98	–	100	100	100	100	–	98	96	97	98	95	96	90	–	–	–	–	–	–
Bahrain	–	100	–	–	100	–	100	–	98	98	97	99	98	97	94	–	–	–	–	–	–
Bangladesh	80	85	78	53	56	52	30	99	99	94	94	89	95	–	93	37	22	68	–	–	–
Barbados	100	100	100	100	100	100	100	–	93	93	93	94	93	93	–	–	–	–	–	–	–
Belarus	100	100	99	93	91	97	75	98	99	98	98	99	98	19	–	90	67	54	–	–	–
Belgium	100	100	100	100	100	100	–	–	98	99	99	94	97	97	–	–	–	–	–	–	–
Belize	99	99	100	90	93	86	100	99	99	97	98	97	97	97	88	71	44	26	–	–	–
Benin	75	84	69	12	24	4	78	99	99	83	83	72	83	83	92	36	–	42	25	20	54
Bhutan	92	99	88	65	87	54	–	96	98	96	96	98	96	–	89	–	–	–	–	–	–
Bolivia (Plurinational State of)	86	96	67	25	34	9	100	88	87	85	84	86	85	85	74	51	–	54 x	–	–	–
Bosnia and Herzegovina	99	100	98	95	99	92	95	97	95	90	90	93	90	80	–	91	73	53	–	–	–
Botswana	95	99	90	60	74	39	1	99	98	96	96	94	93	–	92	14 x	–	7 x	–	–	–
Brazil	97	99	84	80	87	37	100	99	99	99	99	99	98	99	92	50	–	–	–	–	–
Brunei Darussalam	–	–	–	–	–	–	–	99	99	99	99	99	99	99	65	–	–	–	–	–	–
Bulgaria	100	100	100	100	100	100	100	98	98	95	94	96	96	–	–	–	–	–	–	–	–
Burkina Faso	76	95	72	11	33	6	30	92	89	82	84	75	81	81	85	39	15	42	23	10	48
Burundi	72	83	71	46	49	46	8	98	98	92	96	91	92	92	94	38	26	23	8 x	8 x	30 x
Cambodia	61	81	56	29	67	18	22	98	99	94	95	92	91	–	91	48	–	50	5 x	4 x	0 x
Cameroon	74	92	51	47	56	35	34	90	88	80	79	74	80	80	91	35	38	22	4	13	58
Canada	100	100	99	100	100	99	–	–	93	80	80	93	17	80	–	–	–	–	–	–	–
Cape Verde	84	85	82	54	65	38	84	99	98	99	99	96	99	–	78	51	–	–	–	–	–
Central African Republic	67	92	51	34	43	28	74	74	64	54	47	62	54	54	86	32	39	47	16	15	57
Chad	50	67	44	9	23	4	45	40	45	23	36	23	22	22	60	12 x	–	27 x	–	1 x	53 x
Chile	96	99	75	96	98	83	–	99	98	97	97	96	97	97	–	–	–	–	–	–	–
China	89	98	82	55	58	52	100	97	98	97	99	94	95	–	–	–	–	–	–	–	–
Colombia	92	99	73	74	81	55	92	90	97	92	92	95	92	92	78	62	–	39	3 x	–	–
Comoros	95	91	97	36	50	30	4	80	94	83	84	79	83	38	83	56 x	–	31 x	–	9 x	63 x
Congo	71	95	34	30	31	29	100	90	92	91	91	76	91	91	82	48	–	39	8 x	6 x	48 x
Cook Islands	–	98	–	100	100	100	100	99	97	82	82	78	82	82	–	–	–	–	–	–	–
Costa Rica	97	100	91	95	95	96	100	81	98	86	80	81	87	87	–	–	–	–	–	–	–
Côte d'Ivoire	80	93	68	23	36	11	5	95	81	81	77	67	81	81	92	35	19	45	10	3	36
Croatia	99	100	97	99	99	98	–	99	99	96	96	98	97	96	–	–	–	–	–	–	–
Cuba	94	96	89	91	94	81	99	99	98	96	99	96	96	96	–	–	–	–	–	–	–
Cyprus	100	100	100	100	100	100	40	–	99	99	99	87	96	96	–	–	–	–	–	–	–
Czech Republic	100	100	100	98	99	97	1	98	98	99	99	98	99	99	–	–	–	–	–	–	–
Democratic People's Republic of Korea	100	100	100	–	–	–	10	98	94	93	98	98	92	–	91	93 x	–	–	–	–	–
Democratic Republic of the Congo	46	80	28	23	23	23	1	80	91	77	74	76	77	77	85	42	–	42	9	6	30
Denmark	100	100	100	100	100	100	–	–	90	89	89	84	–	89	–	–	–	–	–	–	–
Djibouti	92	98	52	56	63	10	–	90	90	89	89	73	89	89	77	62	43	33	30	20	10
Dominica	–	–	–	–	–	–	100	99	98	99	99	99	99	99	–	–	–	–	–	–	–
Dominican Republic	86	87	84	83	87	74	90	96	85	82	85	79	85	77	86	70	57	55	–	–	–
Ecuador	94	97	88	92	96	84	100	99	93	75	72	66	75	75	73	–	–	–	–	–	–
Egypt	99	100	98	94	97	92	100	98	97	97	97	95	97	–	85	73	58	19	–	–	–
El Salvador	87	94	76	87	89	83	–	87	99	91	91	95	91	91	87	67	51	–	–	–	–
Equatorial Guinea	–	–	–	–	–	–	100	73	65	33	39	51	–	–	75	–	–	36 x	–	1 x	49 x
Eritrea	61	74	57	14	52	4	–	99	99	99	99	95	99	99	86	44 x	–	54 x	–	4 x	4 x
Estonia	98	99	97	95	96	94	–	97	97	95	95	95	95	95	–	–	–	–	–	–	–
Ethiopia	38	98	26	12	29	8	–	76	86	79	76	75	79	79	88	19	5	15	53	33	10
Fiji	–	–	–	–	–	–	100	99	99	99	99	94	99	99	94	–	–	–	–	–	–

	% of population using improved drinking-water sources 2008			% of population using improved sanitation facilities 2008			% of routine EPI vaccines financed by government 2009	Immunization 2009 — 1-year-old children immunized against:							% newborns protected against tetanus	% under-fives with suspected pneumonia taken to an appropriate health-care provider	% under-fives with suspected pneumonia receiving antibiotics	% under-fives with diarrhoea receiving oral rehydration and continued feeding	Malaria 2006–2009*		
								TB	DPT		Polio	Measles	HepB	Hib					% households owning at least one ITN	% under-fives sleeping under ITNs	% under-fives with fever receiving anti-malarial drugs
	total	urban	rural	total	urban	rural	total	BCG	DPT1β	DPT3β	polio3	measles	HepB3	Hib3		2005–2009*		2005–2009*			
Finland	100	100	100	100	100	100	1	–	99	99	99	98	–	98	–	–	–	–	–	–	–
France	100	100	100	100	100	100	10	78	98	99	98	90	42	97	–	–	–	–	–	–	–
Gabon	87	95	41	33	33	30	100	89	69	45	44	55	45	–	75	48 x	–	44 x	–	–	–
Gambia	92	96	86	67	68	65	35	94	98	98	97	96	98	98	91	69	61	38	50	49	63
Georgia	98	100	96	95	96	93	88	95	96	88	92	83	54	–	–	74	56	37	–	–	–
Germany	100	100	100	100	100	100	–	–	97	93	96	96	90	94	–	–	–	–	–	–	–
Ghana	82	90	74	13	18	7	–	99	96	94	94	93	94	94	86	51	24	45	33	28	43
Greece	100	100	99	98	99	97	–	91	98	99	99	99	95	83	–	–	–	–	–	–	–
Grenada	–	97	–	97	96	97	100	–	99	99	99	99	99	99	–	–	–	–	–	–	–
Guatemala	94	98	90	81	89	73	100	93	95	92	92	92	92	92	71	64 x	–	38	–	1 x	–
Guinea	71	89	61	19	34	11	30	81	75	57	53	51	58	58	96	42	–	38	8	5	44 x
Guinea-Bissau	61	83	51	21	49	9	0	89	85	68	72	76	68	68	94	57	42	25	44	39	46
Guyana	94	98	93	81	85	80	–	98	98	98	92	97	98	98	90	64	20	28	–	–	–
Haiti	63	71	55	17	24	10	–	75	83	59	59	59	–	–	70	31	3	43	–	–	5
Holy See	–	–	–	–	–	–	–	–	–	–	–	–	–	–	–	–	–	–	–	–	–
Honduras	86	95	77	71	80	62	71	99	99	98	98	99	98	98	94	56	54	49	–	–	1
Hungary	100	100	100	100	100	100	100	99	99	99	99	99	–	99	–	–	–	–	–	–	–
Iceland	100	100	100	100	100	100	100	–	99	96	96	92	–	97	–	–	–	–	–	–	–
India	88	96	84	31	54	21	–	87	83	66	67	71	21	–	86	69	13	33	–	–	8
Indonesia	80	89	71	52	67	36	100	93	89	82	89	82	82	–	85	66	–	54	3	3	1
Iran (Islamic Republic of)	–	98	–	–	–	–	100	99	99	99	99	99	99	–	83	93 x	–	–	–	–	–
Iraq	79	91	55	73	76	66	1	92	84	65	69	69	58	–	69	82	82	64	–	0 x	1 x
Ireland	100	100	100	99	100	98	–	94	97	93	93	89	–	93	–	–	–	–	–	–	–
Israel	100	100	100	100	100	100	–	–	98	93	94	96	94	93	–	–	–	–	–	–	–
Italy	100	100	100	–	–	–	100	–	96	96	97	91	96	96	–	–	–	–	–	–	–
Jamaica	94	98	89	83	82	84	100	94	98	90	90	88	90	90	62	75	52	39	–	–	–
Japan	100	100	100	100	100	100	–	–	98	98	99	94	–	–	–	–	–	–	–	–	–
Jordan	96	98	91	98	98	97	100	95	98	95	98	95	98	98	87	75	87	32	–	–	–
Kazakhstan	95	99	90	97	97	98	–	96	98	98	99	99	99	97	–	71	32	48	–	–	–
Kenya	59	83	52	31	27	32	–	75	80	75	71	74	75	75	78	56	–	33 x	54	46	23
Kiribati	–	–	–	–	–	–	–	76	92	86	84	82	86	86	–	–	–	–	–	–	–
Kuwait	99	99	99	100	100	100	–	–	99	98	98	97	94	98	84	–	–	–	–	–	–
Kyrgyzstan	90	99	85	93	94	93	64	98	97	95	96	99	96	–	–	62	45	22	–	–	–
Lao People's Democratic Republic	57	72	51	53	86	38	7	67	76	57	67	59	67	–	47	32	52	49	45	41	8
Latvia	99	100	96	78	82	71	100	99	97	95	96	96	94	95	–	–	–	–	–	–	–
Lebanon	100	100	100	–	100	–	100	–	83	74	74	53	74	74	–	74 x	–	–	–	–	–
Lesotho	85	97	81	29	40	25	1	96	93	83	80	85	83	83	83	66	–	53 x	–	–	–
Liberia	68	79	51	17	25	4	–	80	75	64	74	64	64	64	91	62	–	47	47	26	67
Libyan Arab Jamahiriya	–	–	–	97	97	96	100	99	98	98	98	98	98	98	–	–	–	–	–	–	–
Liechtenstein	–	–	–	–	–	–	–	–	–	–	–	–	–	–	–	–	–	–	–	–	–
Lithuania	–	–	–	–	–	–	100	99	98	98	98	96	95	98	–	–	–	–	–	–	–
Luxembourg	100	100	100	100	100	100	100	–	98	99	99	96	95	99	–	–	–	–	–	–	–
Madagascar	41	71	29	11	15	10	51	73	80	78	76	64	78	78	76	42	–	47 x	57	46	20
Malawi	80	95	77	56	51	57	100	95	97	93	93	92	93	93	87	52	30	27	38	25	25
Malaysia	100	100	99	96	96	95	80	98	95	95	95	95	95	95	87	–	–	–	–	–	–
Maldives	91	99	86	98	100	96	100	99	98	98	98	98	98	–	95	22 x	–	–	–	–	–
Mali	56	81	44	36	45	32	–	86	85	74	74	71	75	74	92	38	–	38	50	27	32
Malta	100	100	100	100	100	100	–	–	91	73	73	82	86	73	–	–	–	–	–	–	–
Marshall Islands	94	92	99	73	83	53	–	92	99	93	91	94	93	83	–	–	–	–	–	–	–
Mauritania	49	52	47	26	50	9	100	81	79	64	63	59	64	64	87	45	24	32	12	2 x	21
Mauritius	99	100	99	91	93	90	100	95	99	99	99	99	99	99	87	–	–	–	–	–	–
Mexico	94	96	87	85	90	68	100	90	97	89	89	95	71	89	87	–	–	–	–	–	–
Micronesia (Federated States of)	–	95	–	–	–	–	0	75	97	91	81	86	88	73	–	–	–	–	–	–	–
Monaco	100	100	–	100	100	–	–	90	99	99	99	99	99	99	–	–	–	–	–	–	–
Mongolia	76	97	49	50	64	32	64	98	95	95	96	94	97	97	–	63	71	47	–	–	–
Montenegro	98	100	96	92	96	86	100	95	96	92	91	86	87	87	–	89	57	64	–	–	–
Morocco	81	98	60	69	83	52	100	99	99	99	99	98	98	99	86	38 x	–	46 x	–	–	–
Mozambique	47	77	29	17	38	4	100	87	88	76	75	77	72	74	83	65	22	47	16	23	37
Myanmar	71	75	69	81	86	79	–	93	93	90	90	87	90	–	93	66 x	–	65 x	–	–	–
Namibia	92	99	88	33	60	17	100	85	87	83	83	76	–	–	82	53 x	14	48	20	11	10
Nauru	–	90	–	–	50	–	100	99	98	99	99	99	99	99	–	69	47	68	–	–	–

TABLE 3. HEALTH

	% of population using improved drinking-water sources 2008			% of population using improved sanitation facilities 2008			% of routine EPI vaccines financed by government 2009	Immunization 2009 — 1-year-old children immunized against:							% new-borns protected against tetanus	% under-fives with suspected pneumonia taken to an appropriate health-care provider	% under-fives with suspected pneumonia receiving antibiotics	% under-fives with diarrhoea receiving oral rehydration and continued feeding	Malaria 2006–2009*		
	total	urban	rural	total	urban	rural	total	TB BCG	DPT1	DPT3	polio3	measles	HepB3	Hib3		2005–2009*		2005–2009*	% households owning at least one ITN	% under-fives sleeping under ITNs	% under-fives with fever receiving anti-malarial drugs
Nepal	88	93	87	31	51	27	16	87	84	82	82	79	82	–	81	43	25	37	–	–	0
Netherlands	100	100	100	100	100	100	100	–	98	97	97	96	–	97	–	–	–	–	–	–	–
New Zealand	100	100	100	–	–	–	100	–	99	92	92	89	93	98	–	–	–	–	–	–	–
Nicaragua	85	98	68	52	63	37	–	98	98	98	99	99	98	98	80	58 x	–	49 x	–	–	2 x
Niger	48	96	39	9	34	4	29	78	82	70	71	73	70	70	84	47	–	34	78	43	33
Nigeria	58	75	42	32	36	28	74	53	52	42	54	41	41	–	67	45	23	25	8	6	33
Niue	100	100	100	100	100	100	100	99	99	99	99	99	99	99	–	–	–	–	–	–	–
Norway	100	100	100	100	100	100	74	–	99	92	92	92	–	94	–	–	–	–	–	–	–
Occupied Palestinian Territory	91	91	91	89	91	84	–	99	99	96	97	97	96	96	–	65 x	–	–	–	–	–
Oman	88	92	77	–	97	–	100	99	99	98	97	97	98	98	91	–	–	–	–	–	–
Pakistan	90	95	87	45	72	29	80	90	90	85	85	80	85	85	84	69	50	37	0	–	3
Palau	–	–	–	–	96	–	–	–	99	49	48	75	69	48	–	–	–	–	–	–	–
Panama	93	97	83	69	75	51	100	99	94	84	84	85	84	84	–	–	–	–	–	–	–
Papua New Guinea	40	87	33	45	71	41	61	68	70	52	65	54	56	52	61	63	–	–	–	–	–
Paraguay	86	99	66	70	90	40	100	96	98	92	90	91	94	94	74	–	–	–	–	–	–
Peru	82	90	61	68	81	36	100	99	98	93	92	91	93	93	67	72	55	60	–	–	–
Philippines	91	93	87	76	80	69	100	90	89	87	86	88	85	–	68	50	–	60	–	–	0
Poland	100	100	100	90	96	80	–	93	98	99	99	98	98	88	–	–	–	–	–	–	–
Portugal	99	99	100	100	100	100	–	98	98	96	96	95	96	96	–	–	–	–	–	–	–
Qatar	100	100	100	100	100	100	95	98	99	99	98	99	99	99	–	–	–	–	–	–	–
Republic of Korea	98	100	88	100	100	100	48	96	97	94	95	93	94	–	–	–	–	–	–	–	–
Republic of Moldova	90	96	85	79	89	74	54	96	88	85	87	90	89	47	–	60	–	48	–	–	–
Romania	–	–	–	72	88	54	1	99	98	97	96	97	95	–	–	–	–	–	–	–	–
Russian Federation	96	98	89	87	93	70	–	97	98	98	98	98	–	–	–	–	–	–	–	–	–
Rwanda	65	77	62	54	50	55	–	93	99	97	97	92	97	97	85	28	13	24	56	56	6
Saint Kitts and Nevis	99	99	99	96	96	96	100	95	98	99	98	99	98	97	–	–	–	–	–	–	–
Saint Lucia	98	98	98	–	–	–	100	97	99	95	95	99	95	95	–	–	–	–	–	–	–
Saint Vincent and the Grenadines	–	–	–	–	–	96	–	80	99	99	99	99	99	99	–	–	–	–	–	–	–
Samoa	–	–	–	100	100	100	100	94	95	72	72	49	72	72	–	–	–	–	–	–	–
San Marino	–	–	–	–	–	–	–	–	95	92	92	92	92	92	–	–	–	–	–	–	–
Sao Tome and Principe	89	89	88	26	30	19	25	99	98	92	99	90	98	–	–	75	–	63	61	56	8
Saudi Arabia	–	97	–	–	100	–	100	98	99	98	98	98	98	98	–	–	–	–	–	–	–
Senegal	69	92	52	51	69	38	17	97	94	86	83	79	86	86	88	47	–	43	60	29	9
Serbia	99	99	98	92	96	88	100	98	96	95	97	95	93	94	–	93	57	71	–	–	–
Seychelles	–	100	–	–	97	–	100	96	98	99	99	97	99	–	–	–	–	–	–	–	–
Sierra Leone	49	86	26	13	24	6	–	95	87	75	74	71	75	75	97	46	27	57	37	26	30
Singapore	100	100	–	100	100	–	–	99	98	97	97	95	97	–	–	–	–	–	–	–	–
Slovakia	100	100	100	100	100	99	–	97	99	99	99	99	99	99	–	–	–	–	–	–	–
Slovenia	99	100	99	100	100	100	70	–	98	96	96	95	–	95	–	–	–	–	–	–	–
Solomon Islands	–	–	–	–	98	–	63	81	83	81	82	60	81	77	85	73	23	–	49	40	19
Somalia	30	67	9	23	52	6	0	29	40	31	28	24	–	–	64	13	32	7	12	11	8
South Africa	91	99	78	77	84	65	100	81	77	69	70	62	67	67	75	65 x	–	–	–	–	–
Spain	100	100	100	100	100	100	100	–	98	96	96	98	96	96	–	–	–	–	–	–	–
Sri Lanka	90	98	88	91	88	92	100	98	98	97	97	96	97	–	93	58	–	67	5	3	0
Sudan	57	64	52	34	55	18	3	82	92	84	84	82	76	76	74	90	–	56	18	28	54
Suriname	93	97	81	84	90	66	100	–	91	87	85	88	87	87	93	74	37	28	–	3 x	–
Swaziland	69	92	61	55	61	53	100	99	97	95	96	95	95	95	86	73	24	22	4	1	1
Sweden	100	100	100	100	100	100	–	21	98	98	98	97	–	98	–	–	–	–	–	–	–
Switzerland	100	100	100	100	100	100	5	–	95	95	95	90	–	95	–	–	–	–	–	–	–
Syrian Arab Republic	89	94	84	96	96	95	100	90	88	80	83	81	77	80	94	77	71	34	–	–	–
Tajikistan	70	94	61	94	95	94	17	82	93	93	93	89	93	93	–	64	41	22	2 x	1 x	2 x
Thailand	100	100	99	89	92	82	100	99	99	99	99	98	98	–	91	84	65	46	–	–	–
The former Yugoslav Republic of Macedonia	98	98	98	96	95	96	100	98	98	96	96	96	95	82	–	93	74	45	–	–	–
Timor-Leste	69	86	63	50	76	40	100	71	76	72	78	70	72	–	81	71	–	–	42	42	47 x
Togo	60	87	41	12	24	3	10	91	93	89	89	84	89	89	81	23	26	22	40	38	48
Tonga	100	100	100	96	98	96	95	99	99	99	99	99	99	99	–	–	–	–	–	–	–
Trinidad and Tobago	94	98	93	92	92	92	100	–	95	90	94	94	90	90	–	74	34	–	–	–	–
Tunisia	94	99	84	85	96	64	100	98	98	98	98	98	99	–	96	59	–	62	–	–	–
Turkey	99	100	96	90	97	75	–	96	97	96	96	96	92	96	71	41 x	–	22	–	–	–
Turkmenistan	–	97	–	98	99	97	–	99	99	98	99	99	97	–	–	83	50	25	–	–	–
Tuvalu	97	98	97	84	88	81	<1	99	99	89	99	90	92	84	–	–	–	–	–	–	–

	% of population using improved drinking-water sources 2008			% of population using improved sanitation facilities 2008			% of routine EPI vaccines financed by government 2009	Immunization 2009 — 1-year-old children immunized against:							% new-borns protected against tetanus	% under-fives with suspected pneumonia taken to an appropriate health-care provider	% under-fives with suspected pneumonia receiving antibiotics	% under-fives with diarrhoea receiving oral rehydration and continued feeding	Malaria 2006–2009*		
								TB	DPT		Polio	Measles	HepB	Hib					% households owning at least one ITN	% under-fives sleeping under ITNs	% under-fives with fever receiving anti-malarial drugs
									corresponding vaccines:												
	total	urban	rural	total	urban	rural	total	BCG	DPT1β	DPT3β	polio3	measles	HepB3	Hib3		2005–2009*		2005–2009*			
Uganda	67	91	64	48	38	49	13	90	90	64	59	68	64	64	89	73	47	39	16	10	61
Ukraine	98	98	97	95	97	90	–	95	94	90	91	94	84	81	–	–	–	–	–	–	–
United Arab Emirates	100	100	100	97	98	95	100	98	98	92	94	92	92	92	–	–	–	–	–	–	–
United Kingdom	100	100	100	100	100	100	–	–	97	93	93	86	–	93	–	–	–	–	–	–	–
United Republic of Tanzania	54	80	45	24	32	21	21	93	90	85	88	91	85	85	90	59	–	53	39	26	57
United States	99	100	94	100	100	99	–	–	98	95	93	92	92	93	–	–	–	–	–	–	–
Uruguay	100	100	100	100	100	100	–	99	99	95	95	94	95	95	–	–	–	–	–	–	–
Uzbekistan	87	98	81	100	100	100	58	99	98	98	99	95	98	98	–	68	56	28	–	–	–
Vanuatu	83	96	79	52	66	48	100	81	78	68	67	52	59	–	73	–	–	43	–	–	–
Venezuela (Bolivarian Republic of)	–	–	–	–	–	–	100	87	83	83	73	83	83	83	50	72 x	–	51 x	–	–	–
Viet Nam	94	99	92	75	94	67	80	97	97	96	96	97	94	–	87	83	55	65	19	13 x	3
Yemen	62	72	57	52	94	33	35	58	77	66	65	58	66	67	66	47 x	38	48	–	–	–
Zambia	60	87	46	49	59	43	95	92	92	81	85	85	80	81	90	68	47	56	62	41	43
Zimbabwe	82	99	72	44	56	37	0	91	87	73	69	76	73	73	76	25	16	35	27	17	24

SUMMARY INDICATORS

	total	urban	rural	total	urban	rural	total	BCG	DPT1β	DPT3β	polio3	measles	HepB3	Hib3	tetanus	pneumonia provider	antibiotics	diarrhoea	ITN owning	sleeping under ITNs	fever antimalarial
Africa#	65	85	52	41	55	32	58	80	82	73	74	71	72	59	81	49	28	33	28	20	34
Sub-Saharan Africa#	60	83	47	31	44	24	48	78	80	70	72	68	69	61	81	46	23	35	28	20	34
Eastern and Southern Africa	59	87	47	36	55	28	58	83	86	77	76	76	75	75	84	46	22	32	41	29	31
West and Central Africa	61	82	46	27	35	21	46	73	74	63	67	60	63	47	79	43	24	34	18	12	36
Middle East and North Africa	86	93	76	80	90	66	79	92	93	89	89	87	87	46	79	76	62	39	–	–	–
Asia#	87	96	82	49	63	40	88	92	90	82	83	82	64	9	86	65 **	22 **	41 **	–	–	6 **
South Asia	86	95	83	35	57	26	–	88	86	72	73	74	41	15	86	65	19	37	–	–	7
East Asia and Pacific	88	96	81	60	66	55	95	95	95	93	96	91	92	2	–	66 **	–	56 **	–	–	1 **
Latin America and Caribbean	93	97	80	80	86	55	99	94	96	92	91	93	86	90	82	55	–	–	–	–	–
CEE/CIS	94	98	88	89	93	82	–	96	97	95	96	96	93	53	–	–	–	31	–	–	–
Industrialized countries§	100	100	98	99	100	98	–	–	98	95	95	93	66	85	–	–	–	–	–	–	–
Developing countries§	84	94	76	52	68	40	82	88	89	81	82	80	70	34	83	59 **	27 **	38 **	–	–	17 **
Least developed countries§	62	80	54	36	50	31	30	84	89	79	78	77	78	59	86	45	23	43	34	24	33
World	87	96	78	61	76	45	81	88	90	82	83	82	70	38	83	59 **	27 **	39 **	–	–	17 **

For a complete list of countries and territories in the regions and subregions, see page 124.

§ Includes territories within each country category or regional group. Countries and territories in each country category or regional group are listed on page 124.

DEFINITIONS OF THE INDICATORS

Government funding of vaccines – Percentage of vaccines that are routinely administered in a country to protect children and are financed by the national government (including loans).

EPI – Expanded programme on immunization: The immunizations in this programme include those against tuberculosis (TB); diphtheria, pertussis (whooping cough) and tetanus (DPT); polio; and measles, as well as vaccination of pregnant women to protect babies against neonatal tetanus. Other vaccines, e.g., against hepatitis B (HepB), *Haemophilus influenzae* type b (Hib) or yellow fever, may be included in the programme in some countries.

BCG – Percentage of infants who received bacille Calmette-Guérin (vaccine against tuberculosis).

DPT1 – Percentage of infants who received their first dose of diphtheria, pertussis and tetanus vaccine.

DPT3 – Percentage of infants who received three doses of diphtheria, pertussis and tetanus vaccine.

HepB3 – Percentage of infants who received three doses of hepatitis B vaccine.

Hib3 – Percentage of infants who received three doses of *Haemophilus influenzae* type b vaccine.

% under-fives with suspected pneumonia taken to an appropriate health-care provider – Percentage of children (aged 0–4) with suspected pneumonia in the two weeks preceding the survey who were taken to an appropriate health-care provider.

% under-fives with suspected pneumonia receiving antibiotics – Percentage of children (aged 0–4) with suspected pneumonia in the two weeks preceding the survey who are receiving antibiotics.

% under-fives with diarrhoea receiving oral rehydration and continued feeding – Percentage of children (aged 0–4) with diarrhoea in the two weeks preceding the survey who received oral rehydration therapy (a packet of oral rehydration salts, recommended home-made fluids or increased fluids) and continued feeding.

Malaria:

% households owning at least one ITN – Percentage of households with at least one insecticide-treated net.

% under-fives sleeping under ITNs – Percentage of children (aged 0–4) who slept under an insecticide-treated net the night prior to the survey.

% under-fives with fever receiving antimalarial drugs – Percentage of children (aged 0–4) who were ill with fever in the two weeks preceding the survey and received any antimalarial medicine.

MAIN DATA SOURCES

Use of improved drinking-water sources and improved sanitation facilities – UNICEF and World Health Organization (WHO), Joint Monitoring Programme.

Government funding of vaccines – UNICEF and WHO.

Immunization – UNICEF and WHO.

Suspected pneumonia – Demographic and Health Surveys (DHS), Multiple Indicator Cluster Surveys (MICS) and other national household surveys.

Oral rehydration therapy and continued feeding – DHS, MICS and other national household surveys.

Malaria prevention and treatment – DHS, MICS and malaria indicator surveys.

NOTES

– Data not available.

x Data refer to years or periods other than those specified in the column heading, differ from the standard definition or refer to only part of a country. Such data are not included in the calculation of regional and global averages.

β Coverage for DPT1 should be at least as high as DPT3. Discrepancies where DPT1 coverage is less than DPT3 reflect deficiencies in the data collection and reporting process. UNICEF and WHO are working with national and territorial systems to eliminate these discrepancies.

λ WHO and UNICEF have employed a model to calculate the percentage of births that can be considered as protected against tetanus because pregnant women were given two doses or more of tetanus toxoid (TT) vaccine. The model aims to improve the accuracy of this indicator by capturing or including other potential scenarios where women might be protected (e.g., women who receive doses of TT in supplemental immunization activities). A fuller explanation of the methodology can be found at <www.childinfo.org>.

* Data refer to the most recent year available during the period specified in the column heading.

** Excludes China.

TABLE 4. HIV/AIDS

Countries and territories	Estimated adult HIV prevalence rate (aged 15–49), 2009	Estimated number of people (all ages) living with HIV, 2009 (thousands)			Mother-to-child transmission Estimated number of women (aged 15+) living with HIV, 2009 (thousands)	Paediatric infections Estimated number of children (aged 0–14) living with HIV, 2009 (thousands)	HIV prevalence among young people (aged 15–24), 2009			% who have comprehensive knowledge of HIV, 2005–2009*		% who used condom at last higher-risk sex, 2005–2009*		Urphans Children (aged 0–17)		Orphan school attendance ratio
		estimate	low estimate	high estimate			total	male	female	male	female	male	female	orphaned by AIDS, 2009 estimate (thousands)	orphaned due to all causes, 2009 estimate (thousands)	2005–2009*
Afghanistan	–	–	–	–	–	–	–	–	–	–	–	–	–	–	–	–
Albania	–	–	–	–	–	–	–	–	–	22	36	55	25	–	–	–
Algeria	0.1	18	13	24	5.2	–	<0.1	0.1	<0.1	–	13	–	–	–	550	–
Andorra	–	–	–	–	–	–	–	–	–	–	–	–	–	–	–	–
Angola	2.0	200	160	250	110	22	1.1	0.6	1.6	–	–	–	–	140	1500	–
Antigua and Barbuda	–	–	–	–	–	–	–	–	–	–	–	–	–	–	–	–
Argentina	0.5	110	88	140	36	–	0.2	0.3	0.2	–	–	–	–	–	630	–
Armenia	0.1	1.9	1.5	2.4	<1.0	–	<0.1	<0.1	<0.1	15	23	86	–	–	46	–
Australia	0.1	20	15	25	6.2	–	0.1	0.1	0.1	–	–	–	–	–	80	–
Austria	0.3	15	12	20	4.6	–	0.2	0.3	0.2	–	–	–	–	–	28	–
Azerbaijan	0.1	3.6	2.6	5.2	2.1	–	0.1	<0.1	0.1	5	5	31	–	–	190	–
Bahamas	3.1	6.6	2.6	11	3.7	–	2.2	1.4	3.1	–	–	–	–	–	6.8	–
Bahrain	–	–	–	–	–	–	–	–	–	–	–	–	–	–	–	–
Bangladesh	<0.1	6.3	5.2	8.3	1.9	–	<0.1	<0.1	<0.1	–	15	–	–	–	4800	84
Barbados	1.4	2.1	1.8	2.5	<1.0	–	1.0	0.9	1.1	–	–	–	–	–	2	–
Belarus	0.3	17	13	20	8.3	–	0.1	0.1	0.1	–	34	–	–	–	150	–
Belgium	0.2	14	11	18	4.4	–	<0.1	<0.1	<0.1	–	–	–	–	–	47	–
Belize	2.3	4.8	4.0	5.7	2.6	–	1.3	0.7	1.8	–	40	–	50	–	6.4	–
Benin	1.2	60	52	69	32	5.4	0.5	0.3	0.7	35	16	45	28	30	310	90
Bhutan	0.2	<1.0	<1.0	1.5	<0.5	–	0.1	0.1	<0.1	–	–	–	–	–	21	–
Bolivia (Plurinational State of)	0.2	12	9.0	16	3.6	–	0.1	0.1	0.1	28	24	49	–	–	320	–
Bosnia and Herzegovina	–	–	–	–	–	–	–	–	–	–	44	–	71	–	–	–
Botswana	24.8	320	300	350	170	16	8.5	5.2	11.8	–	–	–	–	93	130	–
Brazil	–	–	460	810	–	–	–	–	–	–	–	–	–	–	–	–
Brunei Darussalam	–	–	–	–	–	–	–	–	–	–	–	–	–	–	–	–
Bulgaria	0.1	3.8	2.8	5.2	1.1	–	<0.1	<0.1	<0.1	15	17	70	57	–	94	–
Burkina Faso	1.2	110	91	140	56	17	0.6	0.5	0.8	–	19	–	64	140	770	61 p
Burundi	3.3	180	160	190	90	28	1.5	1.0	2.1	–	30	–	25	200	610	85
Cambodia	0.5	63	42	90	35	–	0.1	0.1	0.1	45	50	84	–	–	630	83
Cameroon	5.3	610	540	670	320	54	2.7	1.6	3.9	–	32	–	62	330	1200	91
Canada	0.3	68	53	83	21	–	0.1	0.1	0.1	–	–	–	–	–	45	–
Cape Verde	–	–	–	–	–	–	–	–	–	36	36	79	56	–	–	–
Central African Republic	4.7	130	110	140	67	17	1.6	1.0	2.2	26	17	60	41	140	370	96
Chad	3.4	210	170	300	110	23	1.7	1.0	2.5	20 x	8 x	25 x	17 x	120	670	105 x
Chile	0.4	40	32	51	12	–	0.2	0.2	0.1	–	–	–	–	–	140	–
China	0.1	740	540	1000	230	–	–	–	–	–	–	–	–	–	–	–
Colombia	0.5	160	120	210	50	–	0.2	0.2	0.1	–	–	–	36	–	820	85
Comoros	0.1	<0.5	<0.2	<0.5	<0.1	–	<0.1	<0.1	<0.1	–	–	–	–	<0.1	22	–
Congo	3.4	77	68	87	40	7.9	1.9	1.2	2.6	22	8	38	20	51	220	88
Cook Islands	–	–	–	–	–	–	–	–	–	–	–	–	–	–	–	–
Costa Rica	0.3	9.8	7.5	13	2.8	–	0.2	0.2	0.1	–	–	–	–	–	36	–
Côte d'Ivoire	3.4	450	390	510	220	–	1.1	0.7	1.5	28	18	53	39	–	1100	83
Croatia	<0.1	<1.0	<1.0	1.1	<0.5	–	<0.1	<0.1	<0.1	–	–	–	–	–	44	–
Cuba	0.1	7.1	5.7	8.9	2.2	–	0.1	0.1	0.1	–	52	–	–	–	86	–
Cyprus	–	–	–	–	–	–	–	–	–	–	–	–	–	–	–	–
Czech Republic	<0.1	2.0	1.7	2.3	<1.0	–	<0.1	<0.1	<0.1	–	–	–	–	–	92	–
Democratic People's Republic of Korea	–	–	–	–	–	–	–	–	–	–	–	–	–	–	–	–
Democratic Republic of the Congo	–	–	430	560	–	–	–	–	–	21	15	27	17	–	–	77
Denmark	0.2	5.3	4.0	6.3	1.4	–	0.1	0.1	0.1	–	–	–	–	–	51	–
Djibouti	2.5	14	10	18	7.4	–	1.3	0.8	1.9	–	18	51	26	–	47	–
Dominica	–	–	–	–	–	–	–	–	–	–	–	–	–	–	–	–
Dominican Republic	0.9	57	49	66	32	–	0.5	0.3	0.7	34	41	70	44	–	190	77
Ecuador	0.4	37	28	50	11	–	0.2	0.2	0.2	–	–	–	–	–	210	–
Egypt	<0.1	11	8.4	17	2.4	–	<0.1	<0.1	<0.1	18	5.0	–	–	–	1700	–
El Salvador	0.8	34	25	44	11	–	0.3	0.4	0.3	–	27	–	–	–	150	–
Equatorial Guinea	5.0	20	14	26	11	1.6	3.5	1.9	5	–	–	–	–	4.1	45	–
Eritrea	0.8	25	18	33	13	3.1	0.3	0.2	0.4	–	–	–	–	19	240	–
Estonia	1.2	9.9	8.0	12	3.0	–	0.2	0.3	0.2	–	–	–	–	–	19	–
Ethiopia	–	–	–	–	–	–	–	–	–	33	20	50	28	–	–	90
Fiji	0.1	<1.0	<0.5	<1.0	<0.2	–	0.1	0.1	0.1	–	–	–	–	–	23	–
Finland	0.1	2.6	2.2	3.1	<1.0	–	<0.1	0.1	<0.1	–	–	–	–	–	45	–

	Estimated adult HIV prevalence rate (aged 15–49), 2009	Estimated number of people (all ages) living with HIV, 2009 (thousands)			Mother-to-child transmission — Estimated number of women (aged 15+) living with HIV, 2009 (thousands)	Paediatric infections — Estimated number of children (aged 0–14) living with HIV, 2009 (thousands)	HIV prevalence among young people (aged 15–24), 2009			% who have comprehensive knowledge of HIV, 2005–2009*		% who used condom at last higher-risk sex, 2005–2009*		Orphans — Children (aged 0–17) — orphaned by AIDS, 2009 estimate (thousands)	orphaned due to all causes, 2009 estimate (thousands)	Orphan school attendance ratio 2005–2009*
		estimate	low estimate	high estimate			total	male	female	male	female	male	female			
France	0.4	150	120	190	48	–	0.2	0.2	0.1	–	–	–	–	–	<0.1	–
Gabon	5.2	46	37	55	25	3.2	2.4	1.4	3.5	–	–	–	–	18	64	–
Gambia	2.0	18	12	26	9.7	–	1.6	0.9	2.4	–	39	–	54	2.8	72	87
Georgia	0.1	3.5	2.6	4.9	1.5	–	<0.1	<0.1	<0.1	–	15	–	–	–	68	–
Germany	0.1	67	56	75	12	–	0.1	0.1	<0.1	–	–	–	–	–	380	–
Ghana	1.8	260	230	300	140	27	0.9	0.5	1.3	34	28	46	28	160	1100	76
Greece	0.1	8.8	7.3	11	2.7	–	0.1	0.1	0.1	–	–	–	–	–	73	–
Grenada	–	–	–	–	–	–	–	–	–	–	–	–	–	–	–	–
Guatemala	0.8	62	47	82	20	–	0.4	0.5	0.3	–	–	–	–	–	380	–
Guinea	1.3	79	65	95	41	9.0	0.7	0.4	0.9	23	17	37	26	59	440	73
Guinea-Bissau	2.5	22	18	26	12	2.1	1.4	0.8	2.0	–	18	–	39	9.7	110	97
Guyana	1.2	5.9	2.7	8.8	2.8	–	0.7	0.6	0.8	–	50	68	62	–	30	–
Haiti	1.9	120	110	140	67	12	0.9	0.6	1.3	40	34	43	29	–	440	86
Holy See	–	–	–	–	–	–	–	–	–	–	–	–	–	–	–	–
Honduras	0.8	39	26	51	12	–	0.3	0.3	0.2	–	30	–	24	–	150	108
Hungary	<0.1	3.0	2.2	3.9	<1.0	–	<0.1	<0.1	<0.1	–	–	–	–	–	130	–
Iceland	0.3	<1.0	<0.5	<1.0	<0.2	–	0.1	0.1	0.1	–	–	–	–	–	1.8	–
India	0.3	2400	2100	2800	880	–	0.1	0.1	0.1	36	20	37	22	–	31000	72
Indonesia	0.2	310	200	460	88	–	<0.1	0.1	<0.1	15 y	10 y	–	–	–	4700	–
Iran (Islamic Republic of)	0.2	92	74	120	26	–	<0.1	<0.1	<0.1	–	–	–	–	–	1200	–
Iraq	–	–	–	–	–	–	–	–	–	–	3	–	–	–	–	84
Ireland	0.2	6.9	5.2	8.7	2.0	–	0.1	0.1	0.1	–	–	–	–	–	39	–
Israel	0.2	7.5	5.6	9.9	2.2	–	0.1	0.1	<0.1	–	–	–	–	–	7.6	–
Italy	0.3	140	110	180	48	–	<0.1	<0.1	<0.1	–	–	–	–	–	<0.1	–
Jamaica	1.7	32	21	45	10	–	0.9	1.0	0.7	–	60	–	–	–	73	–
Japan	<0.1	8.1	6.3	10	2.7	–	<0.1	<0.1	<0.1	–	–	–	–	–	<0.1	–
Jordan	–	–	–	–	–	–	–	–	–	–	13 y	–	–	–	–	–
Kazakhstan	0.1	13	9.0	19	7.7	–	0.1	0.1	0.2	–	22	–	–	–	420	–
Kenya	6.3	1500	1300	1600	760	180	2.9	1.8	4.1	55	48	64	40	1200	2600	–
Kiribati	–	–	–	–	–	–	–	–	–	–	–	–	–	–	–	–
Kuwait	–	–	–	–	–	–	–	–	–	–	–	–	–	–	–	–
Kyrgyzstan	0.3	9.8	6.5	16	2.8	–	0.1	0.1	0.1	–	20	–	56	–	140	–
Lao People's Democratic Republic	0.2	8.5	6.0	13	3.5	–	0.2	0.1	0.2	–	–	–	–	–	220	–
Latvia	0.7	8.6	6.3	12	2.6	–	0.1	0.2	0.1	–	–	–	–	–	32	–
Lebanon	0.1	3.6	2.7	4.8	1.1	–	0.1	0.1	<0.1	–	–	–	–	–	70	–
Lesotho	23.6	290	260	310	160	28	9.9	5.4	14.2	18 x	26 x	48 x	50 x	130	200	95 x
Liberia	1.5	37	32	43	19	6.1	0.5	0.3	0.7	27	21	22	14	52	340	85
Libyan Arab Jamahiriya	–	–	–	–	–	–	–	–	–	–	–	–	–	–	–	–
Liechtenstein	–	–	–	–	–	–	–	–	–	–	–	–	–	–	–	–
Lithuania	0.1	1.2	<1.0	1.6	<0.5	–	<0.1	<0.1	<0.1	–	–	–	–	–	52	–
Luxembourg	0.3	<1.0	<1.0	1.2	<0.5	–	0.1	0.1	0.1	–	–	–	–	–	3.6	–
Madagascar	0.2	24	19	30	7.3	–	0.1	0.1	0.1	16 x	19 x	12 x	5 x	11	910	75 x
Malawi	11	920	830	1000	470	120	4.9	3.1	6.8	42	42	58	40	650	1000	97
Malaysia	0.5	100	83	120	11	–	0.1	0.1	<0.1	–	–	–	–	–	450	–
Maldives	<0.1	<0.1	<0.1	<0.1	<0.1	–	<0.1	<0.1	<0.1	–	–	–	–	–	7.3	–
Mali	1.0	76	61	96	40	–	0.4	0.2	0.5	22	18	36	17	59	690	87
Malta	0.1	<0.5	<0.5	<0.5	<0.1	–	<0.1	<0.1	<0.1	–	–	–	–	–	2.6	–
Marshall Islands	–	–	–	–	–	–	–	–	–	39	27	22	9	–	–	–
Mauritania	0.7	14	11	17	4.0	–	0.4	0.4	0.3	14	5	–	–	3.6	120	66 p
Mauritius	1.0	8.8	6.4	12	2.5	–	0.3	0.3	0.2	–	–	–	–	<0.1	19	–
Mexico	0.3	220	180	280	59	–	0.2	0.2	0.1	–	–	–	–	–	1500	–
Micronesia (Federated States of)	–	–	–	–	–	–	–	–	–	–	–	–	–	–	–	–
Monaco	–	–	–	–	–	–	–	–	–	–	–	–	–	–	–	–
Mongolia	<0.1	<0.5	<0.5	<1.0	<0.2	–	<0.1	<0.1	<0.1	–	31	–	–	–	67	96 p
Montenegro	–	–	–	–	–	–	–	–	–	–	30	–	66	–	–	–
Morocco	0.1	26	19	34	8.1	–	0.1	0.1	0.1	–	12 x	–	–	–	650	–
Mozambique	11.5	1400	1200	1500	760	130	5.9	3.1	8.6	–	14	–	44	670	2100	89
Myanmar	0.6	240	200	290	81	–	0.3	0.3	0.3	–	–	–	–	–	1600	–
Namibia	13.1	180	150	210	95	16	4.0	2.3	5.8	62	65	81	64	70	120	100
Nauru	–	–	–	–	–	–	–	–	–	10	13	17	10	–	–	–
Nepal	0.4	64	51	80	20	–	0.2	0.2	0.1	44	28	78	–	–	650	–

TABLE 4. HIV/AIDS

| | Estimated adult HIV prevalence rate (aged 15–49), 2009 | Estimated number of people (all ages) living with HIV, 2009 (thousands) | | | Mother-to-child transmission | Paediatric infections | HIV prevalence among young people (aged 15–24), 2009 | | | % who have comprehensive knowledge of HIV, 2005–2009* | | % who used condom at last higher-risk sex, 2005–2009* | | Orphans — Children (aged 0–17) | | Orphan school attendance ratio |
		estimate	low estimate	high estimate	Estimated number of women (aged 15+) living with HIV, 2009 (thousands)	Estimated number of children (aged 0–14) living with HIV, 2009 (thousands)	total	male	female	male	female	male	female	orphaned by AIDS, 2009 estimate (thousands)	orphaned due to all causes, 2009 estimate (thousands)	2005–2009*
Netherlands	0.2	22	17	32	6.9	–	0.1	0.1	<0.1	–	–	–	–	–	82	–
New Zealand	0.1	2.5	2.0	3.2	<1.0	–	<0.1	<0.1	<0.1	–	–	–	–	–	36	–
Nicaragua	0.2	6.9	5.2	9.1	2.1	–	0.1	0.1	0.1	–	–	–	–	–	120	–
Niger	0.8	61	56	66	28	–	0.4	0.2	0.5	16	13	37	18 y	57	970	67
Nigeria	3.6	3300	2900	3600	1700	360	2.0	1.2	2.9	33	22	49	36	2500	12000	117
Niue	–	–	–	–	–	–	–	–	–	–	–	–	–	–	–	–
Norway	0.1	4.0	3.0	5.4	1.2	–	<0.1	<0.1	<0.1	–	–	–	–	–	35	–
Occupied Palestinian Territory	–	–	–	–	–	–	–	–	–	–	–	–	–	–	–	–
Oman	0.1	1.1	<1.0	1.4	<0.5	–	<0.1	<0.1	<0.1	–	–	–	–	–	41	–
Pakistan	0.1	98	79	120	28	–	0.1	0.1	<0.1	–	3	–	–	–	4200	–
Palau	–	–	–	–	–	–	–	–	–	–	–	–	–	–	–	–
Panama	0.9	20	14	36	6.3	–	0.3	0.4	0.3	–	–	–	–	–	53	–
Papua New Guinea	0.9	34	30	39	18	3.1	0.6	0.3	0.8	–	–	50	35	–	260	–
Paraguay	0.3	13	9.8	16	3.8	–	0.2	0.2	0.1	–	–	–	–	–	150	–
Peru	0.4	75	58	100	18	–	0.2	0.2	0.1	–	19	–	36	–	550	–
Philippines	<0.1	8.7	6.1	13	2.6	–	<0.1	<0.1	<0.1	–	21	–	13	–	1900	–
Poland	0.1	27	20	34	8.2	–	<0.1	<0.1	<0.1	–	–	–	–	–	440	–
Portugal	0.6	42	32	53	13	–	0.2	0.3	0.2	–	–	–	–	–	58	–
Qatar	<0.1	<0.2	<0.1	<0.2	<0.1	–	<0.1	<0.1	<0.1	–	–	–	–	–	14	–
Republic of Korea	<0.1	9.5	7.0	13	2.9	–	<0.1	<0.1	<0.1	–	–	–	–	–	280	–
Republic of Moldova	0.4	12	9.9	16	5.1	–	0.1	0.1	0.1	39 y	42 y	76	60	–	79	–
Romania	0.1	16	12	20	4.7	–	<0.1	0.1	<0.1	1 y, x	3 y, x	–	–	–	290	–
Russian Federation	–	–	840	1200	–	–	–	0.2	0.3	–	–	–	–	–	–	–
Rwanda	2.9	170	140	190	88	22	1.6	1.3	1.9	54	51	40	26	130	690	82
Saint Kitts and Nevis	–	–	–	–	–	–	–	–	–	–	–	–	–	–	–	–
Saint Lucia	–	–	–	–	–	–	–	–	–	–	–	–	–	–	–	–
Saint Vincent and the Grenadines	–	–	–	–	–	–	–	–	–	–	–	–	–	–	–	–
Samoa	–	–	–	–	–	–	–	–	–	–	–	–	–	–	–	–
San Marino	–	–	–	–	–	–	–	–	–	–	–	–	–	–	–	–
Sao Tome and Principe	–	–	–	–	–	–	–	–	–	–	44	63	54	–	–	–
Saudi Arabia	–	–	–	–	–	–	–	–	–	–	–	–	–	–	–	–
Senegal	0.9	59	50	69	32	–	0.5	0.3	0.7	24	19	52	36	19	520	83
Serbia	0.1	4.9	3.5	7.1	1.2	–	0.1	0.1	0.1	–	42	–	74	–	94	–
Seychelles	–	–	–	–	–	–	–	–	–	–	–	–	–	–	–	–
Sierra Leone	1.6	49	40	63	28	2.9	1.0	0.6	1.5	28	17	22	10	15	320	62
Singapore	0.1	3.4	2.5	4.4	1.0	–	<0.1	<0.1	<0.1	–	–	–	–	–	17	–
Slovakia	<0.1	<0.5	<0.5	<0.5	<0.1	–	<0.1	<0.1	<0.1	–	–	–	–	–	54	–
Slovenia	<0.1	<1.0	<0.5	<1.0	<0.2	–	<0.1	<0.1	<0.1	–	–	–	–	–	12	–
Solomon Islands	–	–	–	–	–	–	–	–	–	35	29	26	17	–	–	–
Somalia	0.7	34	25	48	15	–	0.5	0.4	0.6	–	4	–	–	–	630	78
South Africa	17.8	5600	5400	5900	3300	330	9.0	4.5	13.6	–	–	–	–	1900	3400	–
Spain	0.4	130	120	150	32	–	0.1	0.2	0.1	–	–	–	–	–	<0.1	–
Sri Lanka	<0.1	2.8	2.1	3.8	<1.0	–	<0.1	<0.1	<0.1	–	–	–	–	–	340	–
Sudan	1.1	260	210	330	140	–	0.9	0.5	1.3	–	–	–	–	–	2000	–
Suriname	1.0	3.7	2.7	5.3	1.1	–	0.5	0.6	0.4	–	41	–	49	–	12	–
Swaziland	25.9	180	170	200	100	14	11	6.5	15.6	52	52	70	54	69	100	97
Sweden	0.1	8.1	6.1	11	2.5	–	<0.1	<0.1	<0.1	–	–	–	–	–	63	–
Switzerland	0.4	18	13	24	5.7	–	0.2	0.2	0.1	–	–	–	–	–	<0.1	–
Syrian Arab Republic	–	–	–	–	–	–	–	–	–	–	7	–	–	–	–	–
Tajikistan	0.2	9.1	6.4	13	2.7	–	<0.1	<0.1	<0.1	–	2	–	–	–	220	–
Thailand	1.3	530	420	660	210	–	–	–	–	–	46	–	–	–	1400	93
The former Yugoslav Republic of Macedonia	–	–	–	–	–	–	–	–	–	–	27	–	70	–	–	–
Timor-Leste	–	–	–	–	–	–	–	–	–	–	–	–	–	–	–	–
Togo	3.2	120	99	150	67	11	1.5	0.9	2.2	–	15	–	50	66	240	94
Tonga	–	–	–	–	–	–	–	–	–	–	–	–	–	–	–	–
Trinidad and Tobago	1.5	15	11	19	4.7	–	0.9	1.0	0.7	–	–	54	–	51	25	–
Tunisia	<0.1	2.4	1.8	3.3	<1.0	–	<0.1	<0.1	<0.1	–	–	–	–	–	130	–
Turkey	<0.1	4.6	3.4	6.1	1.4	–	<0.1	<0.1	<0.1	–	–	–	–	–	1200	–
Turkmenistan	–	–	–	–	–	–	–	–	–	–	5	–	–	–	–	–
Tuvalu	–	–	–	–	–	–	–	–	–	61	39	44 y	–	–	–	–
Uganda	6.5	1200	1100	1300	610	150	3.6	2.3	4.8	38	32	55	38	1200	2700	96
Ukraine	1.1	350	300	410	170	–	0.2	0.2	0.3	43	45	71	68	–	810	98

	Estimated adult HIV prevalence rate (aged 15–49), 2009	Estimated number of people (all ages) living with HIV, 2009 (thousands)			Mother-to-child transmission Estimated number of women (aged 15+) living with HIV, 2009 (thousands)	Paediatric infections Estimated number of children (aged 0–14) living with HIV, 2009 (thousands)	HIV prevalence among young people (aged 15–24), 2009			% who have comprehensive knowledge of HIV, 2005–2009*		% who used condom at last higher-risk sex, 2005–2009*		Orphans Children (aged 0–17) orphaned by AIDS, 2009 estimate (thousands)	orphaned due to all causes, 2009 estimate (thousands)	Orphan school attendance ratio 2005–2009*
		estimate	low estimate	high estimate			total	male	female	male	female	male	female			
United Arab Emirates	–	–	–	–	–	–	–	–	–	–	–	–	–	–	–	–
United Kingdom	0.2	85	66	110	26	–	0.1	0.2	0.1	–	–	–	–	–	490	–
United Republic of Tanzania	5.6	1400	1300	1500	730	160	2.8	1.7	3.9	42	39	49	46	1300	3000	97
United States	0.6	1200	930	1700	310	–	0.2	0.3	0.2	–	–	–	–	–	2100	–
Uruguay	0.5	9.9	8.4	12	3.1	–	0.2	0.3	0.2	–	–	–	–	–	49	–
Uzbekistan	0.1	28	18	46	8.0	–	<0.1	<0.1	<0.1	–	31	–	61	–	780	–
Vanuatu	–	–	–	–	–	–	–	–	–	–	15	–	–	–	–	–
Venezuela (Bolivarian Republic of)	–	–	–	–	–	–	–	–	–	–	–	–	–	–	–	–
Viet Nam	0.4	280	220	350	81	–	0.1	0.1	0.1	–	44	68	–	–	1400	–
Yemen	–	–	–	–	–	–	–	–	–	–	2 y	–	–	–	–	–
Zambia	13.5	980	890	1100	490	120	6.6	4.2	8.9	41	38	39	33	690	1300	92
Zimbabwe	14.3	1200	1100	1300	620	150	5.1	3.3	6.9	–	53	68	42	1000	1400	95

SUMMARY INDICATORS

Africa#	3.9	22900	21300	24600	12300	2300	1.9	1.1	2.7	32	23	48	34	14900	59000	93
Sub-Saharan Africa#	4.7	22900	21200	24500	12300	2300	2.3	1.3	3.3	34	26	48	34	14900	56100	93
Eastern and Southern Africa	7.2	16300	15100	17600	8800	1600	3.4	1.9	4.8	41	33	54	37	10100	27600	92
West and Central Africa	2.7	6200	5700	6800	3300	690	1.4	0.8	2.0	28	20	43	33	4700	26400	94
Middle East and North Africa	0.2	430	370	490	190	19	0.2	0.1	0.2	–	–	–	–	86	6400	–
Asia#	0.2	4900	4500	5500	1700	160	0.1	0.1	0.1	33 **	19 **	–	–	1100	71400	74 **
South Asia	0.3	2600	2200	2900	930	110	0.1	0.1	0.1	36	17	38	22	570	41000	73
East Asia and Pacific	0.2	2300	2000	2800	750	48	<0.1	<0.1	<0.1	–	24 **	–	–	490	30500	–
Latin America and Caribbean	0.5	1900	1700	2100	660	58	0.2	0.2	0.2	–	–	–	–	440	9800	–
CEE/CIS	0.5	1500	1300	1700	690	19	0.1	0.1	0.2	–	–	–	–	75	7300	–
Industrialized countries§	0.3	2100	1800	2500	570	1.3	0.1	0.2	0.1	–	–	–	–	100	4300	–
Developing countries§	0.9	29800	28100	31700	14700	2500	0.5	0.3	0.6	33 **	20 **	–	–	16400	145000	81 **
Least developed countries§	2.0	9700	8600	11000	5000	1100	1.1	0.7	1.5	–	21	–	–	7200	41300	85
World	0.8	33300	31400	35300	15900	2500	0.4	0.3	0.6	–	20 **	–	–	16600	153000	–

For a complete list of countries and territories in the regions and subregions, see page 124.
§ Includes territories within each country category or regional group. Countries and territories in each country category or regional group are listed on page 124.

DEFINITIONS OF THE INDICATORS

Estimated adult HIV prevalence rate – Percentage of adults (aged 15–49) living with HIV as of 2009.

Estimated number of people (all ages) living with HIV – Estimated number of people (all ages) living with HIV as of 2009.

Estimated number of women (aged 15+) living with HIV – Estimated number of women (aged 15+) living with HIV as of 2009.

Estimated number of children (aged 0–14) living with HIV – Estimated number of children (aged 0–14) living with HIV as of 2009.

HIV prevalence among young people – Percentage of young men and women (aged 15–24) living with HIV as of 2009.

Comprehensive knowledge of HIV – Percentage of young men and women (aged 15–24) who correctly identify the two major ways of preventing the sexual transmission of HIV (using condoms and limiting sex to one faithful, uninfected partner), who reject the two most common local misconceptions about HIV transmission and who know that a healthy-looking person can be HIV-infected.

Condom use at last higher-risk sex – Percentage of young men and women (aged 15–24) who say they used a condom the last time they had sex with a non-marital, non-cohabiting partner, of those who have had sex with such a partner during the past 12 months.

Children orphaned by AIDS – Estimated number of children (aged 0–17) who have lost one or both parents to AIDS as of 2009.

Children orphaned due to all causes – Estimated number of children (aged 0–17) who have lost one or both parents due to any cause as of 2009.

Orphan school attendance ratio – Percentage of children (aged 10–14) who have lost both biological parents and who are currently attending school as a percentage of non-orphaned children of the same age who live with at least one parent and who are attending school.

MAIN DATA SOURCES

Estimated adult HIV prevalence rate – Joint United Nations Programme on HIV/AIDS (UNAIDS), Report on the Global AIDS Epidemic, 2010.

Estimated number of people (all ages) living with HIV – UNAIDS, Report on the Global AIDS Epidemic, 2010.

Estimated number of women (aged 15+) living with HIV – UNAIDS, Report on the Global AIDS Epidemic, 2010.

Estimated number of children (aged 0–14) living with HIV – UNAIDS, Report on the Global AIDS Epidemic, 2010.

HIV prevalence among young people – UNAIDS, Report on the Global AIDS Epidemic, 2010.

Comprehensive knowledge of HIV – AIDS Indicator Surveys (AIS), Behavioural Surveillance Surveys (BSS), Demographic and Health Surveys (DHS), Multiple Indicator Cluster Surveys (MICS), Reproductive Health Surveys (RHS) and other national household surveys, 2005–2009; 'HIV/AIDS Survey Indicators Database', <www.measuredhs.com/hivdata>.

Condom use at last higher-risk sex – AIS, BSS, DHS, RHS and other national household surveys, 2005–2009; 'HIV/AIDS Survey Indicators Database', <www.measuredhs.com/hivdata>.

Children orphaned by AIDS – UNAIDS, Report on the Global AIDS Epidemic, 2010.

Children orphaned due to all causes – UNAIDS estimates, 2010.

Orphan school attendance ratio – AIS, DHS, MICS and other national household surveys, 2005–2009; 'HIV/AIDS Survey Indicators Database', <www.measuredhs.com/hivdata>.

NOTES

– Data not available.

y Data differ from the standard definition or refer to only part of a country. Such data are included in the calculation of regional and global averages.

p Proportion of orphans (aged 10–14) attending school is based on small denominators (typically 25–49 unweighted cases).

* Data refer to the most recent year available during the period specified in the column heading.

** Excludes China.

TABLE 5. EDUCATION

Countries and territories	Youth (15–24 years) literacy rate 2004–2008* male	female	Number per 100 population 2008 phones	Internet users	Primary school enrolment ratio 2005–2009* gross male	female	net male	female	Primary school attendance ratio 2005–2009* net male	female	Survival rate to last primary grade (%) 2005–2009* admin. data	survey data	Secondary school enrolment ratio 2005–2009* gross male	female	net male	female	Secondary school attendance ratio 2005–2009* net male	female
Afghanistan	49 x	18 x	29	2	127	84	74	46	66 x	40 x	–	90 x	41	15	38	15	18 x	6 x
Albania	99	100	100	24	102 x	102 x	91 x	91 x	92	92	90 x	100	79 x	76 x	75 x	73 x	79	77
Algeria	94	89	93	12	111	104	96	94	97	96	93	93	80	86	65 x	68 x	57	65
Andorra	–	–	76	70	88	85	81	79	–	–	–	–	78	87	69	75	–	–
Angola	81	65	38	3	141	114	55 x	48 x	58 x	59 x	–	83 x	19 x	16 x	–	–	22 x	20 x
Antigua and Barbuda	–	–	158	75	105	96	90	86	–	–	97	–	119	110	–	–	–	–
Argentina	99	99	117	28	116	115	–	–	–	–	95	–	80	90	75	84	–	–
Armenia	100	100	100	6	104	106	83	86	99	98	98	100	86	90	83	88	93	95
Australia	–	–	105	72	106	105	96	97	–	–	98	–	153	146	87	89	–	–
Austria	–	–	130	71	100	99	97 x	98 x	–	–	98	–	102	98	–	–	–	–
Azerbaijan	100	100	75	28	117	115	97	95	74	72	98	99 x	107	104	99	97	82	80
Bahamas	–	–	106	32	103	103	90	92	–	–	91	–	92	94	83	87	–	–
Bahrain	100	100	186	52	106	104	98	97	86 x	87 x	99 x	99 x	95	99	87	92	77 x	85 x
Bangladesh	73	76	28	0	89	94	85	86	80	83	55	94	43	45	40	43	46	53
Barbados	–	–	159	74	–	–	–	–	–	–	94	–	–	–	–	–	–	–
Belarus	100	100	84	32	98	100	93	96	93	94	100	100	94	96	–	–	95	97
Belgium	–	–	112	69	103	103	98	99	–	–	87	–	110	107	89	85	–	–
Belize	–	89	53	11	122	119	90	98	95	95	90	98	72	78	61	66	58	60
Benin	64	42	42	2	125	108	99	86	72	62	63 x	89	46	26	26 x	13 x	40	27
Bhutan	80	68	37	7	108	110	86	88	74 x	67 x	90	–	62	61	46	49	–	–
Bolivia (Plurinational State of)	100	99	50	11	108	108	93	94	97	97	80	96	83	81	70	70	78	75
Bosnia and Herzegovina	100	99	84	35	109	110	–	–	97	98	–	100	89	91	–	–	89	89
Botswana	94	96	77	6	111	109	86	88	86	88	87	–	78	82	62	67	36 x	44 x
Brazil	97	99	78	38	132	123	95	93	95	95	76 x	88	96	106	78	85	74	80
Brunei Darussalam	100	100	96	55	107	107	93	93	–	–	98	–	96	98	87	90	–	–
Bulgaria	97	97	138	35	101	101	96	96	–	–	94	–	90	87	85	82	–	–
Burkina Faso	47	33	17	1	83	74	67	59	49	44	71	89	23	17	18	13	17	15
Burundi	77	75	6	1	139	132	100	99	72	70	54	82	21	15	–	–	8	6
Cambodia	89	86	29	1	120	112	90	87	84	86	54	92	44	36	36	32	29	26
Cameroon	88	84	32	4	119	102	94	82	86	81	57	87	41	33	–	–	45	42
Canada	–	–	66	75	99	99	99 x	100 x	–	–	98 x	–	102	100	95 x	94 x	–	–
Cape Verde	97	99	56	21	105	98	85	84	97 x	96 x	87	–	65 x	71 x	54 x	60 x	–	–
Central African Republic	72	56	4	0	104	74	77	57	64	54	46	62	18	10	13	8	16	10
Chad	54	37	17	1	97	68	72 x	50 x	41 x	31 x	30	94 x	26	12	16 x	5 x	13 x	7 x
Chile	99	99	88	32	108	103	95	94	–	–	95	–	89	92	84	87	–	–
China	99	99	48	22	111	116	100	100	–	–	100	–	74	78	–	–	–	–
Colombia	98	98	92	39	120	120	90	90	88	92	88	89	86	95	68	75	64	72
Comoros	86	84	15	3	125	114	79 x	67 x	31 x	31 x	72 x	19 x	52	39	15	15	10 x	11 x
Congo	87	78	50	4	118	110	62	56	86	87	70	93	46 x	40 x	–	–	39	40
Cook Islands	–	–	34	25	99 x	94 x	87 x	83 x	–	–	47 x	–	58 x	63 x	57 x	61 x	–	–
Costa Rica	98	99	42	32	110	109	91	93	87	89	94	–	87	92	–	–	59	65
Côte d'Ivoire	72	60	51	3	83	66	62 x	50 x	66	57	90	90	34 x	19 x	27 x	15 x	32	22
Croatia	100	100	133	51	99	98	91	90	–	–	100	–	92	95	87	89	–	–
Cuba	100	100	3	13	104	103	99	99	–	–	96	–	90	89	82	83	–	–
Cyprus	100	100	118	39	104	103	99	98	–	–	98	–	98	99	95	97	–	–
Czech Republic	–	–	134	58	103	103	88	91	–	–	99	–	94	96	–	–	–	–
Democratic People's Republic of Korea	100	100	–	–	–	–	–	–	–	–	–	–	–	–	–	–	–	–
Democratic Republic of the Congo	69	62	14	0	99	82	33 x	32 x	63	60	79	74	45	25	–	–	30	24
Denmark	–	–	126	84	99	99	95	96	–	–	92 x	–	117	121	88	91	–	–
Djibouti	–	48	13	2	49	43	44	39	67	66	–	92	35	24	25	18	45	37
Dominica	–	–	150	41	79	84	69	76	–	–	91	–	109	101	62	74	–	–
Dominican Republic	95	97	72	22	108	101	80	80	87	90	69	78	69	81	52	63	56	68
Ecuador	95	96	86	29	119	118	96	97	–	–	81	–	75	76	61	62	–	–
Egypt	88	82	51	17	102	97	95	92	96	94	97	98	82 x	77 x	73 x	69 x	72	67
El Salvador	95	96	113	11	117	113	93	95	–	–	76	–	63	64	54	56	–	–
Equatorial Guinea	98	98	52	2	101	96	70 x	63 x	61 x	60 x	33 x	–	33 x	19 x	–	–	23 x	22 x
Eritrea	91	84	2	4	57	47	42	36	69 x	64 x	73	–	36	25	30	22	23 x	21 x
Estonia	100	100	188	66	101	99	95	94	–	–	98	–	98	101	88	91	–	–
Ethiopia	62	39	2	0	103	92	81	75	45	45	40	84	39	28	31	20	30	23
Fiji	–	–	71	12	95	94	90	89	–	–	95	–	78	84	76	83	–	–
Finland	–	–	129	83	98	97	96	96	–	–	100	–	108	113	96	97	–	–

| | Youth (15–24 years) literacy rate 2004–2008* | | Number per 100 population 2008 | | Primary school enrolment ratio 2005–2009* | | | | Primary school attendance ratio 2005–2009* net | | Survival rate to last primary grade (%) 2005–2009* | | Secondary school enrolment ratio 2005–2009* | | | | Secondary school attendance ratio 2005–2009* net | |
| | | | | | gross | | net | | | | | | gross | | net | | | |
	male	female	phones	Internet users	male	female	male	female	male	female	admin. data	survey data	male	female	male	female	male	female
France	–	–	93	68	111	109	98	99	–	–	98 x	–	113	113	98	99	–	–
Gabon	98	96	90	6	135 x	134 x	81 x	80 x	94 x	94 x	56 x	–	–	–	–	–	34 x	36 x
Gambia	70	58	70	7	84	89	67	71	60	62	70	95	52	49	42	41	39	34
Georgia	100	100	64	24	109	106	100	98	94	95	95	98	92	88	82	79	89	88
Germany	–	–	128	75	105	105	98	98	–	–	96	–	103	100	–	–	–	–
Ghana	81	78	50	4	106	105	76	77	73	74	60 x	81	58	52	49	45	42	42
Greece	99	99	124	44	101	101	99	100	–	–	98	–	104	99	91	91	–	–
Grenada	–	–	58	23	105	100	94	93	–	–	83 x	–	112	103	93	85	–	–
Guatemala	89	84	109	14	117	110	97	94	80 x	76 x	65	–	58	55	41	39	23 x	24 x
Guinea	67	51	39	1	97	83	76	66	55	48	55	96	45	26	34	21	27	17
Guinea-Bissau	78	62	32	2	–	–	61 x	43 x	54	53	–	76	–	–	12 x	7 x	8	7
Guyana	–	–	37	27	109	108	95	95	96	96	59 x	96	102	102	–	–	66	73
Haiti	–	–	32	10	–	–	–	–	48	52	–	85	–	–	–	–	18	21
Holy See	–																	
Honduras	93	95	85	13	116	116	96	98	77	80	76	–	57	72	–	–	29	36
Hungary	98	99	122	59	100	98	90	89	–	–	99	–	98	97	91	91	–	–
Iceland	–	–	109	91	98	98	97	98	–	–	93	–	108	112	89	91	–	–
India	88	74	29	4	115	111	91	88	85	81	66	95	61	52	–	–	59	49
Indonesia	97	96	62	8	121	118	97	94	86	84	80	–	75	74	69	68	57	59
Iran (Islamic Republic of)	97	96	59	31	107	151	–	–	94 x	91 x	88 x	–	80	79	75	75	–	–
Iraq	85	80	58	1	106	89	93	81	91	80	70 x	93	56	37	46	33	46	34
Ireland	–	–	121	63	105	105	96	98	–	–	–	–	111	119	86	90	–	–
Israel	–	–	127	50	110	111	97	98	–	–	100	–	89	91	85	88	–	–
Italy	100	100	152	42	104	103	99	98	–	–	100	–	100	99	92	93	–	–
Jamaica	92	98	101	57	95	92	82	79	97	98	87 x	99	89	93	75	79	88	92
Japan	–	–	87	75	102	102	–	–	–	–	–	–	101	101	98	98	–	–
Jordan	99	99	87	26	97	97	89	90	99	99	99	–	87	90	80	84	85	89
Kazakhstan	100	100	96	11	108	109	88	90	99	98	99	100	101	98	88	89	97	97
Kenya	92	93	42	9	113	110	81	82	72	75	84 x	96	61	56	50	48	40	42
Kiribati	–	–	1	2	107	109	–	–	–	–	81 x	–	79	95	65	72	–	–
Kuwait	98	99	100	34	96	95	89	87	–	–	100	–	88	91	80	80	–	–
Kyrgyzstan	100	100	63	16	95	94	84	83	91	93	98	99	85	86	80	81	90	92
Lao People's Democratic Republic	89	79	33	9	117	106	84	81	81	77	67	91	48	39	33	33	39	32
Latvia	100	100	99	61	100	96	98 x	96 x	–	–	96	–	97	99	–	–	–	–
Lebanon	98	99	34	23	104	102	91	89	97 x	97 x	93	93 x	78	87	71	79	61 x	68 x
Lesotho	86	98	28	4	108	107	71	74	82	88	46	84	34	45	20	31	16	27
Liberia	70	80	19	1	96	86	85 x	66 x	41	39	–	–	36	27	25 x	14 x	21	18
Libyan Arab Jamahiriya	100	100	77	5	113	108	–	–	–	–	–	–	86	101	–	–	–	–
Liechtenstein	–	–	95	66	107	107	87	92	–	–	82	–	117	100	85	81	–	–
Lithuania	100	100	151	55	97	95	93	91	–	–	98	–	99	99	91	92	–	–
Luxembourg	–	–	147	81	100	101	95	97	–	–	86	–	95	98	82	85	–	–
Madagascar	73	68	25	2	154	149	98	99	74 x	77 x	42	93 x	31	29	23	24	17 x	21 x
Malawi	87	85	12	2	119	122	88	93	86	87	36	71	32	27	26	24	13	13
Malaysia	98	99	103	56	97	96	96	96	–	–	92	–	66	71	66	70	–	–
Maldives	99	99	143	24	115	109	97	95	–	–	–	–	81	86	68	71	–	–
Mali	47	31	27	2	103	86	79	66	46	40	79	90 x	46	30	35	22	23	17
Malta	97	99	95	49	99	99	91	92	–	–	99 x	–	97	99	79	85	–	–
Marshall Islands	94	96	2	4	94	92	67	66	–	–	–	–	66	67	43	47	–	–
Mauritania	71	63	65	2	101	108	74	79	56	59	82	77	26	23	17	15	21	17
Mauritius	95	97	81	22	100	100	93	95	–	–	98	–	86	88	79	81	–	–
Mexico	98	98	69	22	115	113	98	98	97	97	92	–	87	93	71	74	–	–
Micronesia (Federated States of)	94 x	96 x	31	14	110	111	–	–	–	–	–	–	–	–	–	–	–	–
Monaco	–	–	67	67	131	125	–	–	–	–	–	–	153	154	–	–	–	–
Mongolia	93	97	67	12	102	101	89	88	96	98	95	97	92	99	79	85	85	91
Montenegro	–	93	118	47	–	–	–	–	98	97	–	97	–	–	–	–	90	92
Morocco	85	68	72	33	112	102	92	87	91	88	76	–	60	51	37 x	32 x	39 x	36 x
Mozambique	78	62	20	2	121	107	82	77	82	80	44	60	24	18	6	6	21	20
Myanmar	96	95	1	0	117	117	–	–	83 x	84 x	74	100 x	–	–	49	50	51 x	48 x
Namibia	91	95	49	5	113	112	87	91	91	91	77	90 x	61	71	49	60	40	53
Nauru	92	99	–	–	80	84	72	73	–	–	25 x	–	47	58	–	–	–	–
Nepal	86	75	15	2	123 x	106 x	78 x	64 x	86	82	62	95	46	41	–	–	46	38

TABLE 5. EDUCATION

| | Youth (15–24 years) literacy rate 2004–2008* | | Number per 100 population 2008 | | Primary school enrolment ratio 2005–2009* | | | | Primary school attendance ratio 2005–2009* net | | Survival rate to last primary grade (%) 2005–2009* | | Secondary school enrolment ratio 2005–2009* | | | | Secondary school attendance ratio 2005–2009* net | |
| | | | | | gross | | net | | | | | | gross | | net | | | |
	male	female	phones	Internet users	male	female	male	female	male	female	admin. data	survey data	male	female	male	female	male	female
Netherlands	–	–	125	87	108	106	99	98	–	–	98 x	–	122	120	88	89	–	–
New Zealand	–	–	109	72	101	101	99	100	–	–	–	–	115	122	90 x	92 x	–	–
Nicaragua	85	89	55	3	118	116	92	92	77 x	84 x	48	56 x	64	72	42	48	35 x	47 x
Niger	52	23	13	1	69	55	60	48	44	31	67	88	14	9	11	7	13	9
Nigeria	78	65	42	16	99	87	64	58	65	60	75 x	98	34	27	29	22	45	43
Niue	–	–	38	66	107	102	99 x	98 x	–	–	78 x	–	96	102	91 x	96 x	–	–
Norway	–	–	110	83	99	99	99	99	–	–	100	–	113	110	96	96	–	–
Occupied Palestinian Territory	99	99	28	9	80	79	75	75	91 x	92 x	99	–	87	93	85	90	–	–
Oman	98	98	116	20	74	75	67	69	–	–	100	–	90	87	79	78	–	–
Pakistan	79	59	50	10	93	77	72	60	76	67	70 x	–	37	28	37	28	39	33
Palau	100	100	60	27	98	100	98 x	94 x	–	–	–	–	98	96	–	–	–	–
Panama	97	96	115	27	113	109	99	98	–	–	85	–	68	74	63	69	–	–
Papua New Guinea	65	69	9	2	59	50	–	–	–	–	–	–	–	–	–	–	–	–
Paraguay	99	99	95	14	107	104	90	90	87	89	79	–	65	67	57	60	81 x	80 x
Peru	98	97	73	25	109	109	94	95	94 x	94 x	83	94 x	89	89	75	75	70 x	70 x
Philippines	94	96	75	6	111	109	91	93	88 x	89 x	73	90 x	79	86	55	66	55 x	70 x
Poland	100	100	115	49	97	97	95	96	–	–	97	–	100	99	93	95	–	–
Portugal	100	100	140	42	118	112	99	98	–	–	–	–	98	105	84	92	–	–
Qatar	99	99	131	34	109	108	95 x	94 x	–	–	97	–	79	115	67	98	–	–
Republic of Korea	–	–	95	77	106	104	100	98	–	–	98	–	99	95	97	94	–	–
Republic of Moldova	99	100	67	23	95	93	88	87	84	85	96	100	86	89	82	85	82	85
Romania	97	98	115	29	100	99	91	90	–	–	93	–	92	91	74	72	–	–
Russian Federation	100	100	141	32	97	97	–	–	–	–	95	–	86	84	–	–	–	–
Rwanda	77	77	14	3	150	152	95	97	84	87	31 x	76	23	21	–	–	5	5
Saint Kitts and Nevis	–	–	157	31	96	102	91	96	–	–	68	–	95	93	87	85	–	–
Saint Lucia	–	–	100	59	99	97	92	91	–	–	96 x	–	91	95	77	82	–	–
Saint Vincent and the Grenadines	–	–	119	60	111	103	97	92	–	–	64 x	–	107	111	85	95	–	–
Samoa	99	100	69	5	101	99	93	93	–	–	96 x	–	72	81	66	75	–	–
San Marino	–	–	77	55	–	–	–	–	–	–	–	–	–	–	–	–	–	–
Sao Tome and Principe	95	96	31	15	133	134	95	97	94	95	74	83	49	54	36	40	39	41
Saudi Arabia	98	96	143	31	100	96	85	84	–	–	96	–	102	87	70	76	–	–
Senegal	58	45	44	8	83	84	72	74	58	59	58	93	34	27	28	22	20	16
Serbia	99	99	98	34	98	98	95	95	99	98	98	100	87	90	87	89	81	87
Seychelles	99	99	112	40	131	130	99 x	100 x	–	–	98	–	101	120	–	–	–	–
Sierra Leone	66	46	18	0	168	148	–	–	69	69	–	94	42	28	30	20	21	17
Singapore	100	100	138	73	–	–	–	–	–	–	–	–	–	–	–	–	–	–
Slovakia	–	–	102	66	103	102	–	–	–	–	97	–	92	93	–	–	–	–
Slovenia	100	100	102	56	98	97	97	97	–	–	99 x	–	97	97	91	92	–	–
Solomon Islands	90 x	80 x	6	2	109	106	67	67	63	69	–	–	38	32	32	29	29	30
Somalia	–	24	7	1	42	23	–	–	25	21	–	85	11	5	–	–	9	5
South Africa	96	98	91	8	106	103	87	88	80 x	83 x	77 x	–	93	97	70	74	41 x	48 x
Spain	100	100	112	57	107	106	100	100	–	–	100	–	117	123	93	97	–	–
Sri Lanka	97	99	55	6	101	102	99	100	–	–	98	–	86 x	88 x	–	–	–	–
Sudan	89	82	29	10	78	70	43 x	36 x	56	52	93	56 x	40	36	–	–	17	22
Suriname	96	95	81	10	116	111	91	90	95	94	68	92	66	85	55	74	56	67
Swaziland	92	95	46	7	112	104	82	84	83	86	74	80 x	56	50	31	26	31	41
Sweden	–	–	118	88	95	95	95	94	–	–	100	–	104	103	99	99	–	–
Switzerland	–	–	118	77	103	103	94	94	–	–	–	–	98	94	87	83	–	–
Syrian Arab Republic	96	93	33	17	127	122	97 x	92 x	97	96	97	–	75	73	68	67	64	65
Tajikistan	100	100	54	9	104	100	99	95	99	96	99	100	90	78	88	77	89	74
Thailand	98	98	92	24	92	90	91	89	98	98	–	99	73	79	68	77	77	84
The former Yugoslav Republic of Macedonia	99	99	123	42	93	93	86	87	97	93	97	100	85	82	82	81	79	78
Timor-Leste	–	–	9	0	110	103	77	74	76 x	74 x	–	–	55	55	30	33	–	–
Togo	87	80	24	5	119	111	98	89	82	76	45	89	54	28	30 x	15 x	45	32
Tonga	99	100	49	8	113	110	–	–	–	–	91	–	101	105	60	74	–	–
Trinidad and Tobago	100	100	113	17	105	102	92	91	98	98	96	98	86	92	71	76	84	90
Tunisia	98	96	85	28	108	106	97	98	95 x	93 x	94	–	88	96	67	76	–	–
Turkey	99	94	89	34	101	98	96	94	91 x	87 x	94	95 x	87	77	77	70	52 x	43 x
Turkmenistan	100	100	23	1	–	–	–	–	99	99	–	100	–	–	–	–	84	84
Tuvalu	98	99	20	43	106	105	–	–	–	–	63 x	–	87 x	81 x	–	–	–	–
Uganda	89	86	27	8	120	121	96	98	83	82	32	72	27	23	22	21	16	15

| | Youth (15–24 years) literacy rate 2004–2008* | | Number per 100 population 2008 | | Primary school enrolment ratio 2005–2009* | | | | Primary school attendance ratio 2005–2009* net | | Survival rate to last primary grade (%) 2005–2009* | | Secondary school enrolment ratio 2005–2009* | | | | Secondary school attendance ratio 2005–2009* net | |
| | | | | | gross | | net | | | | | | gross | | net | | | |
	male	female	phones	Internet users	male	female	male	female	male	female	admin. data	survey data	male	female	male	female	male	female
Ukraine	100	100	121	11	98	99	89	89	96	98	97	100	95	94	84	85	90	93
United Arab Emirates	94	97	209	65	108	108	92	91	–	–	100	–	93	95	83	85	–	–
United Kingdom	–	–	126	76	106	106	99	100	–	–	–	–	98	100	92	95	–	–
United Republic of Tanzania	79	76	31	1	111	109	100	99	71	75	83	91	7 x	5 x	5 x	5 x	8	8
United States	–	–	87	74	98	99	91	93	–	–	95	–	94	94	88	89	–	–
Uruguay	99	99	105	40	116	113	97	98	–	–	94	–	93	91	64	71	–	–
Uzbekistan	100	100	47	9	94	92	89	87	100	100	99	100	102	101	92	90	91	90
Vanuatu	94	94	15	7	111	106	98	96	80	82	73	89	43 x	37 x	41 x	35 x	38	36
Venezuela (Bolivarian Republic of)	98	99	96	25	104	102	90	90	91 x	93 x	81	82 x	77	85	66	74	30 x	43 x
Viet Nam	97	96	80	24	107 x	101 x	96 x	91 x	94	94	92	98	70 x	64 x	–	–	77	78
Yemen	95	70	16	2	94	76	79	66	75	64	59 x	73	61	30	49	26	48	27
Zambia	82	68	28	6	120	118	95	96	80	80	79	87	50	41	47	39	38	35
Zimbabwe	98	99	13	11	104	103	89	91	90	92	62 x	79	43	39	39	37	46	43

SUMMARY INDICATORS

	male	female	phones	Internet users	male	female	male	female	male	female	admin. data	survey data	male	female	male	female	male	female
Africa#	79	70	38	8	105	96	83	79	69	67	67	87	44	36	33	29	35	32
Sub-Saharan Africa#	77	67	32	6	105	95	81	77	65	63	62	86	40	32	32	28	30	27
Eastern and Southern Africa	81	73	30	4	113	107	88	87	68	69	51	82	44	39	35	33	24	22
West and Central Africa	72	60	34	7	99	86	71	64	64	59	70	89	38	26	29	22	36	31
Middle East and North Africa	92	86	63	19	101	99	91	86	85	81	93	–	72	66	66	62	54	51
Asia#	92	86	44	14	111	108	92	89	84 **	81 **	79	–	64	60	–	–	56 **	50 **
South Asia	86	73	32	5	110	104	88	83	83	80	65	94	56	48	–	–	55	47
East Asia and Pacific	98	98	54	21	112	113	98	97	89 **	88 **	92	–	74	77	65 **	67 **	63 **	65 **
Latin America and Caribbean	97	98	80	29	118	114	95	94	92	93	85	–	87	94	72	77	68	74
CEE/CIS	99	99	109	26	100	98	93	92	–	–	96	–	91	88	82	81	–	–
Industrialized countries§	–	–	104	69	102	102	95	95	–	–	–	–	102	101	91	92	–	–
Developing countries§	91	84	48	15	109	105	90	87	80 **	77 **	77	91	64	60	54 **	53 **	52 **	48 **
Least developed countries§	76	67	21	2	104	96	85	81	67	66	60	83	39	31	33	29	30	28
World	91	85	59	23	108	105	91	88	80 **	77 **	79	91	69	65	61 **	60 **	53 **	48 **

For a complete list of countries and territories in the regions and subregions, see page 124.
§ Includes territories within each country category or regional group. Countries and territories in each country category or regional group are listed on page 124.

DEFINITIONS OF THE INDICATORS

Youth literacy rate – Number of literate persons aged 15–24, expressed as a percentage of the total population in that age group.

Primary school gross enrolment ratio – Number of children enrolled in primary school, regardless of age, expressed as a percentage of the total number of children of official primary school age.

Secondary school gross enrolment ratio – Number of children enrolled in secondary school, regardless of age, expressed as a percentage of the total number of children of official secondary school age.

Primary school net enrolment ratio – Number of children enrolled in primary school who are of official primary school age, expressed as a percentage of the total number of children of official primary school age.

Secondary school net enrolment ratio – Number of children enrolled in secondary school who are of official secondary school age, expressed as a percentage of the total number of children of official secondary school age.

Primary school net attendance ratio – Number of children attending primary or secondary school who are of official primary school age, expressed as a percentage of the total number of children of official primary school age.

Secondary school net attendance ratio – Number of children attending secondary or tertiary school who are of official secondary school age, expressed as a percentage of the total number of children of official secondary school age.

Survival rate to the last grade of primary school – Percentage of children entering the first grade of primary school who eventually reach the last grade of primary school.

MAIN DATA SOURCES

Youth literacy – UNESCO Institute for Statistics (UIS).

Phone and Internet use – International Telecommunications Union, Geneva.

Primary and secondary school enrolment – UIS.

Primary and secondary school attendance – Demographic and Health Surveys (DHS) and Multiple Indicator Cluster Surveys (MICS).

Survival rate to the last grade of primary school – Administrative data: UIS, survey data: DHS and MICS.

NOTES
– Data not available.
x Data refer to years or periods other than those specified in the column heading, differ from the standard definition or refer to only part of a country. Such data are not included in the calculation of regional and global averages.
* Data refer to the most recent year available during the period specified in the column heading.
** Excludes China.

TABLE 6. DEMOGRAPHIC INDICATORS

Countries and territories	Population (thousands) 2009 under 18	under 5	Population annual growth rate (%) 1970–1990	1990–2000	2000–2009	Crude death rate 1970	1990	2009	Crude birth rate 1970	1990	2009	Life expectancy 1970	1990	2009	Total fertility rate 2009	% of population urbanized 2009	Average annual growth rate of urban population (%) 1970–1990	1990–2000	2000–2009
Afghanistan	14897	5031	0.3	4.9	3.9	29	23	19	52	52	46	35	41	44	6.5	22	2.0	6.0	4.7
Albania	929	219	2.2	-0.7	0.4	8	6	6	33	24	15	67	72	77	1.9	51	2.8	0.7	2.5
Algeria	11667	3383	3.0	1.9	1.7	16	7	5	49	32	21	53	67	73	2.3	66	4.4	3.3	2.6
Andorra	15	4	3.9	2.3	3.2	–	–	–	–	–	–	–	–	–	–	88	4.7	2.1	2.3
Angola	9596	3200	2.8	2.9	3.2	27	23	16	52	53	42	37	42	48	5.6	58	7.4	5.7	4.7
Antigua and Barbuda	17	4	-0.6	2.2	1.6	–	–	–	–	–	–	–	–	–	–	30	-0.3	1.2	0.8
Argentina	12181	3383	1.5	1.3	1.1	9	8	8	23	22	17	67	72	76	2.2	92	2.0	1.6	1.2
Armenia	787	224	1.7	-1.4	0.0	5	8	9	23	21	15	70	68	74	1.7	64	2.3	-1.8	-0.1
Australia	4913	1342	1.5	1.1	1.3	9	7	7	20	15	13	71	77	82	1.8	89	1.5	1.4	1.4
Austria	1550	388	0.1	0.4	0.5	13	11	9	15	11	9	70	76	80	1.4	67	0.2	0.4	0.7
Azerbaijan	2671	764	1.7	1.2	1.0	7	7	7	29	27	19	65	66	71	2.2	52	2.0	0.7	1.1
Bahamas	106	28	2.0	1.8	1.4	7	6	6	31	24	17	66	70	74	2.0	84	2.9	2.0	1.5
Bahrain	251	70	4.0	2.8	2.5	9	4	3	40	29	18	62	72	76	2.2	89	4.3	2.8	2.2
Bangladesh	61091	16463	2.6	2.0	1.8	21	12	6	47	35	21	44	54	67	2.3	28	7.4	3.7	3.3
Barbados	55	14	0.4	-0.3	0.2	9	8	8	22	16	11	69	75	78	1.5	44	-0.3	1.3	1.7
Belarus	1785	476	0.6	-0.2	-0.5	7	11	15	16	14	10	71	71	69	1.3	74	2.7	0.4	0.2
Belgium	2171	598	0.2	0.3	0.5	12	11	10	14	12	11	71	76	80	1.8	97	0.3	0.3	0.5
Belize	129	36	2.2	2.8	2.5	8	5	4	40	36	24	66	72	77	2.8	52	1.8	2.9	3.1
Benin	4431	1490	2.8	3.3	3.7	22	15	9	46	46	39	45	54	62	5.4	42	6.4	4.3	4.2
Bhutan	260	70	3.1	0.2	2.7	23	14	7	47	39	21	41	52	66	2.6	34	8.0	4.6	5.6
Bolivia (Plurinational State of)	4225	1244	2.3	2.2	2.1	20	11	7	46	36	27	46	59	66	3.4	66	4.0	3.3	2.6
Bosnia and Herzegovina	717	171	0.9	-1.5	0.2	7	9	10	23	15	9	66	67	75	1.2	48	2.8	-0.6	1.4
Botswana	779	224	3.3	2.4	1.5	13	7	12	46	35	24	55	64	55	2.8	60	11.7	4.8	2.8
Brazil	60134	15655	2.2	1.5	1.3	10	7	6	35	24	16	59	66	73	1.8	86	3.6	2.5	1.8
Brunei Darussalam	128	37	3.4	2.6	2.3	7	3	3	36	28	20	67	74	77	2.1	75	3.7	3.4	2.6
Bulgaria	1255	354	0.2	-1.0	-0.7	9	12	15	16	12	10	71	71	74	1.4	71	1.4	-0.6	-0.3
Burkina Faso	8337	3073	2.3	2.8	3.7	23	17	13	47	48	47	41	47	53	5.8	25	6.6	5.4	7.1
Burundi	3772	1184	2.4	1.3	3.1	20	19	14	44	47	34	44	46	51	4.5	11	7.2	4.1	5.6
Cambodia	6036	1640	1.7	2.8	1.9	20	12	8	42	44	25	44	55	62	2.9	20	0.5	5.7	3.4
Cameroon	9306	3071	2.9	2.6	2.6	19	13	14	45	42	36	46	55	51	4.5	58	6.4	4.6	3.9
Canada	6878	1775	1.2	1.0	1.1	7	7	7	17	14	11	73	77	81	1.6	80	1.3	1.4	1.1
Cape Verde	220	59	1.4	2.1	1.8	12	8	5	40	38	24	56	66	72	2.7	60	5.5	4.1	2.9
Central African Republic	2088	659	2.4	2.5	2.1	23	17	17	43	41	35	42	49	47	4.7	39	3.8	2.7	2.2
Chad	5867	2024	2.5	3.2	3.6	21	16	16	46	48	45	45	51	49	6.1	27	5.5	4.4	4.9
Chile	4747	1243	1.6	1.6	1.2	10	6	5	29	23	15	62	74	79	1.9	89	2.1	1.9	1.4
China	335915	87282	1.7	1.0	0.8	8	7	7	33	22	14	62	68	73	1.8	46	3.8	4.1	3.5
Colombia	15937	4497	2.2	1.8	1.7	9	6	6	38	27	20	61	68	73	2.4	75	3.3	2.3	1.9
Comoros	299	99	3.0	2.3	2.5	18	11	7	47	37	32	48	56	66	3.9	28	4.9	2.4	2.3
Congo	1739	555	3.0	2.2	2.4	14	10	13	43	38	34	54	59	54	4.3	62	4.7	2.9	2.8
Cook Islands	8	2	-0.9	-0.1	1.5	–	–	–	–	–	–	–	–	–	–	74	-0.5	1.1	2.8
Costa Rica	1443	372	2.6	2.4	1.9	7	4	4	33	27	16	67	75	79	1.9	64	4.0	4.0	2.6
Côte d'Ivoire	9953	3178	4.4	3.2	2.5	19	11	11	53	41	34	47	57	58	4.5	50	6.1	4.1	3.7
Croatia	822	209	0.4	0.0	-0.3	10	11	12	15	12	10	69	72	76	1.4	57	1.9	0.3	0.2
Cuba	2441	595	1.0	0.5	0.1	7	7	7	29	17	10	70	75	79	1.5	75	2.0	0.8	0.1
Cyprus	194	49	0.5	1.4	1.3	10	8	7	19	19	12	71	77	80	1.5	70	3.0	1.7	1.4
Czech Republic	1821	535	0.2	-0.1	0.2	12	12	11	16	12	11	70	72	77	1.5	74	1.0	-0.2	0.1
Democratic People's Republic of Korea	6410	1561	1.7	1.3	0.6	7	6	10	35	21	14	62	71	68	1.9	60	2.1	1.4	0.6
Democratic Republic of the Congo	35353	11982	3.0	3.2	3.3	21	18	17	48	51	44	44	48	48	5.9	35	2.6	3.9	4.6
Denmark	1209	318	0.2	0.4	0.3	10	12	10	16	12	11	73	75	79	1.8	87	0.5	0.4	0.5
Djibouti	372	108	6.2	2.6	2.1	21	14	11	49	42	28	43	51	56	3.8	76	7.2	2.7	1.9
Dominica	13	3	0.3	-0.1	-0.3	–	–	–	–	–	–	–	–	–	–	67	2.1	-0.2	-0.2
Dominican Republic	3781	1087	2.4	1.8	1.7	11	6	6	42	30	22	58	68	73	2.6	68	3.9	2.9	2.6
Ecuador	5046	1381	2.7	1.8	1.3	12	6	5	42	29	20	58	69	75	2.5	66	4.4	2.7	2.2
Egypt	31695	9559	2.4	1.9	2.1	16	8	6	40	33	24	50	63	70	2.8	43	2.6	1.8	2.0
El Salvador	2415	607	1.8	1.1	0.4	13	8	7	43	32	20	57	66	72	2.3	64	2.9	2.9	1.3
Equatorial Guinea	322	106	1.3	3.3	3.1	25	20	15	39	49	38	40	47	51	5.3	40	2.6	4.4	2.9
Eritrea	2432	832	2.7	1.5	4.1	21	16	8	47	40	36	43	48	60	4.5	21	3.8	2.6	5.6
Estonia	249	76	0.7	-1.3	-0.3	11	13	13	15	14	12	71	69	73	1.7	69	1.1	-1.6	-0.2
Ethiopia	41831	13581	2.6	3.0	2.9	21	18	12	47	48	38	43	47	56	5.2	17	4.5	4.7	3.8
Fiji	318	87	1.6	1.0	0.7	8	6	7	34	29	21	60	67	69	2.7	51	2.5	2.4	1.4
Finland	1088	293	0.4	0.4	0.4	10	10	9	14	13	11	70	75	80	1.8	85	1.5	0.7	0.7

	Population (thousands) 2009		Population annual growth rate (%)			Crude death rate			Crude birth rate			Life expectancy			Total fertility rate 2009	% of population urbanized 2009	Average annual growth rate of urban population (%)		
	under 10	under 5	1970–1990	1990–2000	2000–2009	1970	1990	2009	1970	1990	2009	1970	1990	2009			1970–1990	1990–2000	2000–2009
France	13698	3859	0.6	0.4	0.7	11	10	9	17	13	12	72	77	81	1.9	85	0.8	0.8	1.6
Gabon	636	183	2.8	2.9	2.2	20	11	10	34	38	27	47	61	61	3.2	86	6.7	4.3	2.7
Gambia	831	271	3.7	3.7	3.4	24	15	11	49	44	36	41	51	56	5.0	57	7.0	6.2	4.7
Georgia	921	245	0.7	-1.4	-1.3	9	9	12	19	17	12	67	71	72	1.6	53	1.4	-1.8	-1.2
Germany	13666	3392	0.1	0.3	0.0	12	11	10	14	11	8	71	76	80	1.3	74	0.1	0.3	0.1
Ghana	10726	3365	2.7	2.7	2.5	17	11	11	47	39	32	49	57	57	4.2	51	3.8	4.5	3.8
Greece	1917	537	0.7	0.7	0.2	8	9	10	17	10	10	72	77	80	1.4	61	1.3	0.9	0.5
Grenada	36	10	0.1	0.5	0.3	9	8	6	28	28	20	64	69	76	2.3	39	0.3	1.3	1.1
Guatemala	6834	2142	2.5	2.3	2.8	15	9	5	44	39	32	52	62	71	4.0	49	3.2	3.2	3.4
Guinea	4972	1667	2.3	3.1	2.3	26	18	11	49	47	39	39	48	58	5.3	35	5.2	4.1	3.4
Guinea-Bissau	787	269	2.6	2.4	2.6	26	20	17	46	42	41	37	44	48	5.7	30	5.7	3.0	2.4
Guyana	269	66	0.3	0.1	0.1	11	9	8	38	25	17	60	62	67	2.3	29	0.3	-0.2	0.0
Haiti	4316	1259	2.1	2.0	1.9	18	13	9	39	37	27	47	55	61	3.4	50	3.9	4.2	5.6
Holy See	–	–	–	–	–	–	–	–	–	–	–	–	–	–	–	100	–	–	–
Honduras	3311	964	3.0	2.4	2.3	15	7	5	47	38	27	52	66	72	3.2	51	4.7	3.6	3.3
Hungary	1840	490	0.0	-0.1	-0.3	11	14	13	15	12	10	69	69	74	1.4	68	0.5	-0.3	0.3
Iceland	81	23	1.1	1.0	1.7	7	7	6	21	17	15	74	78	82	2.1	93	1.4	1.2	1.6
India	447401	126114	2.2	1.9	1.7	16	11	8	38	32	22	49	58	64	2.7	30	3.5	2.7	2.4
Indonesia	74403	20732	2.1	1.5	1.4	17	9	6	41	26	18	48	62	71	2.1	44	5.0	4.6	1.8
Iran (Islamic Republic of)	22221	6555	3.4	1.6	1.3	14	7	6	43	34	19	54	65	72	1.8	70	5.0	3.0	2.1
Iraq	14672	4491	2.9	3.1	2.8	12	7	6	45	38	31	58	64	68	4.0	66	3.9	2.8	2.2
Ireland	1101	343	0.9	0.8	2.1	11	9	6	22	15	16	71	75	80	2.0	62	1.3	1.2	2.4
Israel	2331	697	2.2	3.0	2.1	7	6	5	27	22	20	71	76	81	2.8	92	2.6	3.1	1.9
Italy	10219	2899	0.3	0.0	0.6	10	10	10	17	10	9	71	77	81	1.4	68	0.5	0.1	0.7
Jamaica	973	254	1.2	0.8	0.7	8	7	7	35	26	19	68	71	72	2.4	52	2.1	1.3	0.7
Japan	20551	5304	0.8	0.3	0.0	7	7	9	19	10	8	72	79	83	1.3	67	1.7	0.6	0.3
Jordan	2582	765	3.5	4.0	3.3	16	6	4	52	37	25	54	67	73	3.0	78	4.8	4.8	2.9
Kazakhstan	4540	1441	1.2	-1.0	0.6	9	9	11	26	23	20	62	67	65	2.3	58	1.7	-1.0	0.9
Kenya	19652	6721	3.7	2.9	2.9	15	10	11	51	42	38	52	60	55	4.9	22	6.5	3.7	3.8
Kiribati	36	10	2.5	1.6	1.9	–	–	–	–	–	–	–	–	–	–	44	4.3	3.6	1.9
Kuwait	817	254	5.3	0.4	3.7	6	2	2	48	24	17	66	75	78	2.2	98	6.0	0.4	3.3
Kyrgyzstan	1961	563	2.0	1.2	1.3	11	8	7	31	31	22	60	66	68	2.5	35	2.0	0.5	1.0
Lao People's Democratic Republic	2832	789	2.2	2.5	2.0	18	13	7	43	41	27	46	54	65	3.4	32	4.6	6.0	6.0
Latvia	390	112	0.6	-1.2	-0.7	11	13	14	14	14	10	70	69	73	1.4	68	1.3	-1.3	-0.6
Lebanon	1303	322	1.0	2.4	1.4	9	7	7	33	26	16	65	69	72	1.8	87	2.7	2.7	1.4
Lesotho	955	271	2.2	1.6	1.1	17	11	17	43	36	29	49	59	46	3.3	26	4.6	5.2	4.0
Liberia	1950	640	2.1	2.7	4.2	21	18	10	47	47	38	44	49	59	5.0	47	4.3	3.4	4.5
Libyan Arab Jamahiriya	2258	709	3.9	2.0	2.3	16	4	4	49	26	23	51	68	74	2.6	78	6.0	2.1	2.2
Liechtenstein	7	2	1.5	1.3	1.1	–	–	–	–	–	–	–	–	–	–	14	1.1	0.1	0.4
Lithuania	629	152	0.8	-0.5	-0.8	9	11	13	17	15	10	71	71	72	1.4	67	2.4	-0.6	-0.7
Luxembourg	105	27	0.6	1.3	1.3	12	10	8	13	13	11	70	75	80	1.7	85	1.0	1.7	1.3
Madagascar	9759	3104	2.7	3.0	3.1	21	15	9	48	45	35	44	51	61	4.6	30	5.3	4.4	3.9
Malawi	8106	2634	3.7	2.2	3.2	24	17	12	56	50	40	41	49	54	5.5	19	6.9	5.0	5.5
Malaysia	9700	2727	2.6	2.5	2.1	9	5	5	37	30	20	61	70	75	2.5	71	4.5	4.7	3.4
Maldives	110	27	2.9	2.3	1.6	17	9	5	40	40	19	50	60	72	2.0	39	6.7	3.0	5.2
Mali	6649	2259	1.8	2.0	2.7	27	21	15	48	47	42	38	43	49	5.4	35	4.2	3.9	4.8
Malta	80	18	0.9	0.8	0.6	9	8	8	17	15	9	70	76	80	1.3	94	0.9	1.0	0.8
Marshall Islands	23	6	4.2	1.0	2.2	–	–	–	–	–	–	–	–	–	–	71	5.2	1.5	2.4
Mauritania	1514	481	2.7	2.7	2.9	18	12	10	47	40	33	48	56	57	4.4	41	7.7	2.8	2.9
Mauritius	358	89	1.2	1.2	0.9	7	6	7	28	20	14	62	69	72	1.8	42	1.4	0.9	0.6
Mexico	37564	10163	2.4	1.8	1.2	10	5	5	43	28	18	61	71	76	2.2	78	3.3	2.2	1.5
Micronesia (Federated States of)	49	13	2.2	1.1	0.4	9	7	6	41	34	25	62	66	69	3.5	23	2.4	-0.4	0.5
Monaco	6	2	1.1	0.9	0.3	–	–	–	–	–	–	–	–	–	–	100	1.1	0.9	0.3
Mongolia	862	234	2.8	0.8	1.4	14	9	7	42	33	19	53	61	67	2.0	62	4.0	0.7	2.1
Montenegro	146	38	0.6	1.2	-0.7	3	5	10	10	11	12	69	76	74	1.6	62	3.5	3.2	-0.1
Morocco	10997	3079	2.4	1.5	1.3	17	8	6	47	30	20	52	64	72	2.3	58	4.1	2.5	2.0
Mozambique	11561	3842	1.8	3.0	2.8	25	21	16	48	43	38	39	43	48	5.0	38	8.3	6.7	4.8
Myanmar	16124	4631	2.2	1.3	0.9	15	11	10	40	27	20	51	59	62	2.3	33	2.6	2.5	2.7
Namibia	952	279	3.0	2.5	2.2	15	8	8	43	38	27	53	62	62	3.3	37	4.1	4.1	3.6
Nauru	4	1	1.7	0.9	0.2	–	–	–	–	–	–	–	–	–	–	100	1.7	0.9	0.2
Nepal	12712	3505	2.4	2.5	2.3	21	13	6	44	39	25	43	54	67	2.8	18	6.4	6.6	5.4

TABLE 6. DEMOGRAPHIC INDICATORS

	Population (thousands) 2009		Population annual growth rate (%)			Crude death rate			Crude birth rate			Life expectancy			Total fertility rate 2009	% of population urbanized 2009	Average annual growth rate of urban population (%)		
	under 18	under 5	1970–1990	1990–2000	2000–2009	1970	1990	2009	1970	1990	2009	1970	1990	2009			1970–1990	1990–2000	2000–2009
Netherlands	3562	943	0.7	0.6	0.5	8	9	8	17	13	11	74	77	80	1.7	82	1.2	1.7	1.2
New Zealand	1063	290	0.9	1.3	1.2	9	8	7	22	17	14	71	75	80	2.0	86	1.1	1.4	1.1
Nicaragua	2420	679	2.7	2.1	1.5	13	7	5	46	37	24	54	64	73	2.7	57	3.3	2.5	1.8
Niger	8611	3280	2.9	3.3	4.1	27	24	15	57	56	53	38	42	52	7.1	17	5.7	3.9	4.2
Nigeria	75994	25426	2.7	2.5	2.7	24	20	16	47	46	39	40	45	48	5.2	49	4.9	4.4	4.0
Niue	1	0	–	–	–	–	–	–	–	–	–	–	–	–	–	37	-2.0	-1.3	-1.4
Norway	1108	296	0.4	0.6	0.9	10	11	9	17	14	12	74	77	81	1.9	79	0.9	1.1	1.2
Occupied Palestinian Territory	2204	708	3.4	3.8	3.8	19	7	4	49	46	35	54	68	74	4.9	74	4.5	4.4	3.7
Oman	1067	297	4.5	2.6	2.1	17	4	3	50	38	22	49	70	76	3.0	73	8.5	3.4	2.1
Pakistan	78786	24121	3.1	2.5	2.5	16	10	7	43	40	30	54	61	67	3.9	36	4.2	3.3	3.0
Palau	7	2	1.4	2.6	0.7	–	–	–	–	–	–	–	–	–	–	82	2.2	2.6	2.5
Panama	1196	345	2.4	2.0	2.0	8	5	5	37	26	20	65	72	76	2.5	74	3.0	4.0	3.1
Papua New Guinea	3112	961	2.4	2.7	2.8	19	11	8	42	37	31	43	54	61	4.0	13	4.5	1.4	1.9
Paraguay	2563	739	2.7	2.3	2.1	7	6	6	37	33	24	65	68	72	3.0	61	4.0	3.6	3.0
Peru	10591	2969	2.5	1.8	1.4	14	7	5	42	30	21	53	66	73	2.5	77	3.4	2.4	1.8
Philippines	37033	10800	2.7	2.2	2.1	11	7	5	40	33	24	57	65	72	3.0	49	4.6	2.1	2.1
Poland	7166	1832	0.8	0.1	-0.1	8	10	10	17	15	10	70	71	76	1.3	46	2.9	-1.1	-1.0
Portugal	1971	531	0.7	0.2	0.6	11	10	10	21	11	10	67	74	79	1.4	60	1.8	1.5	1.6
Qatar	272	83	7.2	2.8	10.3	13	3	2	34	23	12	60	69	76	2.4	96	7.4	3.1	9.1
Republic of Korea	10176	2278	1.6	0.8	0.5	10	6	6	32	16	9	59	71	80	1.2	83	4.5	1.5	0.9
Republic of Moldova	786	208	1.0	-0.6	-1.6	10	10	13	18	19	12	65	68	69	1.5	61	1.6	0.2	-0.2
Romania	3961	1057	0.7	-0.5	-0.5	9	11	12	21	14	10	68	69	73	1.3	57	2.1	-0.5	0.3
Russian Federation	25780	7491	0.6	-0.1	-0.5	9	12	15	14	14	11	69	68	67	1.4	73	1.4	-0.1	-0.5
Rwanda	4865	1694	3.2	1.1	2.9	20	32	14	53	45	41	44	33	51	5.3	19	5.8	10.4	5.9
Saint Kitts and Nevis	10	2	-0.5	1.2	1.4	–	–	–	–	–	–	–	–	–	–	32	-0.4	0.7	1.1
Saint Lucia	56	15	1.4	1.3	1.1	8	7	6	41	25	18	64	71	74	2.0	28	2.4	0.8	1.0
Saint Vincent and the Grenadines	36	9	0.9	0.0	0.2	11	7	7	40	25	17	61	69	72	2.1	49	2.4	0.9	1.0
Samoa	84	21	0.6	0.9	0.2	10	7	5	39	34	23	55	65	72	3.9	20	0.8	1.3	-0.7
San Marino	6	2	1.2	1.1	1.9	–	–	–	–	–	–	–	–	–	–	94	3.2	1.4	1.7
Sao Tome and Principe	77	23	2.3	1.9	1.9	13	10	7	47	38	32	55	62	66	3.7	61	4.2	3.9	3.2
Saudi Arabia	9874	2864	5.2	2.5	2.6	18	5	4	48	36	23	52	68	73	3.0	82	7.5	2.9	2.6
Senegal	6333	2094	3.0	2.7	2.9	23	14	11	51	44	38	43	52	56	4.9	42	4.3	3.1	3.1
Serbia	2132	570	0.8	0.6	-0.4	9	10	12	18	15	12	68	72	74	1.6	56	2.0	1.1	0.3
Seychelles	43	14	1.6	1.2	0.5	–	–	–	–	–	–	–	–	–	–	55	2.7	1.5	1.2
Sierra Leone	2827	964	2.1	0.3	3.7	28	24	15	46	42	40	36	40	48	5.2	38	3.8	1.1	4.1
Singapore	993	198	1.9	2.9	2.1	5	5	5	23	18	8	69	75	81	1.3	100	1.9	2.9	1.8
Slovakia	1047	270	0.7	0.2	0.1	10	10	10	19	15	10	70	72	75	1.3	55	2.3	0.2	-0.2
Slovenia	342	96	0.7	0.3	0.2	10	10	10	17	11	10	69	73	79	1.4	50	2.3	0.4	-0.1
Solomon Islands	239	73	3.3	2.8	2.9	10	12	6	46	40	30	54	57	67	3.8	18	5.5	4.2	4.2
Somalia	4667	1637	3.0	1.1	2.6	24	20	16	51	45	44	40	45	50	6.4	37	4.4	2.3	3.6
South Africa	18285	5175	2.5	2.0	1.4	14	8	15	38	29	22	53	61	52	2.5	61	2.9	2.9	2.0
Spain	7956	2422	0.7	0.4	1.4	9	8	9	20	10	11	72	77	81	1.5	77	1.4	0.5	1.3
Sri Lanka	5850	1784	1.6	0.8	0.9	9	7	7	31	21	18	63	69	74	2.3	14	0.8	-0.8	-0.2
Sudan	19352	5880	2.9	2.5	2.4	19	14	10	46	41	31	46	53	58	4.1	39	5.3	4.8	4.0
Suriname	177	48	0.4	1.4	1.3	8	7	8	37	24	19	63	67	69	2.4	69	1.8	2.2	1.9
Swaziland	561	160	3.3	2.2	1.2	18	9	15	49	43	30	48	61	46	3.5	21	7.6	2.1	0.5
Sweden	1907	536	0.3	0.3	0.5	10	11	10	14	14	12	74	78	81	1.9	85	0.4	0.5	0.6
Switzerland	1431	366	0.4	0.7	0.7	9	9	8	16	12	10	73	78	82	1.5	74	1.6	0.7	0.6
Syrian Arab Republic	9001	2868	3.5	2.6	3.5	13	5	3	47	37	27	55	68	74	3.2	55	4.1	3.2	3.8
Tajikistan	3081	879	2.9	1.5	1.5	10	8	6	40	39	28	60	63	67	3.4	26	2.2	-0.3	1.3
Thailand	17902	4847	2.1	1.0	1.0	10	6	9	37	20	14	59	69	69	1.8	34	3.8	1.5	1.8
The former Yugoslav Republic of Macedonia	459	110	1.0	0.5	0.2	8	8	9	24	17	11	66	71	74	1.4	59	2.0	0.8	0.1
Timor-Leste	589	193	1.0	1.0	4.1	22	18	8	46	43	40	40	46	62	6.4	28	3.4	2.5	5.2
Togo	3082	958	3.1	2.9	2.9	18	11	8	48	42	32	49	58	63	4.2	43	4.8	4.8	4.3
Tonga	46	14	-0.2	0.4	0.7	6	6	6	37	30	27	65	70	72	3.9	23	0.4	0.6	0.7
Trinidad and Tobago	340	94	1.1	0.6	0.4	7	7	8	27	21	15	66	69	70	1.6	14	-0.5	3.0	2.9
Tunisia	2961	788	2.4	1.4	1.0	14	6	6	39	27	16	54	69	74	1.8	67	3.8	2.3	1.5
Turkey	24142	6561	2.2	1.7	1.5	12	8	6	39	26	18	56	65	72	2.1	69	4.4	2.6	2.1
Turkmenistan	1848	519	2.6	2.0	1.6	11	8	8	37	35	22	58	63	65	2.4	49	2.3	2.2	2.2
Tuvalu	4	1	1.0	0.7	0.5	–	–	–	–	–	–	–	–	–	–	50	4.0	1.9	1.4
Uganda	18276	6368	3.2	3.2	3.6	16	17	12	49	49	46	50	48	53	6.3	13	5.7	4.1	4.2

	Population (thousands) 2009		Population annual growth rate (%)			Crude death rate			Crude birth rate			Life expectancy			Total fertility rate 2009	% of popula-tion urbanized 2009	Average annual growth rate of urban population (%)		
	under 18	under 5	1970–1990	1990–2000	2000–2009	1970	1990	2009	1970	1990	2009	1970	1990	2009			1970–1990	1990–2000	2000–2009
Ukraine	8024	2193	0.4	-0.5	-0.8	9	13	16	15	13	10	71	70	68	1.4	69	1.4	-0.5	-0.5
United Arab Emirates	1019	307	10.6	5.5	4.4	11	3	2	36	27	14	61	73	78	1.9	84	10.7	5.7	4.3
United Kingdom	13100	3662	0.1	0.3	0.6	12	11	10	16	14	12	72	76	80	1.9	80	0.2	0.4	0.6
United Republic of Tanzania	22416	7792	3.1	2.9	3.1	18	15	11	48	44	41	47	51	56	5.5	26	7.5	4.6	4.5
United States	77319	21823	1.0	1.2	1.1	9	9	8	16	16	14	71	75	79	2.1	82	1.1	1.7	1.4
Uruguay	926	248	0.5	0.7	0.1	10	10	9	21	18	15	69	73	76	2.1	92	0.9	0.9	0.3
Uzbekistan	9977	2585	2.7	1.9	1.3	10	7	7	36	35	20	63	67	68	2.2	36	3.1	1.2	0.8
Vanuatu	109	34	2.8	2.4	2.9	14	7	5	43	37	30	53	64	70	3.9	25	4.9	3.9	4.3
Venezuela (Bolivarian Republic of)	10161	2924	3.1	2.1	2.0	7	5	5	37	29	21	65	71	74	2.5	93	3.8	2.8	2.1
Viet Nam	28172	7238	2.2	1.7	1.4	18	8	5	41	31	17	49	65	75	2.0	30	2.7	3.6	3.4
Yemen	12062	3829	3.3	3.9	3.2	27	13	7	56	51	36	38	54	63	5.1	31	5.5	6.2	4.8
Zambia	6851	2327	3.2	2.8	2.6	17	15	17	49	44	42	49	51	46	5.7	36	4.5	1.6	2.6
Zimbabwe	6001	1717	3.5	1.7	0.1	13	9	15	48	37	30	55	61	46	3.4	38	6.1	3.3	1.4

SUMMARY INDICATORS

Africa#	473927	154528	2.8	2.5	2.6	20	15	12	46	42	35	46	53	56	4.5	40	4.3	3.6	3.4
Sub-Saharan Africa#	414349	137009	2.8	2.6	2.8	21	16	14	47	44	38	45	50	53	5.0	37	4.7	4.1	3.8
Eastern and Southern Africa	192017	62944	2.8	2.6	2.7	19	15	13	47	43	37	46	51	53	4.8	30	4.7	3.9	3.4
West and Central Africa	202608	68077	2.8	2.7	2.9	22	18	15	48	46	40	42	48	51	5.2	43	4.6	4.1	4.1
Middle East and North Africa	156647	46917	3.1	2.2	2.2	16	8	6	45	35	24	52	64	70	2.8	59	4.4	2.9	2.6
Asia#	1172419	323529	2.0	1.5	1.4	13	9	7	37	27	19	55	63	69	2.3	39	3.8	3.4	2.8
South Asia	621106	177114	2.3	2.0	1.9	17	11	8	40	33	23	49	58	64	2.8	30	3.8	2.9	2.6
East Asia and Pacific	551312	146415	1.8	1.2	1.0	10	7	7	35	23	15	59	67	73	1.9	46	3.9	3.7	3.0
Latin America and Caribbean	194445	53079	2.2	1.6	1.4	10	7	6	37	27	18	60	68	74	2.2	79	3.2	2.3	1.8
CEE/CIS	96724	26876	1.0	0.2	0.1	9	11	12	20	18	14	67	68	69	1.7	70	1.9	0.3	0.2
Industrialized countries§	204686	56301	0.7	0.6	0.7	10	9	9	17	13	11	71	76	80	1.7	74	1.0	1.0	1.0
Developing countries§	1970587	569072	2.2	1.7	1.6	13	9	8	38	30	22	55	62	67	2.7	45	3.8	3.1	2.7
Least developed countries§	390642	124367	2.6	2.5	2.6	21	16	11	47	42	34	44	51	57	4.3	29	4.9	4.2	4.0
World	2219545	637723	1.8	1.4	1.4	12	10	8	32	26	20	59	65	69	2.5	50	2.6	2.3	2.1

For a complete list of countries and territories in the regions and subregions, see page 124.
§ Includes territories within each country category or regional group. Countries and territories in each country category or regional group are listed on page 124.

DEFINITIONS OF THE INDICATORS

Life expectancy at birth – Number of years newborn children would live if subject to the mortality risks prevailing for the cross section of population at the time of their birth.

Crude death rate – Annual number of deaths per 1,000 population.

Crude birth rate – Annual number of births per 1,000 population.

Total fertility rate – Number of children who would be born per woman if she lived to the end of her childbearing years and bore children at each age in accordance with prevailing age-specific fertility rates.

Urban population – Percentage of population living in urban areas as defined according to the national definition used in the most recent population census.

MAIN DATA SOURCES

Child population – United Nations Population Division.

Crude death and birth rates – United Nations Population Division.

Life expectancy – United Nations Population Division.

Fertility – United Nations Population Division.

Urban population – United Nations Population Division.

NOTES — Data not available.

TABLE 7. ECONOMIC INDICATORS

Countries and territories	GNI per capita (US$) 2009	GDP per capita average annual growth rate (%) 1970–1990	GDP per capita average annual growth rate (%) 1990–2009	Average annual rate of inflation (%) 1990–2009	% of population below international poverty line of US$1.25 per day 1994–2008*	% of central government expenditure (1998–2008*) allocated to: health	% of central government expenditure (1998–2008*) allocated to: education	% of central government expenditure (1998–2008*) allocated to: defence	ODA inflow in millions US$ 2008	ODA inflow as a % of recipient GNI 2008	Debt service as a % of exports of goods and services 1990	Debt service as a % of exports of goods and services 2008
Afghanistan	370 x	–	–	–	–	–	–	–	4865	–	–	–
Albania	3950	-0.7 x	5.4	15	<2	4	2	4	386	3	4 x	2
Algeria	4420	1.6	1.5	12	7	4	24	17	316	0	62	–
Andorra	41130	–	–	3 x	–	–	–	–	–	–	–	–
Angola	3490	–	3.8	253	54	6 x	15 x	34 x	369	1	7	2
Antigua and Barbuda	12130	8.3 x	2	2	–	–	–	–	8	1	–	–
Argentina	7600	-0.7	1.9	7	3	5	5	3	131	0	30	9
Armenia	3100	–	6.2	56	4	–	–	–	303	3	–	11
Australia	43770	1.5	2.3	3	–	15	9	6	–	–	–	–
Austria	46850	2.4	1.9	2	–	16	9	2	–	–	–	–
Azerbaijan	4840	–	4.9	58	<2	1	4	12	235	1	–	1
Bahamas	21390 x	1.9	1.1 x	3 x	–	16	20	3	–	–	–	–
Bahrain	25420 x	-1.3 x	2.8 x	3 x	–	8	15	14	–	–	–	–
Bangladesh	590	0.4	3.4	4	50	7	15	10	2061	2	17	4
Barbados	d	1.7	2.2 x	3 x	–	–	–	–	5	–	–	–
Belarus	5540	–	4.2	133	<2	2	4	3	110	0	–	3
Belgium	45310	2.2	1.7	2	–	16	3	3	–	–	–	–
Belize	3740 x	2.9	2.2 x	1 x	13	8 x	20 x	5 x	25	2	5	10
Benin	750	0.3	1.2	6	47	6 x	31 x	1/ x	641	11	7	7x
Bhutan	2020	–	5.2	7	26	9	13	–	87	7	–	–
Bolivia (Plurinational State of)	1630	-1.1	1.6	7	12	9	24	6	628	4	31	11
Bosnia and Herzegovina	4700	–	9.6 x	5 x	<2	–	–	–	482	3	–	4
Botswana	6260	8.2	3.6	9	31	5 x	26 x	8 x	716	6	4	1
Brazil	8070	2.3	1.4	59	5	6	6	3	460	0	19	22
Brunei Darussalam	d	-2.2 x	-0.3 x	5 x	–	–	–	–	–	–	–	–
Bulgaria	5770	3.4 x	2.8	43	<2	11	5	6	–	–	19	12
Burkina Faso	510	1.4	2.4	3	57	7 x	17 x	14 x	998	14	6	–
Burundi	150	1.1	-1.8	12	81	2	15	23	509	47	41	28
Cambodia	650	–	6.3 x	4 x	26	–	–	–	743	8	0 x	1
Cameroon	1170	3.4	0.7	4	33	3	12	10	525	2	18	5
Canada	42170	2	2.1	2	–	9	2	6	–	–	–	–
Cape Verde	3010	–	4.1	3	21	–	–	–	219	14	5	3
Central African Republic	450	-1.3	-0.8	3	62	–	–	–	256	14	8	–
Chad	620	-1	3	6	62	8 x	8 x	–	416	7	2	–
Chile	9460	1.5	3.5	6	<2	16	18	5	73	0	20	18
China	3620	6.6	9	5	16	0	1	7	1489	0	10	2
Colombia	4950	1.9	1.4	14	16	9	20	13	972	0	39	16
Comoros	870	0.1 x	-0.2	4	46	–	–	–	37	8	2	–
Congo	1830	3.1	0.5	8	54	4	4	10	505	7	31	1x
Cook Islands	–	–	–	–	–	–	–	–	6	–	–	0
Costa Rica	6260	0.7	2.6	12	<2	20	24	–	66	0	21	10
Côte d'Ivoire	1060	-1.9	-1	5	23	4 x	21 x	4 x	617	3	26	9
Croatia	13810	–	2.9	29	<2	16	9	4	397	1	–	32x
Cuba	c	–	3.6 x	4 x	–	23 x	10 x	–	127	–	–	–
Cyprus	26940 x	5.9 x	2.2 x	4 x	–	6	12	4	–	–	–	–
Czech Republic	17310	–	2.5	7	<2	16	9	3	–	–	–	–
Democratic People's Republic of Korea	a	–	–	–	–	–	–	–	218	–	–	–
Democratic Republic of the Congo	160	-2.3	-3.5	261	59	0 x	0 x	18 x	1610	16	–	–
Denmark	58930	2	1.7	2	–	0	10	4	–	–	–	–
Djibouti	1280	–	-1.4	3	19	–	–	–	121	13	4 x	5
Dominica	4900	4.7 x	1.7	2	–	–	–	–	22	6	4	10
Dominican Republic	4530	2.1	3.8	11	4	10	13	4	153	0	7	7
Ecuador	3940	1.3	1.6	5	5	11 x	18 x	13 x	231	0	27	11
Egypt	2070	4.1	2.6	7	<2	4	12	7	1348	1	18	5
El Salvador	3370	-1.9	2.7	4	6	15	14	3	233	1	14	10
Equatorial Guinea	12420	–	19.8	12	–	–	–	–	38	0	–	–
Eritrea	300 x	–	-0.8 x	14 x	–	–	–	–	143	10	–	–
Estonia	14060	1.5 x	5.3	20	<2	16	7	5	–	–	–	–
Ethiopia	330	–	2.7	6	39	1	5	17	3327	15	33	3
Fiji	3950	0.7	4	1	–	9 x	18 x	6 x	45	1	12	1
Finland	45680	2.8	2.7	2	–	3	10	4	–	–	–	–
France	43990	2.2	1.4	2	–	16 x	7 x	6 x	–	–	–	–
Gabon	7370	0.2	-0.9	6	5	–	–	–	55	1	4	1x

	GNI per capita (US$) 2009	GDP per capita average annual growth rate (%)		Average annual rate of inflation (%) 1990–2009	% of population below international poverty line of US$1.25 per day 1994–2008*	% of central government expenditure (1998–2008*) allocated to:			ODA inflow in millions US$ 2008	ODA inflow as a % of recipient GNI 2008	Debt service as a % of exports of goods and services	
		1970–1990	1990–2009			health	education	defence			1990	2008
Gambia	440	0.7	0.6	8	34	7 x	12 x	4 x	94	14	18	7
Georgia	2530	–	–	82	13	6	9	36	888	8	–	3
Germany	42560	2.3	1.3	1	–	20	1	4	–	–	–	–
Ghana	700	-2	2.2	23	30	7 x	22 x	5 x	1293	8	21	3
Greece	28630	1.3	2.7	6	–	7	11	8	–	–	–	–
Grenada	5580	4.2 x	3.1	3	–	10 x	17 x	–	33	5	2	10
Guatemala	2630	0.2	1.4	7	12	11 x	17 x	11 x	536	1	11	12
Guinea	370	0.2 x	3.3	7	70	3 x	11 x	29 x	319	–	18	8
Guinea-Bissau	510	0.1	-9.6	29	49	1 x	3 x	4 x	132	34	21	–
Guyana	1450 x	-1.6	3 x	8 x	8	–	–	–	166	15	20 x	2
Haiti	a	–	-1.1 x	15 x	55	–	–	–	912	14	5	2
Holy See	–	–	–	–	–	–	–	–	–	–	–	0
Honduras	1820	0.8	1.6	14	18	10 x	19 x	7 x	564	4	30	4
Hungary	12980	3	3.2	12	<2	11	8	3	–	–	–	–
Iceland	43220	3.2	2.4	4	–	17	8	0	–	–	–	–
India	1170	2.1	4.8	6	42	2	5	12	2108	0	25	8
Indonesia	2230	4.7	2.5	15	29	1	4	7	1225	0	31	13
Iran (Islamic Republic of)	4530	-2.3	2.7	22	<2	7	8	10	98	–	1	–
Iraq	2210	–	-2.6 x	14 x	–	–	–	–	9870	–	–	–
Ireland	44310	2.8	5.2	4	–	16 x	14 x	3 x	–	–	–	–
Israel	25740	1.9	1.8	6	–	13	16	18	–	–	–	–
Italy	35080	2.8	1	3	–	14	11	4	–	–	–	–
Jamaica	5020	-1.3	0.7	16	<2	6	17	2	79	1	20	14
Japan	37870	3	0.9	-1	–	2 x	6 x	4 x	–	–	–	–
Jordan	3740	2.5 x	2.5	3	<2	10	16	19	742	4	18	15
Kazakhstan	6740	–	3.8	63	<2	5	7	8	333	0	–	42
Kenya	770	1.2	0.2	10	20	7	26	6	1360	5	26	4
Kiribati	1890	-5.3	1.8	3	–	–	–	–	27	14	–	–
Kuwait	43930 x	-6.8 x	2 x	5 x	–	5	8	6	–	–	–	–
Kyrgyzstan	870	–	0.3	40	3	12	11	7	360	9	–	8
Lao People's Democratic Republic	880	–	4.2	23	44	–	–	–	496	11	8	19x
Latvia	12390	3.4	4.7	19	<2	11	13	5	–	–	0 x	35
Lebanon	7970	–	2.2	8	–	2	7	11	1076	4	–	13
Lesotho	1020	2.8	1.6	8	43	9	18	4	143	7	4	2
Liberia	160	-4.2	1.8	37	84	5 x	11 x	9 x	1250	197	–	12
Libyan Arab Jamahiriya	12020	–	2.9 x	18 x	–	–	–	–	60	0	–	–
Liechtenstein	113210 x	2.2	3.1 x	1 x	–	–	–	–	–	–	–	–
Lithuania	11410	–	3.5	24	<2	11	7	4	–	–	–	30
Luxembourg	74430	2.7	3	3	–	13	10	1	–	–	–	–
Madagascar	420 x	-2.3	-0.1	14	68	7	18	6	841	11	32	5x
Malawi	280	-0.1	0.5	28	74	7 x	12 x	5 x	913	22	23	–
Malaysia	7230	4	3.2	4	<2	6 x	23 x	11 x	158	0	12	3
Maldives	3870	–	5.9 x	1 x	–	13	15	6	54	5	4	5
Mali	680	0.2	2.9	5	51	2 x	9 x	8 x	964	13	8	3x
Malta	16690 x	6.5	2.6 x	3 x	–	14	13	2	–	–	–	–
Marshall Islands	3060	–	-1.1	4	–	–	–	–	53	27	–	–
Mauritania	960	-1	0.8	8	21	4 x	23 x	–	311	–	24	–
Mauritius	7240	3.2 x	3.5	6	–	8	15	1	110	1	6	3
Mexico	8960	1.6	1.5	13	4	5	25	3	149	0	16	12
Micronesia (Federated States of)	2220	–	0.1	2	–	–	–	–	94	36	–	–
Monaco	203900 x	1.6	2 x	2 x	–	–	–	–	–	–	–	–
Mongolia	1630	–	2.9	27	2	6	9	9	246	6	17 x	2x
Montenegro	6550	–	3.8 x	–	<2	–	–	–	106	3	–	–
Morocco	2790	1.9	2.3	3	3	3	18	13	1217	2	18	10
Mozambique	440	-1	4.3	18	75	5 x	10 x	35 x	1994	25	21	1
Myanmar	a	1.4	8.2 x	24 x	–	3	13	23	534	–	17	1x
Namibia	4310	-2.1 x	2	10	49	10 x	22 x	7 x	207	2	–	–
Nauru	–	–	–	–	–	–	–	–	31	–	–	0
Nepal	440	1	1.9	7	55	7	18	9	716	6	12	4
Netherlands	49350	1.6	2.1	2	–	14	11	3	–	–	–	–
New Zealand	26830 x	0.8	2	2	–	17	17	3	–	–	–	–
Nicaragua	1010	-3.7	1.9	19	16	13 x	15 x	6 x	741	12	2	7
Niger	340	-2.1	-0.2	4	66	–	–	–	605	13	12	10x

TABLE 7. ECONOMIC INDICATORS

Countries and territories	GNI per capita (US$) 2009	GDP per capita average annual growth rate (%) 1970–1990	GDP per capita average annual growth rate (%) 1990–2009	Average annual rate of inflation (%) 1990–2009	% of population below international poverty line of US$1.25 per day 1994–2008*	% of central government expenditure (1998–2008*) allocated to: health	education	defence	ODA inflow in millions US$ 2008	ODA inflow as a % of recipient GNI 2008	Debt service as a % of exports of goods and services 1990	Debt service 2008
Nigeria	1140	-1.4	1.7	21	64	1 x	3 x	3 x	1290	1	22	0
Niue	–	–	–	–	–	–	–	–	18	–	–	0
Norway	86440	3.2	2.3	4	–	16	6	5	–	–	–	–
Occupied Palestinian Territory	b	–	-2.4 x	4 x	–	–	–	–	2593	–	–	–
Oman	17890 x	3.3	2 x	4 x	–	7	15	33	32	–	–	–
Pakistan	1020	3	1.7	10	23	1	2	13	1539	1	16	8
Palau	8940	–	-0.1 x	3 x	–	–	–	–	43	24	–	–
Panama	6740	0.3	3	2	10	18	16	–	29	0	3	9
Papua New Guinea	1180	-0.7	-0.4	8	36	7	22	4	304	5	37	9x
Paraguay	2280	3.1	-0.1	11	7	7 x	22 x	11 x	134	1	12	5
Peru	4160	-0.6	2.9	11	8	13	7	–	466	0	6	12
Philippines	1790	0.6	1.9	7	23	2	19	5	61	0	23	15
Poland	12260	–	4.4	11	<2	12	11	4	–	–	4	24
Portugal	20940	2.6	1.7	4	–	16	16	3	–	–	–	–
Qatar	d	–	–	–	–	–	–	–	–	–	–	–
Republic of Korea	19830	6.2	4.3	4	–	1	16	11	–	–	–	–
Republic of Moldova	1590	–	-1	44	2	14	8	2	299	6	–	10
Romania	8330	0.9 x	2.7	50	<2	12	6	5	–	–	0	24
Russian Federation	9370	–	1.9	60	<2	5	3	8	–	–	–	11
Rwanda	460	1.2	1.7	10	77	5 x	26 x	–	931	24	9	3
Saint Kitts and Nevis	10150	6.3 x	2.5	3	–	–	–	–	46	9	3	17
Saint Lucia	5190	5.3 x	1.1	2	21	–	–	–	19	2	2	7
Saint Vincent and the Grenadines	5130	3.3	3.8	2	–	12	16	–	27	5	3	13
Samoa	2840	–	3.1	6	–	–	–	–	39	8	5	8x
San Marino	50670 x	–	–	3 x	–	18	9	–	–	–	–	–
Sao Tome and Principe	1140	–	–	–	28	–	–	–	47	29	28	34x
Saudi Arabia	17700 x	-1.4	0.3	4	–	6 x	14 x	36 x	–	–	–	–
Senegal	1040	-0.7	1.1	4	34	3	14	7	1058	9	14	4x
Serbia	5990	–	1.3	26 x	<2	–	–	–	1047	2	–	25
Seychelles	8480	2.9	1.7	5	<2	9	8	3	12	1	7	8x
Sierra Leone	340	-0.5	0.9	17	53	10 x	13 x	10 x	367	21	8	1
Singapore	37220	5.6	3.9	1	–	6	19	25	–	–	–	–
Slovakia	16130	–	3.7	7	<2	20	4	4	–	–	–	–
Slovenia	23520	–	3.5	13	<2	15	12	4	–	–	–	–
Solomon Islands	910	–	-1.3	7	–	–	–	–	224	38	10	2x
Somalia	a	-0.8	–	–	–	1 x	2 x	38 x	758	–	25 x	–
South Africa	5770	0.1	1.2	8	26	–	–	–	1125	0	–	4
Spain	31870	1.9	2.2	4	–	2	1	4	–	–	–	–
Sri Lanka	1990	3	4	10	14	6	10	18	730	2	10	8
Sudan	1230	0.1	3.8	29	–	1	8	28	2384	5	4	2
Suriname	4760 x	-2.2 x	1.4 x	51 x	16	–	–	–	102	4	–	–
Swaziland	2350	3	1.7	8	63	8	20	8	67	2	5	2x
Sweden	48930	1.8	2.2	2	–	4	6	5	–	–	–	–
Switzerland	56370 x	1.2	0.9 x	1 x	–	0	5	5	–	–	–	–
Syrian Arab Republic	2410	2	1.4	7	–	2	9	24	136	0	–	–
Tajikistan	700	–	-0.9	84	22	2	4	9	291	7	–	2
Thailand	3760	4.7	2.9	3	<2	15	21	6	-621	0	14	7
The former Yugoslav Republic of Macedonia	4400	–	0.9	26	<2	–	–	–	221	3	–	7
Timor-Leste	2460 x	–	-1.3 x	4 x	37	–	–	–	278	10	–	–
Togo	440	-0.6	–	4	39	5 x	20 x	11 x	330	13	8	2x
Tonga	3260	–	2.9	5	–	7 x	13 x	–	26	10	2	3x
Trinidad and Tobago	16560	0.5	5.1	6	4	7	14	2	12	0	–	–
Tunisia	3720	2.5	3.5	4	3	5	20	4	479	1	22	7
Turkey	8730	2	2.3	50	3	3	10	8	2024	0	27	27
Turkmenistan	3420	–	4.7	104	25	–	–	–	18	0	–	–
Tuvalu	–	–	–	–	–	–	–	–	17	–	–	0
Uganda	460	–	3.6	8	52	2 x	15 x	26 x	1657	13	47	2
Ukraine	2800	–	0.1	78	<2	3	6	3	618	0	–	18
United Arab Emirates	d	-4.9 x	0.5	6	–	7	17	30	–	–	–	–
United Kingdom	41520	2	2.3	3	–	15	4	7	–	–	–	–
United Republic of Tanzania	500	–	2	14	89	6 x	8 x	16 x	2331	13	25	1
United States	47240	2.2	1.8	2	–	24	2	20	–	–	–	–
Uruguay	9400	0.9	1.8	17	<2	7	8	4	33	0	31	14

	GNI per capita (US$) 2009	GDP per capita average annual growth rate (%) 1970–1990	GDP per capita average annual growth rate (%) 1990–2009	Average annual rate of inflation (%) 1990–2009	% of population below international poverty line of US$1.25 per day 1994–2008*	% of central government expenditure (1998–2008*) allocated to: health	% of central government expenditure (1998–2008*) allocated to: education	% of central government expenditure (1998–2008*) allocated to: defence	ODA inflow in millions US$ 2008	ODA inflow as a % of recipient GNI 2008	Debt service as a % of exports of goods and services 1990	Debt service as a % of exports of goods and services 2008
Uzbekistan	1100	–	1.9	90	46	–	–	–	187	1	–	–
Vanuatu	2620	1.1 x	6.7	-3	–	–	–	–	92	17	2	1x
Venezuela (Bolivarian Republic of)	10200	-1.6	0.2	33	4	8	21	5	59	0	22	5
Viet Nam	1010	–	6	10	22	4	14	–	2552	3	–	2
Yemen	1060	–	1.5	17	18	4	22	19	305	1	4	2
Zambia	970	-2.3	0.3	30	64	13	14	4	1086	9	13	3
Zimbabwe	a	-0.4	-1.9 x	62 x	–	8 x	24 x	7 x	611	–	19	–

SUMMARY INDICATORS

	GNI per capita (US$) 2009	GDP per capita average annual growth rate (%) 1970–1990	GDP per capita average annual growth rate (%) 1990–2009	Average annual rate of inflation (%) 1990–2009	% of population below international poverty line of US$1.25 per day 1994–2008*	% of central government expenditure (1998–2008*) allocated to: health	% of central government expenditure (1998–2008*) allocated to: education	% of central government expenditure (1998–2008*) allocated to: defence	ODA inflow in millions US$ 2008	ODA inflow as a % of recipient GNI 2008	Debt service as a % of exports of goods and services 1990	Debt service as a % of exports of goods and services 2008
Africa#	1500	0.9	2.0	24	44	–	–	–	39109	3	24	4
Sub-Saharan Africa#	1147	0	1.8	33	53	–	–	–	35689	4	17	3
Eastern and Southern Africa	1496	–	1.8	40	51	–	–	–	19247	4	14	3
West and Central Africa	841	-0.5	1.6	23	55	–	–	–	13937	4	19	2
Middle East and North Africa	3029	-0.2	2.4	14	4	5	13	13	20778	3	21	–
Asia#	2550	4.2	6.6	6	28	1	5	9	20559	0	17	4
South Asia	1092	2.1	4.4	6	40	2	5	12	12161	1	21	8
East Asia and Pacific	3748	5.4	7.2	5	18	1	5	8	8398	0	16	4
Latin America and Caribbean	7195	1.4	1.6	32	7	7	14	4	7240	0	20	14
CEE/CIS	6854	–	2.2	59	6	5	5	7	8303	0	–	17
Industrialized countries§	40463	2.3	1.7	2	–	18	4	12	–	–	–	–
Developing countries§	2988	2.1	4.6	17	28	3	8	8	86398	1	19	8
Least developed countries§	638	-0.2	3.0	53	54	5	13	15	38427	9	12	3
World	8686	2.3	2.5	8	26	13	5	11	90064	0	18	9

For a complete list of countries and territories in the regions and subregions, see page 124.

§ Includes territories within each country category or regional group. Countries and territories in each country category or regional group are listed on page 124.

DEFINITIONS OF THE INDICATORS

GNI per capita – Gross national income (GNI) is the sum of value added by all resident producers plus any product taxes (less subsidies) not included in the valuation of output plus net receipts of primary income (compensation of employees and property income) from abroad. GNI per capita is gross national income divided by midyear population. GNI per capita in US dollars is converted using the World Bank Atlas method.

GDP per capita – Gross domestic product (GDP) is the sum of value added by all resident producers plus any product taxes (less subsidies) not included in the valuation of output. GDP per capita is gross domestic product divided by midyear population. Growth is calculated from constant price GDP data in local currency.

% of population below international poverty line of US$1.25 per day – Percentage of population living on less than US$1.25 per day at 2005 prices, adjusted for purchasing power parity. The new poverty threshold reflects revisions to purchasing power parity exchange rates based on the results of the 2005 International Comparison Program. The revisions reveal that the cost of living is higher across the developing world than previously estimated. As a result of these revisions, poverty rates for individual countries cannot be compared with poverty rates reported in previous editions. More detailed information on the definition, methodology and sources of the data presented is available at <www.worldbank.org>.

ODA – Net official development assistance.

Debt service – Sum of interest payments and repayments of principal on external public and publicly guaranteed long-term debts.

MAIN DATA SOURCES

GNI per capita – World Bank.

GDP per capita – World Bank.

Rate of inflation – World Bank.

% of population below international poverty line of US$1.25 per day – World Bank.

Expenditure on health, education and defence – International Monetary Fund (IMF).

ODA – Organisation for Economic Co-operation and Development (OECD).

Debt service – World Bank.

NOTES

a: low income ($995 or less).
b: lower-middle income ($996 to $3,945).
c: upper-middle income ($3,946 to $12,195).
d: high income ($12,196 or more).

– Data not available.

x Data refer to years or periods other than those specified in the column heading, differ from the standard definition or refer to only part of a country. Such data are not included in the calculation of regional and global averages.

y Data refer to years or periods other than those specified in the column heading, differ from the standard definition or refer to only part of a country. Such data are included in the calculation of regional and global averages.

* Data refer to the most recent year available during the period specified in the column heading.

TABLE 8. WOMEN

Countries and territories	Life expectancy: females as a % of males 2009	Adult literacy rate: females as a % of males 2005–2008*	Net primary school 2005–2009* enrolled	attending	Net secondary school 2005–2009* enrolled	attending	Contraceptive prevalence (%) 2005–2009*	At least once	At least four times	Skilled attendant at birth	Institutional delivery	C-section	2005–2009* reported	2008 adjusted	2008 Lifetime risk of maternal death: 1 in:
Afghanistan	100	–	63	60 x	38	33 x	10 x	16 x	–	14 x	13 x	–	1600 x	1400	11
Albania	108	99	100 x	100	98 x	97	69	97	67	99	97	19	21	31	1700
Algeria	104	79	99	99	106 x	112	61	89	–	95	95	–	120 x	120	340
Andorra	–	–	98	–	109	–	–	–	–	–	–	–	–	–	–
Angola	109	69	86 x	102 x	–	90 x	6 x	80	32 x	47	46	–	–	610	29
Antigua and Barbuda	–	101	94	–	–	–	53 x	100	–	100	–	–	–	–	–
Argentina	111	100	–	–	112	–	78	99	89	95	99	–	40	70	600
Armenia	109	100	103	99	106	102	53	93	71	100	100	15	27	29	1900
Australia	106	–	101	–	102	–	71 x	100 x	–	100 x	–	30	–	8	7400
Austria	107	–	101 x	–	–	–	51 x	100 x	–	100 x	–	24	–	5	14300
Azerbaijan	107	99	99	98	98	98	51	77	45	88	78	5	26	38	1200
Bahamas	108	–	102	–	105	–	45 x	98	–	99	–	–	–	49	1000
Bahrain	104	97	99	100 x	105	111 x	62 x	97 x	–	98 x	98 x	–	46 x	19	2200
Bangladesh	103	83	102	103	105	116	53	51	21	24	15	8	350	340	110
Barbados	107	–	–	–	–	–	55 x	100	–	100	–	–	–	64	1100
Belarus	119	100	102	101	–	102	73	99	–	100	100	–	3	15	5100
Belgium	108	–	101	–	96	–	75 x	–	–	–	–	18	–	5	10900
Belize	105	–	100	100	109	103	34	94	76 x	95	88	–	57	94	330
Benin	104	53	87	87	49 x	66	17	84	61	74	78	4	400	410	43
Bhutan	106	59	103	91 x	107	–	35	88	–	71	55	9	260 x	200	170
Bolivia (Plurinational State of)	107	90	101	100	99	96	61	86	72	71	68	19	310	180	150
Bosnia and Herzegovina	107	96	–	101	–	100	36	99	–	100	100	–	3	9	9300
Botswana	99	100	102	103	109	122 x	53	94	73 y	95	94	–	200	190	180
Brazil	111	101	98	101	110	108	81	97	89	97	98	44	75	58	860
Brunei Darussalam	106	97	100	–	104	–	–	100 x	–	99 x	–	–	–	21	2000
Bulgaria	110	99	100	–	97	–	63 x	–	–	100	100	29	6	13	5800
Burkina Faso	105	59	89	90	74	91	17	85	18 x	54	51	1 x	310	560	28
Burundi	106	83	99	97	–	79	9	92	–	34	29	–	620	970	25
Cambodia	106	83	96	102	88	90	40	69	27	44	22	2	460	290	110
Cameroon	102	81	87	94	–	93	29	82	60 x	63	61	2 x	670 x	600	35
Canada	106	–	100 x	–	100 x	–	74 x	–	–	98 x	–	26	–	12	5600
Cape Verde	106	89	98	100 x	112 x	–	61	98	72	78	78	11	16	94	350
Central African Republic	106	60	74	84	58	64	19	69	40 x	44	56	2 x	540	850	27
Chad	105	50	70 x	76 x	33 x	51 x	3 x	39	18 x	14 x	13 x	0 x	1100 x	1200	14
Chile	108	100	99	–	103	–	58	95 x	–	100	98	–	18	26	2000
China	105	94	100	–	–	–	85	91	–	99	95	27	34	38	1500
Colombia	111	100	99	102	109	111	78	94	83	96	92	27	76	85	460
Comoros	107	85	85 x	100 x	101	103 x	26 x	75 x	52 x	62 x	43 x	–	380 x	340	71
Congo	104	–	91	101	–	104	44	86	75	83	82	3	780	580	39
Cook Islands	–	–	96 x	–	107 x	–	44 x	–	–	98 x	–	–	6 x	–	–
Costa Rica	106	101	102	102	–	110	80	90	86	99	99	21 y	27	44	1100
Côte d'Ivoire	105	69	80 x	87	57 x	69	13	85	45	57	54	6	540	470	44
Croatia	109	98	99	–	102	–	–	–	–	100	–	–	7	14	5200
Cuba	105	100	100	–	101	–	78	100	99	100	100	–	47	53	1400
Cyprus	106	98	99	–	102	–	–	–	–	–	–	–	–	10	6600
Czech Republic	108	–	103	–	–	–	72 x	99 x	97 x	100	–	20	6	8	8500
Democratic People's Republic of Korea	106	100	–	–	–	–	69 x	97 x	–	97 x	–	–	77	250	230
Democratic Republic of the Congo	107	72	95 x	95	–	80	21	85	47	74	70	4	550	670	24
Denmark	106	–	101	–	103	–	–	–	–	–	–	21	10 x	5	10900
Djibouti	105	–	89	99	71	82	23	92	7 x	93	87	12	550 x	300	93
Dominica	–	–	109	–	121	–	50 x	100	–	100	–	–	–	–	–
Dominican Republic	108	100	101	103	122	122	73	99	95	98	98	42	160	100	320
Ecuador	108	94	101	–	103	–	73 x	84 x	58 x	98 x	85	26 x	60	140	270
Egypt	105	77	96	97	95 x	93	60	74	66	79	72	28	55	82	380
El Salvador	114	93	101	–	103	–	73	94	78	96	85	25	59	110	350
Equatorial Guinea	105	92	91 x	98 x	–	95 x	–	86 x	–	65 x	–	–	–	280	73
Eritrea	108	71	87	93 x	71	92 x	8 x	70 x	41 x	28 x	26 x	3 x	1000 x	280	72
Estonia	116	100	99	–	103	–	70 x	–	–	100	–	–	7	12	5300
Ethiopia	105	46	93	101	64	77	15	28	12	6	5	1	670	470	40
Fiji	107	–	99	–	110	–	35 x	–	–	99 x	–	–	34 x	26	1300
Finland	109	–	100	–	101	–	–	100 x	–	100 x	100 x	16	6 x	8	7600

	Life expectancy: females as a % of males 2009	Adult literacy rate: females as a % of males 2005–2008*	Enrolment and attendance ratios: females as a % of males Net primary school 2005–2009* enrolled	attending	Net secondary school 2005–2009* enrolled	attending	Contraceptive prevalence (%) 2005–2009*	Antenatal care coverage (%) 2005–2009* At least once	At least four times	Delivery care coverage (%) 2005–2009* Skilled attendant at birth	Institutional delivery	C-section	Maternal mortality ratio† 2005–2009* reported	2008 adjusted	2008 Lifetime risk of maternal death: 1 in:
France	109	–	100	–	102	–	71	99 x	–	99 x	–	21	10 x	8	6600
Gabon	104	92	99 x	100 x	–	106 x	33 x	94 x	63 x	86 x	85 x	6 x	520 x	260	110
Gambia	106	60	107	103	98	87	18 x	98	–	57	55	–	730 x	400	49
Georgia	110	100	98	101	96	98	47	96	75	98	96	13	14	48	1300
Germany	107	–	100	–	–	–	75 x	–	–	–	–	29	8 x	7	11100
Ghana	103	82	101	101	92	101	24	90	78	57	57	7	450	350	66
Greece	106	98	100	–	99	–	61 x	–	–	–	–	–	1 x	2	31800
Grenada	104	–	98	–	91	–	54	100	–	99	–	–	–	–	–
Guatemala	111	86	97	94 x	94	103 x	54	93	–	51	52	16	130	110	210
Guinea	107	53	87	87	61	66	9	88	50	46	39	2	980	680	26
Guinea-Bissau	107	55	72 x	97	56 x	88	10	78	–	39	36	–	410	1000	18
Guyana	109	–	100	100	–	110	43	92	–	92	89	–	110	270	150
Haiti	106	–	–	107	–	117	32	85	54	26	25	3	630	300	93
Holy See	–	–	–	–	–	–	–	–	–	–	–	–	–	–	–
Honduras	107	100	102	104	–	123	65	92	81	67	67	13	110 x	110	240
Hungary	112	100	98	–	99	–	77 x	–	–	100	–	31	17	13	5500
Iceland	104	–	100	–	102	–	–	–	–	–	–	17	–	5	9400
India	105	68	96	96	–	83	54	75	51 y	53	47	9	250	230	140
Indonesia	106	93	97	98	99	103	57	93	82	75	46	7	230	240	190
Iran (Islamic Republic of)	104	89	–	97 x	100	–	79	98	94	97	96	40	25	30	1500
Iraq	111	80	87	88	72	75	50	84	–	80	65	21	84	75	300
Ireland	106	–	102	–	105	–	89 x	–	–	100 x	100 x	25	6 x	3	17800
Israel	105	–	101	–	102	–	–	–	–	–	–	–	5 x	7	5100
Italy	108	99	99	–	102	–	60 x	–	68 x	–	–	40	7 x	5	15200
Jamaica	110	113	97	100	105	105	69 x	91	87 x	97	94	–	95 x	89	450
Japan	109	–	–	–	100	–	54	–	–	100 x	–	–	8 x	6	12200
Jordan	105	93	102	100	105	104	59	99	94	99	99	19	19	59	510
Kazakhstan	121	100	102	99	101	100	51	100	70 x	100	100	–	31	45	950
Kenya	102	92	101	104	96	105	46	92	47	44	43	6	490	530	38
Kiribati	–	–	–	–	111	–	22 x	88 x	–	63	–	–	56 x	–	–
Kuwait	105	98	98	–	101	–	52 x	95 x	–	98 x	98 x	–	5 x	9	4500
Kyrgyzstan	112	100	99	103	101	103	48	97	81 x	98	97	–	55	81	450
Lao People's Democratic Republic	105	77	96	95	87	82	38	35	–	20	17	–	410	580	49
Latvia	114	100	98 x	–	–	–	48 x	–	–	100	–	–	8	20	3600
Lebanon	106	92	98	99 x	111	113 x	58 x	96 x	–	98 x	–	–	100 x	26	2000
Lesotho	102	115	104	108	158	171	47	92	70 x	62	59	5 x	760 x	530	62
Liberia	105	86	77 x	93	56 x	84	11	79	66	46	37	4	990	990	20
Libyan Arab Jamahiriya	107	84	–	–	–	–	45 x	81 x	–	94 x	–	–	77 x	64	540
Liechtenstein	–	–	105	–	96	–	–	–	–	–	–	–	–	–	–
Lithuania	118	100	98	–	102	–	47 x	–	–	100	–	–	9	13	5800
Luxembourg	107	–	102	–	104	–	–	–	–	100 x	–	29	–	17	3800
Madagascar	106	85	101	104 x	105	125 x	40	86	49	44	35	2	500	440	45
Malawi	103	82	106	101	93	98	41	92	57 x	54	54	3 x	810	510	36
Malaysia	107	95	100	–	107	–	55 x	79	–	99	98	–	29	31	1200
Maldives	105	100	98	–	104	–	39 x	81 x	91 x	84 x	–	–	140 x	37	1200
Mali	103	52	84	86	63	72	8	70	35	49	45	2	460	830	22
Malta	105	103	101	–	107	–	86 x	–	–	98 x	–	–	–	8	9200
Marshall Islands	–	–	99	–	108	–	45	81	77	86	85	9	74 x	–	–
Mauritania	107	77	107	105	88	82	9	75	16 x	61	48	3 x	690	550	41
Mauritius	111	94	101	–	102	–	76 x	–	–	98 x	98 x	–	22 x	36	1600
Mexico	107	97	100	100	103	–	73	94	–	93	86	40	63	85	500
Micronesia (Federated States of)	103	–	–	–	–	–	45 x	–	–	88 x	–	–	270 x	–	–
Monaco	–	–	–	–	–	–	–	–	–	–	–	–	–	–	–
Mongolia	110	101	98	102	108	106	55	100	–	99	98	17	81	65	730
Montenegro	107	–	–	99	–	101	39	97	–	99	100	–	13	15	4000
Morocco	107	64	95	97	85 x	93 x	63 x	68 x	31 x	63	61 x	5 x	130	110	360
Mozambique	103	58	94	97	93	98	16	92	53 x	55	58	2 x	410 x	550	37
Myanmar	107	94	–	102 x	101	94 x	41	80	73 y	64	23	–	320	240	180
Namibia	103	99	105	101	123	132	55	95	70	81	81	13	450	180	160
Nauru	–	–	101	–	–	–	36	95	40	97	99	8	–	–	–
Nepal	102	64	82 x	95	–	83	48	44	29	19	18	3	280	380	80

TABLE 8. WOMEN

Countries and territories	Life expectancy: females as a % of males 2009	Adult literacy rate: females as a % of males 2005–2008*	Enrolment and attendance ratios: females as a % of males Net primary school 2005–2009* enrolled	attending	Net secondary school 2005–2009* enrolled	attending	Contraceptive prevalence (%) 2005–2009*	Antenatal care coverage (%) 2005–2009* At least once	At least four times	Delivery care coverage (%) 2005–2009* Skilled attendant at birth	Institutional delivery	C-section	Maternal mortality ratio† 2005–2009* reported	2008 adjusted	2008 Lifetime risk of maternal death: 1 in:
Netherlands	105	–	99	–	101	–	69	–	–	100 x	–	14	7 x	9	7100
New Zealand	105	–	101	–	103 x	–	75 x	95 x	–	100 x	–	23	–	14	3800
Nicaragua	109	100	100	108 x	116	132 x	72	90	78	74	74	20	77	100	300
Niger	104	35	79	70	62	65	11	46	15	33	17	1	650	820	16
Nigeria	102	68	90	92	77	96	15	58	45	39	35	2	550	840	23
Niue	–	–	100 x	–	105 x	–	23 x	–	–	100	–	–	–	–	–
Norway	105	–	100	–	100	–	88	–	–	–	–	16	6 x	7	7600
Occupied Palestinian Territory	104	94	100	101 x	107	–	50	99	–	99	97	15	–	–	–
Oman	104	90	103	–	99	–	32 x	100 x	86	99	99	14	17	20	1600
Pakistan	101	60	83	88	76	83	30	61	28	39	34	7	280	260	93
Palau	–	–	96 x	–	–	–	21	100	88	100	–	–	–	–	–
Panama	107	99	99	–	110	–	–	72 x	–	92	92 x	–	60	71	520
Papua New Guinea	107	87	–	–	–	–	32	79	55	53	52	–	730	250	94
Paraguay	106	98	100	103	107	99 x	79	96	91	82	85	33	120	95	310
Peru	108	89	100	101 x	100	100 x	73	94	93	83	82	21	190 x	98	370
Philippines	106	101	102	102 x	119	127 x	51	91	78	62	44	10	160	94	320
Poland	112	100	101	–	102	–	49 x	–	–	100	–	21	5	6	13300
Portugal	109	96	99	–	109	–	67	–	–	100 x	–	31	8 x	7	9800
Qatar	103	96	99 x	–	147	–	43 x	–	–	99 x	98 x	–	10 x	8	4400
Republic of Korea	109	–	98	–	96	–	80	–	–	100 x	–	32	20 x	18	4700
Republic of Moldova	112	99	98	102	104	103	68	98	89	100	99	9	38	32	2000
Romania	110	99	99	–	97	–	70 x	94 x	76 x	99	98 x	19 x	14	27	2700
Russian Federation	121	100	–	–	–	–	80	–	–	100	–	–	21	39	1900
Rwanda	107	88	103	103	–	88	36	96	24	52	45	3	750 x	540	35
Saint Kitts and Nevis	–	–	106	–	99	–	54	100	–	100	–	–	–	–	–
Saint Lucia	105	–	99	–	106	–	47 x	99	–	100	–	–	–	–	–
Saint Vincent and the Grenadines	106	–	95	–	112	–	48	100	–	99	–	–	–	–	–
Samoa	109	99	100	–	113	–	25 x	–	–	100 x	–	–	29 x	–	–
San Marino	–	–	–	–	–	–	–	–	–	–	–	–	–	–	–
Sao Tome and Principe	106	89	103	101	111	105	38	98	–	82	79	–	150	–	–
Saudi Arabia	106	90	99	–	108	–	24	90 x	–	91 x	91 x	–	–	24	1300
Senegal	106	63	102	102	76	78	12	87	40	52	62	3	400	410	46
Serbia	106	97	100	100	103	108	41	98	–	99	99	19	6	8	7500
Seychelles	–	101	101 x	–	–	–	–	–	–	–	–	–	57 x	–	–
Sierra Leone	106	56	–	101	69	79	8	87	56	42	25	2	860	970	21
Singapore	106	94	–	–	–	–	62 x	–	–	100 x	–	–	6 x	9	10000
Slovakia	111	–	–	–	–	–	80 x	–	–	100	–	24	4	6	13300
Slovenia	110	100	99	–	101	–	74 x	98 x	–	100	–	–	26	18	4100
Solomon Islands	103	82 x	100	110	90	104	27	74	65	70	85	6	140 x	100	230
Somalia	106	–	–	83	–	49	15	26	6	33	9	–	1000	1200	14
South Africa	106	98	100	104 x	106	117 x	60 x	92 x	56 x	91 x	89 x	21 x	170 x	410	100
Spain	108	98	100	–	103	–	66	–	–	–	–	26	6 x	6	11400
Sri Lanka	111	97	101	–	–	–	68	99	93	99	98	24	39	39	1100
Sudan	105	75	83 x	93	–	133	8	64	–	49	19	5	1100	750	32
Suriname	111	95	99	100	134	121	46	90	–	90	88	–	180	100	400
Swaziland	97	98	102	103	86	132	51	85	79	69	74	8	590	420	75
Sweden	105	–	99	–	100	–	–	–	–	–	–	–	5 x	5	11400
Switzerland	106	–	100	–	96	–	82 x	–	–	–	–	30	5 x	10	7600
Syrian Arab Republic	105	86	95 x	100	98	101	58	84	–	93	70	–	65 x	46	610
Tajikistan	108	100	96	98	88	83	37	89	49	88	73	–	38	64	430
Thailand	109	96	99	100	113	109	77	98	–	97	97	–	12	48	1200
The former Yugoslav Republic of Macedonia	107	97	100	96	98	99	14	94	–	100	99	–	4	9	7300
Timor-Leste	103	–	96	98 x	110	–	22	61 x	30 x	18 x	22	–	–	370	44
Togo	106	70	91	93	48 x	70	17	84	46 x	62	63	–	480 x	350	67
Tonga	108	100	–	–	124	–	23 x	–	–	95 x	–	–	140	–	–
Trinidad and Tobago	111	99	99	100	107	107	43	96	–	98	97	–	45 x	55	1100
Tunisia	106	82	101	98 x	113	–	60	96	68	95	89 x	21	–	60	860
Turkey	107	84	98	96 x	91	83 x	73	92	74	91	90	37	29	23	1900
Turkmenistan	113	100	–	100	–	100	48	99	83 x	100	98	3 x	15	77	500
Tuvalu	–	–	–	–	–	–	31	97	67	98	93	7	–	–	–
Uganda	102	81	103	99	92	94	24	94	47	42	41	3	440	430	35
Ukraine	117	100	100	102	101	102	67	99	75	99	99	10	16	26	3000

	Life expectancy: females as a % of males 2009	Adult literacy rate: females as a % of males 2005–2008*	Enrolment and attendance ratios: females as a % of males				Contraceptive prevalence (%) 2005–2009*	Antenatal care coverage (%) 2005–2009*		Delivery care coverage (%) 2005–2009*			Maternal mortality ratio†		
			Net primary school 2005–2009*		Net secondary school 2005–2009*			At least once	At least four times	Skilled attendant at birth	Institutional delivery	C-section	2005–2009* reported	2008 adjusted	2008 Lifetime risk of maternal death: 1 in:
			enrolled	attending	enrolled	attending									
United Arab Emirates	103	102	99	–	102	–	28 x	97 x	–	99 x	99 x	–	3 x	10	4200
United Kingdom	106	–	100	–	103	–	84 x	–	–	99 x	–	26	7 x	12	4700
United Republic of Tanzania	103	84	100	106	95 x	108	26	76	62	43	47	3	580	790	23
United States	106	–	101	–	101	–	73 x	–	–	99 x	–	31	13	24	2100
Uruguay	110	101	100	–	111	–	78	96	90	100 x	–	34	34	27	1700
Uzbekistan	110	99	98	100	98	98	65	99	79 x	100	97	–	21	30	1400
Vanuatu	106	96	98	102	87 x	96	38	84	–	74	80	–	150	–	–
Venezuela (Bolivarian Republic of)	108	100	100	102 x	112	147 x	77 x	94 x	–	95 x	95 x	–	61	68	540
Viet Nam	105	95	95 x	100	–	102	80	91	29 x	88	64	10 x	75	56	850
Yemen	105	54	83	86	53	56	28	47	14 x	36	24	9 x	370 x	210	91
Zambia	102	76	101	100	82	93	41	94	60	47	48	3	590	470	38
Zimbabwe	101	94	101	102	96	93	65	93	71	60	59	5	560	790	42

SUMMARY INDICATORS

Africa#	104	75	96	97	87	92	28	72	45	48	44	5	–	590	36
Sub-Saharan Africa#	104	75	96	97	86	90	21	72	43	45	41	3	–	640	31
Eastern and Southern Africa	104	80	99	101	93	91	29	72	39	37	35	3	–	550	38
West and Central Africa	104	69	90	93	77	88	17	72	46	51	48	3	–	720	26
Middle East and North Africa	105	80	94	95	94	93	54	78	–	77	65	24	–	170	190
Asia#	105	85	97	96 **	–	89 **	66	79	51 **	66	58	14	–	200	210
South Asia	104	69	95	95	–	86	51	70	45	48	42	8	–	290	110
East Asia and Pacific	105	94	99	99 **	103 **	103 **	77	90	76 **	90	78	22	–	88	600
Latin America and Caribbean	109	98	99	101	107	108	75	95	86	89	87	34	–	85	480
CEE/CIS	114	97	99	–	99	–	69	95	–	97	93	–	–	34	1700
Industrialized countries§	107	–	101	–	102	–	–	–	–	–	–	28	–	14	4300
Developing countries§	105	86	97	96 **	98 **	92 **	61	79	53 **	64	58	14	–	290	120
Least developed countries§	104	75	95	98	87	94	31	68	37	41	35	3	–	590	37
World	106	87	97	97 **	99 **	92 **	61	79	53 **	65	58	15	–	260	140

\# For a complete list of countries and territories in the regions and subregions, see page 124.

§ Includes territories within each country category or regional group. Countries and territories in each country category or regional group are listed on page 124

DEFINITIONS OF THE INDICATORS

Life expectancy – Number of years newborn children would live if subject to the mortality risks prevailing for the cross section of population at the time of their birth.

Adult literacy rate – Number of literate persons aged 15 and above, expressed as a percentage of the total population in that age group.

Enrolment and attendance ratios: females as a % of males – Girls' net enrolment and attendance ratios divided by those of boys, as a percentage.

Primary or secondary school net enrolment ratio – Number of children enrolled in primary or secondary school who are of official primary or secondary school age, expressed as a percentage of the total number of children of official primary or secondary school age.

Primary school net attendance ratio – Number of children attending primary or secondary school who are of official primary school age, expressed as a percentage of the total number of children of official primary school age.

Secondary school net attendance ratio – Number of children attending secondary or tertiary school who are of official secondary school age, expressed as a percentage of the total number of children of official secondary school age.

Contraceptive prevalence – Percentage of women in union 15–49 years old currently using contraception.

Antenatal care coverage – Percentage of women 15–49 years old attended at least once during pregnancy by skilled health personnel (doctors, nurses or midwives) and the percentage attended by any provider at least four times.

Skilled attendant at birth – Percentage of births attended by skilled health personnel (doctors, nurses or midwives).

Institutional delivery – Percentage of women 15–49 years old who gave birth during the two years preceding the survey and delivered in a health facility.

Caesarean section (C-section) – Percentage of births delivered by Caesarean section (C-section rates between 5 per cent and 15 per cent expected with adequate levels of emergency obstetric care).

Maternal mortality ratio – Number of deaths of women from pregnancy-related causes per 100,000 live births during the same time period. The 'reported' column shows country-reported figures that are not adjusted for under-reporting and misclassification.

Lifetime risk of maternal death – Lifetime risk of maternal death takes into account both the probability of becoming pregnant and the probability of dying as a result of that pregnancy accumulated across a woman's reproductive years.

MAIN DATA SOURCES

Life expectancy – United Nations Population Division.

Adult literacy – UNESCO Institute for Statistics (UIS).

Primary and secondary school enrolment – UIS.

Primary and secondary school attendance – Demographic and Health Surveys (DHS) and Multiple Indicator Cluster Surveys (MICS).

Contraceptive prevalence – MICS, DHS and other nationally representative sources; United Nations Population Division.

Antenatal care coverage – MICS, DHS and other nationally representative sources.

Skilled attendant at birth – MICS, DHS and other nationally representative sources.

Institutional delivery – MICS, DHS and other nationally representative sources.

C-section – DHS and other nationally representative sources.

Maternal mortality ratio (reported) – Nationally representative sources, including household surveys and vital registration.

Maternal mortality ratio (adjusted) – WHO, UNICEF, UNFPA and the World Bank.

Lifetime risk – WHO and UNICEF.

† The maternal mortality data in the column headed 'reported' refer to data reported by national authorities. The data in the column headed 'adjusted' refer to the 2008 United Nations Interagency maternal mortality estimates that were released in late 2010. Periodically, the United Nations Interagency Group (WHO, UNICEF, UNFPA and the World Bank) produces internationally comparable sets of maternal mortality data which account for the well-documented problems of under-reporting and misclassification of maternal deaths, also including estimates for countries with no data. Please note that due to an evolving methodology these values are not comparable with previously reported MMR 'adjusted' values. Comparable time series on maternal mortality ratios for the years 1990, 1995, 2000, 2005 and 2008 are available at <www.childinfo.org>.

NOTES

– Data not available.

x Data refer to years or periods other than those specified in the column heading, differ from the standard definition or refer to only part of a country. Such data are not included in the calculation of regional and global averages.

y Data refer to years or periods other than those specified in the column heading, differ from the standard definition or refer to only part of a country. Such data are included in the calculation of regional and global averages.

* Data refer to the most recent year available during the period specified in the column heading.

** Excludes China.

TABLE 9. CHILD PROTECTION

Countries and territories	Child labour 2000–2009* total	male	female	Child marriage 2000–2009* total	urban	rural	Birth registration 2000–2009* total	urban	rural	Female genital mutilation/ cutting women[a] 1997–2009* total	daughters[b] 1997–2008* total	Attitudes towards domestic violence 2002–2009* total	Child discipline[c] 2005–2008* total
Afghanistan	13 y	17 y	9 y	39	–	–	6	12	4	–	–	–	–
Albania	12	14	9	10	–	–	99	99	98	–	–	30	52
Algeria	5	6	4	2	2	2	99	99	99	–	–	68	88
Andorra	–	–	–	–	–	–	–	–	–	–	–	–	–
Angola	24	22	25	–	–	–	29	34	19	–	–	–	–
Antigua and Barbuda	–	–	–	–	–	–	–	–	–	–	–	–	–
Argentina	7 y	8 y	5 y	–	–	–	91 y	–	–	–	–	–	–
Armenia	4 y	–	–	10	7	16	96	97	95	–	–	22	–
Australia	–	–	–	–	–	–	–	–	–	–	–	–	–
Austria	–	–	–	–	–	–	–	–	–	–	–	–	–
Azerbaijan	7 y	8 y	5 y	12	10	15	94	96	92	–	–	49	75
Bahamas	–	–	–	–	–	–	–	–	–	–	–	–	–
Bahrain	5	6	3	–	–	–	–	–	–	–	–	–	–
Bangladesh	13	18	8	66	53	70	10	13	9	–	–	36	–
Barbados	–	–	–	–	–	–	–	–	–	–	–	–	–
Belarus	5	6	4	7	6	10	–	–	–	–	–	–	84
Belgium	–	–	–	–	–	–	–	–	–	–	–	–	–
Belize	40	39	42	–	–	–	94	92	97	–	–	12	71
Benin	46	47	45	34	19	47	60	68	56	13	2	47	–
Bhutan	19 y	16 y	22 y	–	–	–	–	–	–	–	–	–	–
Bolivia (Plurinational State of)	22	22	22	26	22	37	74	76	72	–	–	16	–
Bosnia and Herzegovina	5	7	4	6	2	7	100	99	100	–	–	5	38
Botswana	9 y	11 y	7 y	–	–	–	72	78	67	–	–	–	–
Brazil	4 y	5 y	3 y	36	–	–	91 y	–	–	–	–	–	–
Brunei Darussalam	–	–	–	–	–	–	–	–	–	–	–	–	–
Bulgaria	–	–	–	–	–	–	–	–	–	–	–	–	–
Burkina Faso	47 y	46 y	48 y	48	29	61	64	86	58	73	25	71	83
Burundi	19	19	19	18	14	18	60	62	60	–	–	–	–
Cambodia	45 y	45 y	45 y	23	18	25	66	71	66	–	–	55	–
Cameroon	31	31	30	36	23	57	70	86	58	1	1	56	93
Canada	–	–	–	–	–	–	–	–	–	–	–	–	–
Cape Verde	3 y	4 y	3 y	18	–	–	–	–	–	–	–	17	–
Central African Republic	47	44	49	61	57	64	49	72	36	26	7	–	89
Chad	53	54	51	72	65	73	9	36	3	45	21	–	–
Chile	3	3	2	–	–	–	99 y	–	–	–	–	–	–
China	–	–	–	–	–	–	–	–	–	–	–	–	–
Colombia	7 y	9 y	4 y	23	19	38	90	97	77	–	–	–	–
Comoros	27	26	28	–	–	–	83	87	83	–	–	–	–
Congo	25	24	25	31	24	40	81 y	88 y	75 y	–	–	76	–
Cook Islands	–	–	–	–	–	–	–	–	–	–	–	–	–
Costa Rica	5	6	3	–	–	–	–	–	–	–	–	–	–
Côte d'Ivoire	35	36	34	35	27	43	55	79	41	36	9	65	91
Croatia	–	–	–	–	–	–	–	–	–	–	–	–	–
Cuba	–	–	–	–	–	–	100 y	100 y	100 y	–	–	–	–
Cyprus	–	–	–	–	–	–	–	–	–	–	–	–	–
Czech Republic	–	–	–	–	–	–	–	–	–	–	–	–	–
Democratic People's Republic of Korea	–	–	–	–	–	–	99	99	99	–	–	–	–
Democratic Republic of the Congo	32	29	34	39	31	45	31	33	30	–	–	76	–
Denmark	–	–	–	–	–	–	–	–	–	–	–	–	–
Djibouti	8	8	8	5	5	13	89	90	82	93	49	–	72
Dominica	–	–	–	–	–	–	–	–	–	–	–	–	–
Dominican Republic	10	12	7	40	36	50	78	82	70	–	–	4	83
Ecuador	8	7	8	22	–	–	85	85	85	–	–	–	–
Egypt	7	8	5	17	9	22	99	99	99	91	24 y	39 y	92
El Salvador	6 y	9 y	4 y	25	–	–	99	99	99	–	–	–	–
Equatorial Guinea	28	28	28	–	–	–	32	43	24	–	–	–	–
Eritrea	–	–	–	47	31	60	–	–	–	89	63	70	–
Estonia	–	–	–	–	–	–	–	–	–	–	–	–	–
Ethiopia	53	59	46	49	27	55	7	29	5	74	38	81	–
Fiji	–	–	–	–	–	–	–	–	–	–	–	–	72 y
Finland	–	–	–	–	–	–	–	–	–	–	–	–	–
France	–	–	–	–	–	–	–	–	–	–	–	–	–
Gabon	–	–	–	34	30	49	89	90	87	–	–	–	–

120 THE STATE OF THE WORLD'S CHILDREN 2011

| | Child labour 2000–2009* | | | Child marriage 2000–2009* | | | Birth registration 2000–2009* | | | Female genital mutilation/ cutting | | Attitudes towards domestic violence 2002–2009* | Child discipline◊ 2005–2008* |
| | | | | | | | | | | women[a] 1997–2009* | daughters[b] 1997–2008* | | |
	total	male	female	total	urban	rural	total	urban	rural	total	total	total	total
Gambia	25	20	29	36	74	45	55	57	54	78	64	74	87
Georgia	18	20	17	17	12	23	92	97	87	–	–	7	67
Germany	–	–	–	–	–	–	–	–	–	–	–	–	–
Ghana	34	34	34	25	13	38	71	82	65	4	1	37	90
Greece	–	–	–	–	–	–	–	–	–	–	–	–	–
Grenada	–	–	–	–	–	–	–	–	–	–	–	–	–
Guatemala	21 y	–	–	35	–	–	–	–	–	–	–	–	–
Guinea	25	26	24	63	45	75	43	78	33	96	57	86	–
Guinea-Bissau	39	41	37	24	14	32	39	53	33	45	35	52	82
Guyana	16	17	16	20	15	22	93	96	92	–	–	18	76
Haiti	21	22	19	30	27	33	81	87	78	–	–	29	–
Holy See	–	–	–	–	–	–	–	–	–	–	–	–	–
Honduras	16	16	15	39	33	46	94	95	93	–	–	16	–
Hungary	–	–	–	–	–	–	–	–	–	–	–	–	–
Iceland	–	–	–	–	–	–	–	–	–	–	–	–	–
India	12	12	12	47	29	56	41	59	35	–	–	54	–
Indonesia	7 y	8 y	6 y	22	13	30	53	71	41	–	–	31	–
Iran (Islamic Republic of)	–	–	–	–	–	–	–	–	–	–	–	–	–
Iraq	11	12	9	17	16	19	95	95	96	–	–	59	86
Ireland	–	–	–	–	–	–	–	–	–	–	–	–	–
Israel	–	–	–	–	–	–	–	–	–	–	–	–	–
Italy	–	–	–	–	–	–	–	–	–	–	–	–	–
Jamaica	6	7	5	9	7	11	89	89	88	–	–	6	89
Japan	–	–	–	–	–	–	–	–	–	–	–	–	–
Jordan	–	–	–	10	10	7	–	–	–	–	–	90 y	–
Kazakhstan	2	2	2	7	6	9	99	99	99	–	–	10	54
Kenya	26	27	25	26	–	–	60	76	57	27	–	53	–
Kiribati	–	–	–	–	–	–	92	100	80	–	–	–	81 y
Kuwait	–	–	–	–	–	–	–	–	–	–	–	–	–
Kyrgyzstan	4	4	3	10	7	14	94	96	93	–	–	38	54
Lao People's Democratic Republic	11	10	13	–	–	–	72	84	68	–	–	81	74
Latvia	–	–	–	–	–	–	–	–	–	–	–	–	–
Lebanon	7	8	6	11	–	–	–	–	–	–	–	–	–
Lesotho	23	25	21	23	13	26	26	39	24	–	–	48	–
Liberia	21	21	21	38	25	49	4 y	5 y	3 y	58	–	59	–
Libyan Arab Jamahiriya	–	–	–	–	–	–	–	–	–	–	–	–	–
Liechtenstein	–	–	–	–	–	–	–	–	–	–	–	–	–
Lithuania	–	–	–	–	–	–	–	–	–	–	–	–	–
Luxembourg	–	–	–	–	–	–	–	–	–	–	–	–	–
Madagascar	28 y	29 y	27 y	39	29	42	75	87	72	–	–	28	–
Malawi	26	25	26	50	38	53	–	–	–	–	–	28	–
Malaysia	–	–	–	–	–	–	–	–	–	–	–	–	–
Maldives	–	–	–	–	–	–	73	–	–	–	–	70	–
Mali	34	35	33	71	60	77	53	75	45	85	69	75	–
Malta	–	–	–	–	–	–	–	–	–	–	–	–	–
Marshall Islands	–	–	–	26	–	–	96	96	96	–	–	–	–
Mauritania	16	18	15	35	27	44	56	75	42	72	66	–	–
Mauritius	–	–	–	–	–	–	–	–	–	–	–	–	–
Mexico	6 y	7 y	5 y	23	–	–	–	–	–	–	–	–	–
Micronesia (Federated States of)	–	–	–	–	–	–	–	–	–	–	–	–	–
Monaco	–	–	–	–	–	–	–	–	–	–	–	–	–
Mongolia	18	19	17	4	–	–	98	98	99	–	–	20	81
Montenegro	10	12	8	5	5	5	98	98	99	–	–	11	63
Morocco	8	9	8	16	12	21	85	92	80	–	–	64	–
Mozambique	22	21	24	52	–	–	31	39	28	–	–	36	–
Myanmar	–	–	–	–	–	–	65 y	88 y	59 y	–	–	–	–
Namibia	13 y	15 y	12 y	9	6	11	67	83	59	–	–	35	–
Nauru	–	–	–	27	–	–	83	–	–	–	–	–	–
Nepal	34 y	30 y	38 y	51	41	54	35	42	34	–	–	23	–
Netherlands	–	–	–	–	–	–	–	–	–	–	–	–	–
New Zealand	–	–	–	–	–	–	–	–	–	–	–	–	–
Nicaragua	15	18	11	41	–	–	81	90	73	–	–	14	–
Niger	43	43	43	75	42	84	32	71	25	2	1	70	–

TABLE 9. CHILD PROTECTION

| | Child labour 2000–2009* | | | Child marriage 2000–2009* | | | Birth registration 2000–2009* | | | Female genital mutilation/cutting | | Attitudes towards domestic violence 2002–2009* | Child discipline 2005–2009* |
| | | | | | | | | | | women[a] 1997–2009* | daughters[b] 1997–2008[x] | | |
	total	male	female	total	urban	rural	total	urban	rural	total	total	total	total
Nigeria	13 y	–	–	39	22	50	30	49	22	30	30	43	–
Niue	–	–	–	–	–	–	–	–	–	–			–
Norway	–	–	–	–	–	–	–	–	–				
Occupied Palestinian Territory	–	–	–	19	–	–	96 y	97 y	96 y	–	–	–	95
Oman	–	–	–	–	–	–	–	–	–				
Pakistan	–	–	–	24	16	29	27	32	24	–	–	–	–
Palau	–	–	–	–	–	–	–	–	–				
Panama	11 y	–	–	–	–	–	–	–	–				
Papua New Guinea	–	–	–	21	–	–	–	–	–				
Paraguay	15	17	12	18	–	–	–	–	–				
Peru	34 y	31 y	36 y	19	–	–	93	–	–				
Philippines	12	13	11	14	11	19	83	87	78	–	–	14	–
Poland	–	–	–	–	–	–	–	–	–				
Portugal	3 y	4 y	3 y	–	–	–	–	–	–				
Qatar	–	–	–	–	–	–	–	–	–				
Republic of Korea	–	–	–	–	–	–	–	–	–				
Republic of Moldova	32	32	33	19	16	22	98	98	98	–	–	21	–
Romania	1	1	1	–	–	–	–	–	–				
Russian Federation	–	–	–	–	–	–	–	–	–				
Rwanda	35	36	35	13	9	14	82	79	83	–	–	48	–
Saint Kitts and Nevis	–	–	–	–	–	–	–	–	–				
Saint Lucia	–	–	–	–	–	–	–	–	–				
Saint Vincent and the Grenadines	–	–	–	–	–	–	–	–	–				
Samoa	–	–	–	–	–	–	–	–	–				
San Marino	–	–	–	–	–	–	–	–	–				
Sao Tome and Principe	8	8	7	33	31	37	69	70	67	–	–	32	–
Saudi Arabia	–	–	–	–	–	–	–	–	–				
Senegal	22	24	21	39	23	55	55	75	44	28	20	65	–
Serbia	4	5	4	6	4	8	99	99	99	–	–	6	75
Seychelles	–	–	–	–	–	–	–	–	–				
Sierra Leone	48	49	48	48	30	61	51	59	48	91	33	65	92
Singapore	–	–	–	–	–	–	–	–	–				
Slovakia	–	–	–	–	–	–	–	–	–				
Slovenia	–	–	–	–	–	–	–	–	–				
Solomon Islands	–	–	–	22	–	–	80	70	81	–	–	69	72 y
Somalia	49	45	54	45	35	52	3	6	2	98	46	76 y	–
South Africa	–	–	–	6	–	–	92 y	–	–	–	–	–	–
Spain	–	–	–	–	–	–	–	–	–				
Sri Lanka	8	9	7	12	–	–	97	97	98	–	–	53 y	–
Sudan	13	14	12	34	24	40	33	53	22	89	43 y	–	–
Suriname	6	7	5	19	14	33	97	98	95	–	–	13	86
Swaziland	9	9	9	5	1	6	30	38	28	–	–	38	–
Sweden	–	–	–	–	–	–	–	–	–				
Switzerland	–	–	–	–	–	–	–	–	–				
Syrian Arab Republic	4	5	3	13	15	12	95	96	95	–	–	–	89
Tajikistan	10	9	11	13	13	13	88	85	90	–	–	74 y	78
Thailand	8	8	8	20	12	23	99	100	99	–	–	–	–
The former Yugoslav Republic of Macedonia	6	7	5	4	3	4	94	95	93	–	–	21	72
Timor-Leste	4	4	4	–	–	–	53 y	–	–	–	–	–	–
Togo	29	29	30	24	15	36	78	93	69	6	1	53	91
Tonga	–	–	–	–	–	–	–	–	–				
Trinidad and Tobago	1	1	1	8	–	–	96	–	–	–	–	8	77
Tunisia	–	–	–	–	–	–	–	–	–				
Turkey	3 y	3 y	2 y	14	13	17	94	95	92	–	–	25	–
Turkmenistan	–	–	–	7	9	6	96	96	95	–	–	38 y	–
Tuvalu	–	–	–	–	–	–	50	60	38	–	–	70	–
Uganda	36	37	36	46	27	52	21	24	21	1	–	70	–
Ukraine	7	8	7	10	8	18	100	100	100	–	–	4	70
United Arab Emirates	–	–	–	–	–	–	–	–	–				
United Kingdom	–	–	–	–	–	–	–	–	–				
United Republic of Tanzania	21 y	23 y	19 y	38	–	–	22	48	16	15	4	60	–
United States	–	–	–	–	–	–	–	–	–				
Uruguay	8 y	8 y	8 y	–	–	–	–	–	–				

	Child labour 2000–2009*			Child marriage 2000–2009*			Birth registration 2000–2009*			Female genital mutilation/cutting		Attitudes towards domestic violence 2002–2009*	Child discipline◊ 2005–2008*
										women[a] 1997–2009*	daughters[b] 1997–2008*		
	total	male	female	total	urban	rural	total	urban	rural	total	total	total	total
Uzbekistan	–	–	–	7	9	7	100	100	100	–	–	70	–
Vanuatu	–	–	–	27	–	–	26	39	23	–	–	–	78 y
Venezuela													
(Bolivarian Republic of)	8	9	6	–	–	–	92	–	–	–	–	–	–
Viet Nam	16	15	16	10	3	13	88	94	86	–	–	64	94
Yemen	23	21	24	32	28	35	22	38	16	23	20	–	95
Zambia	41 y	42 y	40 y	42	26	53	14	28	9	1	–	62	–
Zimbabwe	13 y	12 y	14 y	30	–	–	74	83	71	–	–	48	–

SUMMARY INDICATORS

	total	male	female	total	urban	rural	total	urban	rural	total	total	total	total
Africa#	29 n	30 n	28 n	34	21	45	45	61	36	47	26	56	–
Sub-Saharan Africa#	33 n	34 n	32 n	38	26	50	38	54	30	40	27	58	–
Eastern and Southern Africa	34	36	32	35	26	48	36	46	27	42	–	59	–
West and Central Africa	35 n	34 n	35 n	42	26	53	41	57	33	33	24	56	–
Middle East and North Africa	10	11	9	18	12	24	77	87	68	–	–	–	90
Asia#	12 **	13 **	12 **	40 **	24 **	48 **	44 **	59 **	38 **	–	–	48 **	–
South Asia	12	13	12	46	30	55	36	50	31	–	–	51	–
East Asia and Pacific	11 **	11 **	10 **	18 **	11 **	23 **	71 **	82 **	66 **	–	–	36 **	–
Latin America and Caribbean	9	9	7	29	–	–	90	–	–	–	–	–	–
CEE/CIS	5	5	4	11	10	13	96	96	95	–	–	27	–
Industrialized countries§	–	–	–	–	–	–	–	–	–	–	–	–	–
Developing countries§	16 ***	17 ***	15 ***	35 **	22 **	45 **	51 **	64 **	39 **	–	–	49 **	–
Least developed countries§	29	30	27	48	36	55	30	44	25	–	–	54	–
World	–	–	–	–	–	–	–	–	–	–	–	–	–

\# For a complete list of countries and territories in the regions and subregions, see page 124.

§ Includes territories within each country category or regional group. Countries and territories in each country category or regional group are listed on page 124.

DEFINITIONS OF THE INDICATORS

Child labour – Percentage of children 5–14 years old involved in child labour at the moment of the survey. A child is considered to be involved in child labour under the following conditions: (a) children 5–11 years old who, during the week preceding the survey, did at least one hour of economic activity or at least 28 hours of household chores, or (b) children 12–14 years old who, during the week preceding the survey, did at least 14 hours of economic activity or at least 28 hours of household chores.

Child marriage – Percentage of women 20–24 years old who were married or in union before they were 18 years old.

Birth registration – Percentage of children less than five years old who were registered at the moment of the survey. The numerator of this indicator includes children whose birth certificate was seen by the interviewer or whose mother or caretaker says the birth has been registered.

Female genital mutilation/cutting – (a) Women – the percentage of women 15–49 years old who have been mutilated/cut. (b) Daughters – the percentage of women 15–49 years old with at least one mutilated/cut daughter.

Attitudes towards domestic violence – Percentage of women 15–49 years old who consider a husband to be justified in hitting or beating his wife for at least one of the specified reasons. Women were asked whether a husband is justified in hitting or beating his wife under a series of circumstances, i.e., if his wife burns the food, argues with him, goes out without telling him, neglects the children or refuses sexual relations.

Child discipline – Percentage of children 2–14 years old who experience any violent discipline methods (psychological aggression and/or physical punishment).

MAIN DATA SOURCES

Child labour – Multiple Indicator Cluster Surveys (MICS), Demographic and Health Surveys (DHS) and other national surveys.

Child marriage – MICS, DHS and other national surveys.

Birth registration – MICS, DHS, other national surveys and vital registration systems.

Female genital mutilation/cutting – MICS, DHS and other national surveys.

Attitudes towards domestic violence – MICS, DHS and other national surveys.

Child discipline – MICS, DHS and other national surveys.

NOTES
- – Data not available.
- y Data refer to years or periods other than those specified in the column heading, differ from the standard definition or refer to only part of a country. Such data are included in the calculation of regional and global averages.
- n Excludes Nigeria.
- ◊ A more detailed explanation of the methodology and the recent changes in calculating these estimates can be found in the General Note on the Data, page 83.
- * Data refer to the most recent year available during the period specified in the column heading.
- ** Excludes China.
- *** Excludes China and Nigeria.

Averages presented at the end of each of the 12 statistical tables are calculated using data from the countries and territories as classified below.

UPDATES OF UNICEF REGIONAL AND COUNTRY CLASSIFICATIONS

Beginning with last year's special edition of *The State of the World's Children*, UNICEF has been reporting statistical indicators for two continents – Africa and Asia – as well for regional and country groupings.

Africa includes all countries and territories of Eastern and Southern Africa and West and Central Africa, as well as the following countries and territories of the Middle East and North Africa: Algeria, Djibouti, Egypt, the Libyan Arab Jamahiriya, Morocco, the Sudan and Tunisia.

Sub-Saharan Africa now includes Djibouti and the Sudan, as well as all the countries and territories of Eastern and Southern Africa and West and Central Africa. As a consequence of these changes, regional estimates for sub-Saharan Africa published in 2009 and earlier editions of *The State of the World's Children* are not strictly comparable with those published in this issue.

Asia includes all countries and territories of South Asia, and East Asia and the Pacific.

Industrialized countries/territories are defined as those not included in the UNICEF Regional Classification.

Developing countries/territories are classified as such for purposes of statistical analysis only. There is no established convention for the designation of 'developed' and 'developing' countries or areas in the United Nations system.

Least developed countries/territories are those countries and territories classified as such by the United Nations.

UNICEF REGIONAL CLASSIFICATION
Africa
Sub-Saharan Africa; North Africa (Algeria, Egypt, Libyan Arab Jamahiriya, Morocco, Tunisia)

Sub-Saharan Africa
Eastern and Southern Africa; West and Central Africa; Djibouti and the Sudan

Eastern and Southern Africa
Angola; Botswana; Burundi; Comoros; Eritrea; Ethiopia; Kenya; Lesotho; Madagascar; Malawi; Mauritius; Mozambique; Namibia; Rwanda; Seychelles; Somalia; South Africa; Swaziland; Uganda; United Republic of Tanzania; Zambia; Zimbabwe

West and Central Africa
Benin; Burkina Faso; Cameroon; Cape Verde; Central African Republic; Chad; Congo; Côte d'Ivoire; Democratic Republic of the Congo; Equatorial Guinea; Gabon; Gambia; Ghana; Guinea; Guinea-Bissau; Liberia; Mali; Mauritania; Niger; Nigeria; Sao Tome and Principe; Senegal; Sierra Leone; Togo

Middle East and North Africa
Algeria; Bahrain; Djibouti; Egypt; Iran (Islamic Republic of); Iraq; Jordan; Kuwait; Lebanon; Libyan Arab Jamahiriya; Morocco; Occupied Palestinian Territory; Oman; Qatar; Saudi Arabia; Sudan; Syrian Arab Republic; Tunisia; United Arab Emirates; Yemen

Asia
South Asia; East Asia and the Pacific

South Asia
Afghanistan; Bangladesh; Bhutan; India; Maldives; Nepal; Pakistan; Sri Lanka

East Asia and Pacific
Brunei Darussalam; Cambodia; China; Cook Islands; Democratic People's Republic of Korea; Fiji; Indonesia; Kiribati; Lao People's Democratic Republic; Malaysia; Marshall Islands; Micronesia (Federated States of); Mongolia; Myanmar; Nauru; Niue; Palau; Papua New Guinea; Philippines; Republic of Korea; Samoa; Singapore; Solomon Islands; Thailand; Timor-Leste; Tonga; Tuvalu; Vanuatu; Viet Nam

Latin America and Caribbean
Antigua and Barbuda; Argentina; Bahamas; Barbados; Belize; Bolivia (Plurinational State of); Brazil; Chile; Colombia; Costa Rica; Cuba; Dominica; Dominican Republic; Ecuador; El Salvador; Grenada; Guatemala; Guyana; Haiti; Honduras; Jamaica; Mexico; Nicaragua; Panama; Paraguay; Peru; Saint Kitts and Nevis; Saint Lucia; Saint Vincent and the Grenadines; Suriname; Trinidad and Tobago; Uruguay; Venezuela (Bolivarian Republic of)

CEE/CIS
Albania; Armenia; Azerbaijan; Belarus; Bosnia and Herzegovina; Bulgaria; Croatia; Georgia; Kazakhstan; Kyrgyzstan; Montenegro; Republic of Moldova; Romania; Russian Federation; Serbia; Tajikistan; The former Yugoslav Republic of Macedonia; Turkey; Turkmenistan; Ukraine; Uzbekistan

UNICEF COUNTRY CLASSIFICATION
Industrialized countries/territories
Andorra; Australia; Austria; Belgium; Canada; Cyprus; Czech Republic; Denmark; Estonia; Finland; France; Germany; Greece; Holy See; Hungary; Iceland; Ireland; Israel; Italy; Japan; Latvia; Liechtenstein; Lithuania; Luxembourg; Malta; Monaco; Netherlands; New Zealand; Norway; Poland; Portugal; San Marino; Slovakia; Slovenia; Spain; Sweden; Switzerland; United Kingdom; United States

Developing countries/territories
Afghanistan; Algeria; Angola; Antigua and Barbuda; Argentina; Armenia; Azerbaijan; Bahamas; Bahrain; Bangladesh; Barbados; Belize; Benin; Bhutan; Bolivia (Plurinational State of); Botswana; Brazil; Brunei Darussalam; Burkina Faso; Burundi; Cambodia; Cameroon; Cape Verde; Central African Republic; Chad; Chile; China; Colombia; Comoros; Congo; Cook Islands; Costa Rica; Côte d'Ivoire; Cuba; Cyprus; Democratic Republic of the Congo; Democratic People's Republic of Korea; Djibouti; Dominica; Dominican Republic; Ecuador; Egypt; El Salvador; Equatorial Guinea; Eritrea; Ethiopia; Fiji; Gabon; Gambia; Georgia; Ghana; Grenada; Guatemala; Guinea; Guinea-Bissau; Guyana; Haiti; Honduras; India; Indonesia; Iran (Islamic Republic of); Iraq; Israel; Jamaica; Jordan; Kazakhstan; Kenya; Kiribati; Kuwait; Kyrgyzstan; Lao People's Democratic Republic; Lebanon; Lesotho; Liberia; Libyan

Arab Jamahiriya; Madagascar; Malawi; Malaysia; Maldives; Mali; Marshall Islands; Mauritania; Mauritius; Mexico; Micronesia (Federated States of); Mongolia; Morocco; Mozambique; Myanmar; Namibia; Nauru; Nepal; Nicaragua; Niger; Nigeria; Niue; Occupied Palestinian Territory; Oman; Pakistan; Palau; Panama; Papua New Guinea; Paraguay; Peru; Philippines; Qatar; Republic of Korea; Rwanda; Saint Kitts and Nevis; Saint Lucia; Saint Vincent and the Grenadines; Samoa; Sao Tome and Principe; Saudi Arabia; Senegal; Seychelles; Sierra Leone; Singapore; Solomon Islands; Somalia; South Africa; Sri Lanka; Sudan; Suriname; Swaziland; Syrian Arab Republic; Tajikistan; Thailand; Timor-Leste; Togo; Tonga; Trinidad and Tobago; Tunisia; Turkey; Turkmenistan; Tuvalu; Uganda; United Arab Emirates; United Republic of Tanzania; Uruguay; Uzbekistan; Vanuatu; Venezuela (Bolivarian Republic of); Viet Nam; Yemen; Zambia; Zimbabwe

Least developed countries/territories
Afghanistan; Angola; Bangladesh; Benin; Bhutan; Burkina Faso; Burundi; Cambodia; Central African Republic; Chad; Comoros; Democratic Republic of the Congo; Djibouti; Equatorial Guinea; Eritrea; Ethiopia; Gambia; Guinea; Guinea-Bissau; Haiti; Kiribati; Lao People's Democratic Republic; Lesotho; Liberia; Madagascar; Malawi; Maldives; Mali; Mauritania; Mozambique; Myanmar; Nepal; Niger; Rwanda; Samoa; Sao Tome and Principe; Senegal; Sierra Leone; Solomon Islands; Somalia; Sudan; Timor-Leste; Togo; Tuvalu; Uganda; United Republic of Tanzania; Vanuatu; Yemen; Zambia

Measuring human development
An introduction to Table 10

If development is to be measured using a comprehensive and inclusive assessment, it is necessary to appraise human as well as economic progress. From UNICEF's point of view, there is a need for an agreed method of measuring the level of child well-being and its rate of change.

The under-five mortality rate (U5MR) is used in Table 10 (pages 126–129) as the principal indicator of such progress. In 1970, around 16.3 million children were dying every year. In 2009, by comparison, the estimated number of children who died before their fifth birthday stood at 8.1 million – highlighting a significant long-term decline in the global number of under-five deaths.

The U5MR has several advantages as a gauge of child well-being:

• First, the U5MR measures an end result of the development process rather than an 'input' such as school enrolment level, per capita calorie availability or number of doctors per thousand population – all of which are means to an end.

• Second, the U5MR is known to be the result of a wide variety of inputs: for example, antibiotics to treat pneumonia; insecticide-treated mosquito nets to prevent malaria; the nutritional well-being and health knowledge of mothers; the level of immunization and oral rehydration therapy use; the availability of maternal and child health services, including antenatal care; income and food availability in the family; the availability of safe drinking water and basic sanitation; and the overall safety of the child's environment.

• Third, the U5MR is less susceptible to the fallacy of the average than, for example, per capita gross national income (GNI). This is because the natural scale does not allow the children of the rich to be one thousand times more likely to survive, even if the human-made scale does permit them to have one thousand times as much income. In other words, it

is much more difficult for a wealthy minority to affect a nation's U5MR, and this indicator therefore presents a more accurate, if far from perfect, picture of the health status of the majority of children and of society as a whole.

The speed of progress in reducing the U5MR can be assessed by calculating its average annual rate of reduction (AARR). Unlike the comparison of absolute changes, the AARR reflects the fact that the lower limits to the U5MR are approached only with increasing difficulty.

As lower levels of under-five mortality are reached, the same absolute reduction represents a greater percentage reduction. The AARR therefore shows a higher rate of progress for a 10-point reduction, for example, if that reduction happens at a lower level of under-five mortality. A 10-point decrease in the U5MR from 100 to 90 represents a reduction of 10 per cent, whereas the same 10-point decrease from 20 to 10 represents a reduction of 50 per cent. (A negative value for the percentage reduction indicates an increase in the U5MR during the period specified.)

When used in conjunction with gross domestic product (GDP) growth rates, the U5MR and its rate of reduction can therefore give a picture of the progress being made by any country, territory or region, over any period of time, towards the satisfaction of some of the most essential human needs.

As Table 10 shows, there is no fixed relationship between the annual reduction rate of the U5MR and the annual rate of growth in per capita GDP. Such comparisons help shed light on the relationship between economic advances and human development.

Finally, the table gives the total fertility rate for each country and territory and the corresponding AARR. It is clear that many of the nations that have achieved significant reductions in their U5MR have also achieved significant reductions in fertility.

TABLE 10. THE RATE OF PROGRESS

Countries and territories	Under-5 mortality rank	Under-5 mortality rate				Average annual rate of reduction (%)				Reduction since 1990 (%)	Reduction since 2000 (%)	GDP per capita average annual growth rate (%)		Total fertility rate			Average annual rate of reduction (%)	
		1970	1990	2000	2009	1970–1990	1990–2000	2000–2009	1990–2009			1970–1990	1990–2009	1970	1990	2009	1970–1990	1990–2009
Afghanistan	2	319	250	222	199	1.2	1.2	1.2	1.2	20	10	–	–	7.7	8.0	6.5	-0.2	1.1
Albania	118	112	51	27	15	3.9	6.4	6.5	6.4	71	44	-0.7 x	5.4	4.9	2.9	1.9	2.6	2.4
Algeria	79	199	61	46	32	5.9	2.8	4.0	3.4	48	30	1.6	1.5	7.4	4.7	2.3	2.3	3.7
Andorra	169	–	9	5	4	–	5.9	2.5	4.3	56	20	–	–	–	–	–	–	–
Angola	11	–	258	212	161	–	2.0	3.1	2.5	38	24	–	3.8	7.3	7.2	5.6	0.1	1.3
Antigua and Barbuda	130	–	–	19	12	–	–	5.1	–	–	37	8.3 x	2	–	–	–	–	–
Argentina	125	69	28	21	14	4.5	2.9	4.5	3.6	50	33	-0.7	1.9	3.1	3.0	2.2	0.1	1.6
Armenia	97	94	56	36	22	2.6	4.4	5.5	4.9	61	39	–	6.2	3.2	2.5	1.7	1.2	1.7
Australia	165	21	9	6	5	4.2	4.1	2.0	3.1	44	17	1.5	2.3	2.7	1.9	1.8	1.9	0.1
Austria	169	29	9	5	4	5.9	5.9	2.5	4.3	56	20	2.4	1.9	2.3	1.5	1.4	2.4	0.2
Azerbaijan	76	117	98	69	34	0.9	3.5	7.9	5.6	65	51	–	4.9	4.6	3.0	2.2	2.2	1.7
Bahamas	130	–	25	20	12	–	2.2	5.7	3.9	52	40	1.9	1.1 x	3.6	2.6	2.0	1.6	1.4
Bahrain	130	80	16	13	12	8.0	2.1	0.9	1.5	25	8	-1.3 x	2.8 x	6.5	3.7	2.2	2.8	2.7
Bangladesh	57	236	148	90	52	2.3	5.0	6.1	5.5	65	42	0.4	3.4	6.9	4.4	2.3	2.2	3.4
Barbados	140	–	18	15	11	–	1.8	3.4	2.6	39	27	1.7	2.2 x	3.1	1.7	1.5	3.1	0.4
Belarus	130	28	24	18	12	0.8	2.9	4.5	3.6	50	33	–	4.2	2.3	1.9	1.3	1.0	2.0
Belgium	165	24	10	6	5	4.4	5.1	2.0	3.6	50	17	2.2	1.7	2.2	1.6	1.8	1.7	-0.6
Belize	109	101	43	27	18	4.3	4.7	4.5	4.6	58	33	2.9	2.2 x	6.3	4.5	2.8	1.7	2.4
Benin	22	256	184	144	118	1.7	2.5	2.2	2.3	36	18	0.3	1.2	6.6	6.7	5.4	-0.1	1.2
Bhutan	41	288	148	106	79	3.3	3.3	3.3	3.3	47	25	–	5.2	6.7	5.9	2.6	0.6	4.4
Bolivia (Plurinational State of)	58	241	122	86	51	3.4	3.5	5.8	4.6	58	41	-1.1	1.6	6.6	4.9	3.4	1.5	2.0
Bosnia and Herzegovina	125	–	23	17	14	–	3.0	2.2	2.6	39	18	–	9.6 x	2.9	1.7	1.2	2.6	1.8
Botswana	54	132	60	99	57	3.9	-5.0	6.1	0.3	5	42	8.2	3.6	6.6	4.7	2.8	1.7	2.7
Brazil	98	135	56	34	21	4.4	5.0	5.4	5.2	63	38	2.3	1.4	5.0	2.8	1.8	2.9	2.3
Brunei Darussalam	151	–	11	8	7	–	3.2	1.5	2.4	36	13	-2.2 x	-0.3 x	5.7	3.2	2.1	2.8	2.4
Bulgaria	144	33	18	18	10	3.0	0.0	6.5	3.1	44	44	3.4 x	2.8	2.2	1.7	1.4	1.1	1.0
Burkina Faso	9	280	201	188	166	1.7	0.7	1.4	1.0	17	12	1.4	2.4	6.6	6.8	5.8	-0.2	0.8
Burundi	9	229	189	178	166	1.0	0.6	0.8	0.7	12	7	1.1	-1.8	6.8	6.6	4.5	0.1	2.1
Cambodia	36	–	117	106	88	–	1.0	2.1	1.5	25	17	–	6.3 x	5.9	5.8	2.9	0.1	3.7
Cameroon	13	214	148	156	154	1.8	-0.5	0.1	-0.2	-4	1	3.4	0.7	6.2	5.9	4.5	0.2	1.4
Canada	157	22	8	6	6	5.1	2.9	0.0	1.5	25	0	2	2.1	2.2	1.7	1.6	1.5	0.3
Cape Verde	88	151	63	41	28	4.4	4.3	4.2	4.3	56	32	–	4.1	7.0	5.3	2.7	1.4	3.6
Central African Republic	8	239	175	184	171	1.6	-0.5	0.8	0.1	2	7	-1.3	-0.8	6.0	5.8	4.7	0.1	1.1
Chad	1	–	201	205	209	–	-0.2	-0.2	-0.2	-4	-2	-1	3	6.5	6.7	6.1	-0.1	0.5
Chile	147	83	22	11	9	6.6	6.9	2.2	4.7	59	18	1.5	3.5	4.0	2.6	1.9	2.1	1.6
China	105	117	46	36	19	4.7	2.5	7.1	4.7	59	47	6.6	9	5.5	2.3	1.8	4.3	1.5
Colombia	105	104	35	26	19	5.4	3.0	3.5	3.2	46	27	1.9	1.4	5.6	3.1	2.4	2.9	1.3
Comoros	29	197	128	114	104	2.2	1.2	1.0	1.1	19	9	0.1 x	-0.2	7.1	5.5	3.9	1.2	1.8
Congo	19	142	104	116	128	1.6	-1.1	-1.1	-1.1	-23	-10	3.1	0.5	6.3	5.4	4.3	0.8	1.2
Cook Islands	118	63	18	17	15	6.3	0.6	1.4	1.0	17	12	–	–	–	–	–	–	–
Costa Rica	140	80	18	13	11	7.5	3.3	1.9	2.6	39	15	0.7	2.6	5.0	3.2	1.9	2.3	2.6
Côte d'Ivoire	21	236	152	142	119	2.2	0.7	2.0	1.3	22	16	-1.9	-1	7.9	6.3	4.5	1.2	1.7
Croatia	165	–	13	8	5	–	4.9	5.2	5.0	62	38	–	2.9	2.0	1.7	1.4	0.9	0.8
Cuba	157	40	14	9	6	5.2	4.4	4.5	4.5	57	33	–	3.6 x	4.0	1.8	1.5	4.2	0.8
Cyprus	169	–	10	6	4	–	5.1	4.5	4.8	60	33	5.9 x	2.2 x	2.6	2.4	1.5	0.4	2.5
Czech Republic	169	–	12	5	4	–	8.8	2.5	5.8	67	20	–	2.5	2.0	1.8	1.5	0.5	1.2
Democratic People's Republic of Korea	77	–	45	58	33	–	-2.5	6.3	1.6	27	43	–	–	4.0	2.4	1.9	2.6	1.3
Democratic Republic of the Congo	2	240	199	199	199	0.9	0.0	0.0	0.0	0	0	-2.3	-3.5	6.2	7.1	5.9	-0.7	1.0
Denmark	169	17	9	6	4	3.2	4.1	4.5	4.3	56	33	2	1.7	2.1	1.7	1.8	1.2	-0.6
Djibouti	33	–	123	106	94	–	1.5	1.3	1.4	24	11	–	-1.4	7.4	6.2	3.8	0.9	2.6
Dominica	144	73	18	16	10	7.0	1.2	5.2	3.1	44	38	4.7 x	1.7	–	–	–	–	–
Dominican Republic	79	125	62	39	32	3.5	4.6	2.2	3.5	48	18	2.1	3.8	6.2	3.5	2.6	2.9	1.5
Ecuador	93	138	53	34	24	4.8	4.4	3.9	4.2	55	29	1.3	1.6	6.3	3.7	2.5	2.7	2.0
Egypt	98	236	90	47	21	4.8	6.5	9.0	7.7	77	55	4.1	2.6	5.9	4.6	2.8	1.3	2.5
El Salvador	112	163	62	33	17	4.8	6.3	7.4	6.8	73	48	-1.9	2.7	6.2	4.0	2.3	2.3	2.9
Equatorial Guinea	14	–	198	168	145	–	1.6	1.6	1.6	27	14	–	19.8	5.7	5.9	5.3	-0.2	0.6
Eritrea	56	–	150	89	55	–	5.2	5.3	5.3	63	38	–	-0.8 x	6.6	6.2	4.5	0.3	1.7
Estonia	157	–	17	11	6	–	4.4	6.7	5.5	65	45	1.5 x	5.3	2.1	1.9	1.7	0.4	0.7
Ethiopia	29	230	210	148	104	0.5	3.5	3.9	3.7	50	30	–	2.7	6.8	7.1	5.2	-0.2	1.6
Fiji	109	–	22	19	18	–	1.5	0.6	1.1	18	5	0.7	4	4.5	3.4	2.7	1.5	1.2
Finland	184	16	7	4	3	4.1	5.6	3.2	4.5	57	25	2.8	2.7	1.9	1.7	1.8	0.3	-0.3

	Under-5 mortality rank	Under-5 mortality rate				Average annual rate of reduction (%)[e]				Reduction since 1990 (%)[o]	Reduction since 2000 (%)[o]	GDP per capita average annual growth rate (%)		Total fertility rate			Average annual rate of reduction (%)	
		1970	1990	2000	2009	1970–1990	1990–2000	2000–2009	1990–2009			1970–1990	1990–2009	1970	1990	2009	1970–1990	1990–2009
France	169	18	9	5	4	3.5	5.9	2.5	4.3	56	20	2.2	1.4	2.5	1.8	1.9	1.7	-0.4
Gabon	45	–	93	83	69	–	1.1	2.1	1.6	26	17	0.2	-0.9	4.7	5.2	3.2	-0.5	2.5
Gambia	31	311	153	131	103	3.5	1.6	2.7	2.1	33	21	0.7	0.6	6.1	6.1	5.0	0.0	1.1
Georgia	85	–	47	35	29	–	2.9	2.1	2.5	38	17	–	–	2.6	2.2	1.6	0.9	1.7
Germany	169	26	9	5	4	5.3	5.9	2.5	4.3	56	20	2.3	1.3	2.0	1.4	1.3	1.9	0.2
Ghana	45	183	120	106	69	2.1	1.2	4.8	2.9	43	35	-2	2.2	7.0	5.6	4.2	1.1	1.5
Greece	184	32	11	7	3	5.3	4.5	9.4	6.8	73	57	1.3	2.7	2.4	1.4	1.4	2.5	0.1
Grenada	118	–	40	20	15	–	6.9	3.2	5.2	63	25	4.2 x	3.1	4.6	3.8	2.3	0.9	2.8
Guatemala	65	165	76	48	40	3.9	4.6	2.0	3.4	47	17	0.2	1.4	6.2	5.6	4.0	0.6	1.7
Guinea	15	326	231	185	142	1.7	2.2	2.9	2.6	39	23	0.2 x	3.3	6.8	6.7	5.3	0.1	1.2
Guinea-Bissau	4	–	240	218	193	–	1.0	1.4	1.1	20	11	0.1	-9.6	6.1	5.9	5.7	0.2	0.2
Guyana	72	79	61	45	35	1.3	3.0	2.8	2.9	43	22	-1.6	3 x	5.6	2.6	2.3	3.8	0.6
Haiti	37	222	152	113	87	1.9	3.0	2.9	2.9	43	23	–	-1.1 x	5.8	5.4	3.4	0.3	2.4
Holy See	–																	
Honduras	83	172	55	40	30	5.7	3.2	3.2	3.2	45	25	0.8	1.6	7.3	5.1	3.2	1.7	2.5
Hungary	157	39	17	10	6	4.2	5.3	5.7	5.5	65	40	3	3.2	2.0	1.8	1.4	0.6	1.4
Iceland	184	15	7	4	3	3.8	5.6	3.2	4.5	57	25	3.2	2.4	3.0	2.2	2.1	1.6	0.2
India	48	186	118	93	66	2.3	2.4	3.8	3.1	44	29	2.1	4.8	5.5	4.0	2.7	1.5	2.1
Indonesia	66	170	86	56	39	3.4	4.3	4.0	4.2	55	30	4.7	2.5	5.5	3.1	2.1	2.8	2.0
Iran (Islamic Republic of)	81	190	73	48	31	4.8	4.2	4.9	4.5	58	35	-2.3	2.7	6.6	4.8	1.8	1.6	5.2
Iraq	63	125	53	48	44	4.3	1.0	1.0	1.0	17	8	–	-2.6 x	7.4	6.0	4.0	1.0	2.2
Ireland	169	22	9	7	4	4.5	2.5	6.2	4.3	56	43	2.8	5.2	3.9	2.1	2.0	3.1	0.4
Israel	169	–	11	7	4	–	4.5	6.2	5.3	64	43	1.9	1.8	3.8	3.0	2.8	1.2	0.4
Italy	169	33	10	6	4	6.0	5.1	4.5	4.8	60	33	2.8	1	2.5	1.3	1.4	3.2	-0.3
Jamaica	81	61	33	32	31	3.1	0.3	0.4	0.3	6	3	-1.3	0.7	5.5	2.9	2.4	3.1	1.2
Japan	184	17	6	4	3	5.2	4.1	3.2	3.6	50	25	3	0.9	2.1	1.6	1.3	1.5	1.2
Jordan	91	103	39	30	25	4.9	2.6	2.0	2.3	36	17	2.5 x	2.5	7.9	5.5	3.0	1.8	3.2
Kazakhstan	85	–	60	44	29	–	3.1	4.6	3.8	52	34	–	3.8	3.5	2.8	2.3	1.1	1.1
Kenya	39	152	99	105	84	2.1	-0.6	2.5	0.9	15	20	1.2	0.2	8.1	6.0	4.9	1.5	1.1
Kiribati	61	156	89	63	46	2.8	3.5	3.5	3.5	48	27	-5.3	1.8	–	–	–	–	–
Kuwait	144	58	17	13	10	6.1	2.7	2.9	2.8	41	23	-6.8 x	2 x	7.2	3.5	2.2	3.6	2.6
Kyrgyzstan	69	–	75	51	37	–	3.9	3.6	3.7	51	27	–	0.3	4.9	3.9	2.5	1.2	2.2
Lao People's Democratic Republic	52	211	157	86	59	1.5	6.0	4.2	5.2	62	31	–	4.2	6.0	6.0	3.4	0.0	3.0
Latvia	149	–	16	14	8	–	1.3	6.2	3.6	50	43	3.4	4.7	1.9	1.9	1.4	0.0	1.5
Lebanon	130	56	40	24	12	1.7	5.1	7.7	6.3	70	50	–	2.2	5.1	3.1	1.8	2.4	2.8
Lesotho	39	175	93	124	84	3.2	-2.9	4.3	0.5	10	32	2.8	1.6	5.8	4.9	3.3	0.8	2.2
Liberia	24	260	247	198	112	0.3	2.2	6.3	4.2	55	43	-4.2	1.8	6.8	6.5	5.0	0.2	1.4
Libyan Arab Jamahiriya	105	142	36	25	19	6.9	3.6	3.0	3.4	47	24	–	2.9 x	7.6	4.8	2.6	2.3	3.2
Liechtenstein	193	–	10	6	2	–	5.1	12.2	8.5	80	67	2.2	3.1 x	–	–	–	–	–
Lithuania	157	–	15	10	6	–	4.1	5.7	4.8	60	40	–	3.5	2.3	2.0	1.4	0.7	2.0
Luxembourg	184	22	9	5	3	4.5	5.9	5.7	5.8	67	40	2.7	3	2.0	1.6	1.7	1.1	-0.3
Madagascar	53	179	167	100	58	0.3	5.1	6.1	5.6	65	42	-2.3	-0.1	7.3	6.3	4.6	0.8	1.6
Malawi	26	323	218	164	110	2.0	2.8	4.4	3.6	50	33	-0.1	0.5	7.3	7.0	5.5	0.2	1.3
Malaysia	157	52	18	10	6	5.3	5.9	5.7	5.8	67	40	4	3.2	5.6	3.7	2.5	2.0	2.1
Maldives	128	–	113	53	13	–	7.6	15.6	11.4	88	75	–	5.9 x	7.0	6.1	2.0	0.7	5.8
Mali	6	374	250	217	191	2.0	1.4	1.4	1.4	24	12	0.2	2.9	6.7	6.4	5.4	0.2	0.9
Malta	151	28	11	7	7	4.7	4.5	0.0	2.4	36	0	6.5	2.6 x	2.1	2.0	1.3	0.0	2.6
Marshall Islands	72	103	49	39	35	3.7	2.3	1.2	1.8	29	10	–	-1.1	–	–	–	–	–
Mauritania	23	224	129	122	117	2.8	0.6	0.5	0.5	9	4	-1	0.8	6.8	5.9	4.4	0.7	1.5
Mauritius	112	88	24	19	17	6.5	2.3	1.2	1.8	29	11	3.2 x	3.5	3.7	2.2	1.8	2.5	1.1
Mexico	112	110	45	26	17	4.5	5.5	4.7	5.1	62	35	1.6	1.5	6.7	3.4	2.2	3.4	2.4
Micronesia (Federated States of)	66	–	58	47	39	–	2.1	2.1	2.1	33	17	–	0.1	6.9	5.0	3.5	1.7	1.8
Monaco	169	–	8	5	4	–	4.7	2.5	3.6	50	20	1.6	2 x	–	–	–	–	–
Mongolia	85	194	101	63	29	3.3	4.7	8.6	6.6	71	54	–	2.9	7.5	4.2	2.0	2.9	3.9
Montenegro	147	–	17	14	9	–	1.9	4.9	3.3	47	36	–	3.8 x	2.4	2.1	1.6	0.6	1.3
Morocco	68	183	89	55	38	3.6	4.8	4.1	4.5	57	31	1.9	2.3	7.1	4.0	2.3	2.8	2.9
Mozambique	15	276	232	183	142	0.9	2.4	2.8	2.6	39	22	-1 x	4.3	6.6	6.2	5.0	0.3	1.2
Myanmar	44	179	118	85	71	2.1	3.3	2.0	2.7	40	16	1.4	8.2 x	6.1	3.4	2.3	2.9	2.1
Namibia	59	103	73	76	48	1.7	-0.4	5.1	2.2	34	37	-2.1 x	2.4	6.5	5.2	3.3	1.1	2.4
Nauru	63	–	–	51	44	–	–	1.6	–	–	14	–	–	–	–	–	–	–
Nepal	59	237	142	85	48	2.6	5.1	6.3	5.7	66	44	1	1.9	6.1	5.2	2.8	0.9	3.2
Netherlands	169	16	8	6	4	3.5	2.9	4.5	3.6	50	33	1.6	2.1	2.4	1.6	1.7	2.2	-0.6
New Zealand	157	21	11	7	6	3.2	4.5	1.7	3.2	45	14	0.8	2	3.1	2.1	2.0	2.0	0.1

TABLE 10. THE RATE OF PROGRESS

	Under-5 mortality rank	Under-5 mortality rate				Average annual rate of reduction (%)[e]				Reduction since 1990 (%)[e]	Reduction since 2000 (%)[e]	GDP per capita average annual growth rate (%)		Total fertility rate			Average annual rate of reduction (%)		
		1970	1990	2000	2009	1970–1990	1990–2000	2000–2009	1990–2009			1970–1990	1990–2009	1970	1990	2009	1970 1990	1990 2009
Nicaragua	89	161	68	42	26	4.3	4.8	5.3	5.1	62	38	-3.7	1.9	6.9	4.8	2.7	1.9	3.0
Niger	12	309	305	227	160	0.1	3.0	3.9	3.4	48	30	-2.1	-0.2	7.6	7.9	7.1	-0.2	0.6
Nigeria	18	–	212	190	138	–	1.1	3.6	2.3	35	27	-1.4	1.7	6.6	6.6	5.2	0.0	1.3
Niue	–	–	–	–	–	–	–	–	–	–	–	–	–	–	–	–	–	–
Norway	184	16	9	5	3	2.9	5.9	5.7	5.8	67	40	3.2	2.3	2.5	1.9	1.9	1.5	-0.1
Occupied Palestinian Territory	83	–	43	30	30	–	3.6	0.0	1.9	30	0	–	-2.4 x	7.9	6.4	4.9	1.0	1.4
Oman	130	206	48	22	12	7.3	7.8	6.7	7.3	75	45	3.3	2 x	7.2	6.6	3.0	0.4	4.2
Pakistan	37	180	130	108	87	1.6	1.9	2.4	2.1	33	19	3	1.7	7.0	6.1	3.9	0.7	2.4
Palau	118	–	21	16	15	–	2.7	0.7	1.8	29	6	–	-0.1 x	–	–	–	–	–
Panama	95	70	31	26	23	4.1	1.8	1.4	1.6	26	12	0.3	3	5.3	3.0	2.5	2.8	1.0
Papua New Guinea	47	155	91	77	68	2.7	1.7	1.4	1.5	25	12	-0.7	-0.4	6.2	4.8	4.0	1.2	0.9
Paraguay	95	76	42	30	23	3.0	3.4	3.0	3.2	45	23	3.1	-0.1	5.7	4.5	3.0	1.2	2.2
Peru	98	170	78	40	21	3.9	6.7	7.2	6.9	73	48	-0.6	2.9	6.3	3.8	2.5	2.5	2.2
Philippines	77	89	59	38	33	2.1	4.4	1.6	3.1	44	13	0.6	1.9	6.3	4.3	3.0	1.8	1.9
Poland	151	36	17	9	7	3.8	6.4	2.8	4.7	59	22	–	4.4	2.2	2.0	1.3	0.4	2.5
Portugal	169	67	15	7	4	7.5	7.6	6.2	7.0	73	43	2.6	1.7	2.8	1.5	1.4	3.1	0.5
Qatar	140	83	19	14	11	7.4	3.1	2.7	2.9	42	21	–	–	6.9	4.4	2.4	2.3	3.3
Republic of Korea	165	52	9	6	5	8.8	4.1	2.0	3.1	44	17	6.2	4.3	4.5	1.6	1.2	5.2	1.5
Republic of Moldova	112	–	37	24	17	–	4.3	3.8	4.1	54	29	–	-1	2.6	2.4	1.5	0.3	2.5
Romania	130	52	32	22	12	2.4	3.7	6.7	5.2	63	45	0.9 x	2.7	2.9	1.9	1.3	2.0	1.9
Russian Federation	130	40	27	24	12	2.0	1.2	7.7	4.3	56	50	–	1.9	2.0	1.9	1.4	0.3	1.5
Rwanda	25	212	171	180	111	1.1	-0.5	5.4	2.3	35	38	1.2	1.7	8.2	6.8	5.3	0.9	1.3
Saint Kitts and Nevis	118	–	26	21	15	–	2.1	3.7	2.9	42	29	6.3 x	2.5	–	–	–	–	–
Saint Lucia	103	–	20	17	20	–	1.6	-1.8	0.0	0	-18	5.3 x	1.1	6.1	3.4	2.0	2.9	2.8
Saint Vincent and the Grenadines	130	–	24	23	12	–	0.4	7.2	3.6	50	48	3.3	3.8	6.0	3.0	2.1	3.6	1.8
Samoa	91	–	50	34	25	–	3.9	3.4	3.6	50	26	–	3.1	6.1	4.8	3.9	1.2	1.1
San Marino	193	–	15	6	2	–	9.2	12.2	10.6	87	67	–	–	–	–	–	–	–
Sao Tome and Principe	42	117	95	86	78	1.0	1.0	1.1	1.0	18	9	–	–	6.5	5.4	3.7	0.9	2.0
Saudi Arabia	98	–	43	23	21	–	6.3	1.0	3.8	51	9	-1.4	0.3	7.3	5.8	3.0	1.1	3.4
Senegal	34	276	151	120	93	3.0	2.3	2.8	2.6	38	23	-0.7	1.1	7.4	6.7	4.9	0.5	1.7
Serbia	151	–	29	12	7	–	8.8	6.0	7.5	76	42	–	1.3	2.4	1.9	1.6	1.2	0.8
Seychelles	130	66	15	14	12	7.4	0.7	1.7	1.2	20	14	2.9	1.7	–	–	–	–	–
Sierra Leone	5	372	285	250	192	1.3	1.3	2.9	2.1	33	23	-0.5	0.9	5.8	5.5	5.2	0.3	0.4
Singapore	184	27	8	4	3	6.1	6.9	3.2	5.2	63	25	5.6	3.9	3.0	1.8	1.3	2.7	1.7
Slovakia	151	–	15	10	7	–	4.1	4.0	4.0	53	30	–	3.7	2.5	2.0	1.3	1.0	2.4
Slovenia	184	–	10	5	3	–	6.9	5.7	6.3	70	40	–	3.5	2.3	1.5	1.4	2.0	0.4
Solomon Islands	70	101	38	37	36	4.9	0.3	0.3	0.3	5	3	–	-1.3	6.9	5.9	3.8	0.9	2.3
Somalia	7	–	180	180	180	–	0.0	0.0	0.0	0	0	-0.8	–	7.2	6.6	6.4	0.4	0.2
South Africa	50	–	62	77	62	–	-2.2	2.4	0.0	0	19	0.1	1.2	5.6	3.7	2.5	2.1	2.0
Spain	169	25	9	5	4	5.1	5.9	2.5	4.3	56	20	1.9	2.2	2.9	1.3	1.5	3.9	-0.5
Sri Lanka	118	84	28	21	15	5.5	2.9	3.7	3.3	46	29	3	4	4.3	2.5	2.3	2.7	0.5
Sudan	27	169	124	115	108	1.5	0.8	0.7	0.7	13	6	0.1	3.8	6.6	6.0	4.1	0.5	2.0
Suriname	89	71	51	38	26	1.7	2.9	4.2	3.5	49	32	-2.2 x	1.4 x	5.7	2.7	2.4	3.6	0.7
Swaziland	43	179	92	105	73	3.3	-1.3	4.0	1.2	21	30	3	1.7	6.9	5.7	3.5	0.9	2.7
Sweden	184	13	7	4	3	3.1	5.6	3.2	4.5	57	25	1.8	2.2	2.0	2.0	1.9	0.1	0.4
Switzerland	169	18	8	6	4	4.1	2.9	4.5	3.6	50	33	1.2	0.9 x	2.0	1.5	1.5	1.4	0.3
Syrian Arab Republic	116	123	36	22	16	6.1	4.9	3.5	4.3	56	27	2	1.4	7.6	5.5	3.2	1.6	2.9
Tajikistan	51	–	117	94	61	–	2.2	4.8	3.4	48	35	–	-0.9	6.9	5.2	3.4	1.4	2.3
Thailand	125	98	32	20	14	5.6	4.7	4.0	4.4	56	30	4.7	2.9	5.6	2.1	1.8	4.8	0.8
The former Yugoslav Republic of Macedonia	140	–	36	19	11	–	6.4	6.1	6.2	69	42	–	0.9	3.1	2.1	1.4	1.9	2.1
Timor-Leste	55	–	184	106	56	–	5.5	7.1	6.3	70	47	–	-1.3 x	6.3	5.3	6.4	0.8	-0.9
Togo	32	219	150	124	98	1.9	1.9	2.6	2.2	35	21	-0.6	–	7.1	6.3	4.2	0.6	2.2
Tonga	105	42	23	20	19	3.0	1.4	0.6	1.0	17	5	–	2.9	5.9	4.6	3.9	1.3	0.8
Trinidad and Tobago	72	54	34	34	35	2.3	0.0	-0.3	-0.2	-3	-3	0.5	5.1	3.5	2.4	1.6	1.8	2.1
Tunisia	98	187	50	27	21	6.6	6.2	2.8	4.6	58	22	2.5	3.5	6.6	3.6	1.8	3.0	3.6
Turkey	103	200	84	42	20	4.3	6.9	8.2	7.6	76	52	2	2.3	5.6	3.1	2.1	3.0	2.0
Turkmenistan	62	–	99	71	45	–	3.3	5.1	4.1	55	37	–	4.7	6.3	4.3	2.4	1.9	3.1
Tuvalu	72	–	53	43	35	–	2.1	2.3	2.2	34	19	–	–	–	–	–	–	–
Uganda	19	193	184	154	128	0.2	1.8	2.1	1.9	30	17	–	3.6	7.1	7.1	6.3	0.0	0.7
Ukraine	118	34	21	19	15	2.4	1.0	2.6	1.8	29	21	–	0.1	2.1	1.9	1.4	0.6	1.7
United Arab Emirates	151	84	17	11	7	8.0	4.4	5.0	4.7	59	36	-4.9 x	0.5	6.6	4.4	1.9	2.0	4.4

	Under-5 mortality rank	Under-5 mortality rate				Average annual rate of reduction (%)[⊖]				Reduction since 1990 (%)[⊖]	Reduction since 2000 (%)[⊖]	GDP per capita average annual growth rate (%)		Total fertility rate			Average annual rate of reduction (%)	
		1970	1990	2000	2009	1970–1990	1990–2000	2000–2009	1990–2009			1970–1990	1990–2009	1970	1990	2009	1970–1990	1990–2009
United Kingdom	157	21	10	7	6	3.7	3.6	1.7	2.7	40	14	2	2.3	2.3	1.8	1.9	1.2	-0.1
United Republic of Tanzania	27	210	162	139	108	1.3	1.5	2.8	2.1	33	22	–	2	6.8	6.2	5.5	0.4	0.6
United States	149	23	11	8	8	3.7	3.2	0.0	1.7	27	0	2.2	1.8	2.2	2.0	2.1	0.6	-0.2
Uruguay	128	53	24	18	13	4.0	2.9	3.6	3.2	46	28	0.9	1.8	2.9	2.5	2.1	0.7	1.0
Uzbekistan	70	–	74	62	36	–	1.8	6.0	3.8	51	42	–	1.9	6.5	4.2	2.2	2.2	3.3
Vanuatu	116	103	40	25	16	4.7	4.7	5.0	4.8	60	36	1.1 x	6.7	6.3	4.9	3.9	1.2	1.3
Venezuela (Bolivarian Republic of)	109	63	32	23	18	3.4	3.3	2.7	3.0	44	22	-1.6	0.2	5.4	3.4	2.5	2.2	1.7
Viet Nam	93	–	55	29	24	–	6.4	2.1	4.4	56	17	–	6	7.0	3.7	2.0	3.2	3.1
Yemen	48	308	125	100	66	4.5	2.2	4.6	3.4	47	34	–	1.5	8.6	8.1	5.1	0.3	2.4
Zambia	17	178	179	166	141	0.0	0.8	1.8	1.3	21	15	-2.3	0.3	7.4	6.5	5.7	0.7	0.6
Zimbabwe	35	121	81	116	90	2.0	-3.6	2.8	-0.6	-11	22	-0.4	-1.9 x	7.4	5.2	3.4	1.8	2.3

SUMMARY INDICATORS

		1970	1990	2000	2009	1970–1990	1990–2000	2000–2009	1990–2009			1970–1990	1990–2009	1970	1990	2009	1970–1990	1990–2009
Africa[#]		223	165	147	118	1.5	1.2	2.4	1.8	28	20	0.9	2.0	6.7	5.9	4.5	0.6	1.4
Sub-Saharan Africa[#]		226	180	160	129	1.1	1.2	2.4	1.8	28	19	0	1.8	6.7	6.3	5.0	0.3	1.2
Eastern and Southern Africa		210	166	141	108	1.2	1.6	3.0	2.3	35	23	–	1.8	6.8	6.0	4.8	0.6	1.2
West and Central Africa		258	199	181	150	1.3	0.9	2.1	1.5	25	17	-0.5	1.6	6.6	6.6	5.2	0.1	1.2
Middle East and North Africa		192	77	56	41	4.6	3.2	3.5	3.3	47	27	-0.2	2.4	6.8	5.0	2.8	1.5	3.0
Asia[#]		150	87	70	50	2.7	2.2	3.7	2.9	43	29	4.2	6.6	5.6	3.2	2.3	2.8	1.8
South Asia		194	125	97	71	2.2	2.5	3.5	3.0	43	27	2.1	4.4	5.7	4.3	2.8	1.5	2.2
East Asia and Pacific		121	53	40	26	4.1	2.8	4.8	3.7	51	35	5.4	7.2	5.6	2.6	1.9	3.8	1.6
Latin America and Caribbean		121	52	33	23	4.2	4.5	4.0	4.3	56	30	1.4	1.6	5.3	3.2	2.2	2.5	2.0
CEE/CIS		89	51	37	21	2.8	3.2	6.3	4.7	59	43	–	2.2	2.8	2.3	1.7	1.1	1.5
Industrialized countries[§]		24	10	7	6	4.4	3.6	1.7	2.7	40	14	2.3	1.7	2.3	1.7	1.7	1.4	0.0
Developing countries[§]		157	99	84	66	2.3	1.6	2.7	2.1	33	21	2.1	4.6	5.8	3.7	2.7	2.3	1.6
Least developed countries[§]		239	178	146	121	1.5	2.0	2.1	2.0	32	17	-0.2	3.0	6.8	5.9	4.3	0.7	1.6
World		138	89	77	60	2.2	1.4	2.8	2.1	33	22	2.3	2.5	4.7	3.2	2.5	2.0	1.2

For a complete list of countries and territories in the regions and subregions, see page 124.
§ Includes territories within each country category or regional group. Countries and territories in each country category or regional group are listed on page 124.

DEFINITIONS OF THE INDICATORS

Under-five mortality rate – Probability of dying between birth and exactly 5 years of age, expressed per 1,000 live births.

Reduction since 1990 (%) – Percentage reduction in the under-five mortality rate (U5MR) from 1990 to 2009. The United Nations Millennium Declaration in 2000 established a goal of a two-thirds (67 per cent) reduction in U5MR from 1990 to 2015. This indicator provides a current assessment of progress towards this goal.

GDP per capita – Gross domestic product (GDP) is the sum of value added by all resident producers plus any product taxes (less subsidies) not included in the valuation of output. GDP per capita is gross domestic product divided by midyear population. Growth is calculated from constant price GDP data in local currency.

Total fertility rate – Number of children who would be born per woman if she lived to the end of her childbearing years and bore children at each age in accordance with prevailing age-specific fertility rates.

MAIN DATA SOURCES

Under-five mortality rate – Inter-agency Group for Child Mortality Estimation (UNICEF, World Health Organization, United Nations Population Division and the World Bank).

GDP per capita – World Bank.

Fertility – United Nations Population Division.

NOTES
– Data not available.
x Data refer to years or periods other than those specified in the column heading, differ from the standard definition or refer to only part of a country. Such data are not included in the calculation of regional and global averages.
⊖ A negative value indicates an increase in the under-five mortality rate since 1990.

TABLE 11. ADOLESCENTS

Countries and territories	Adolescents population (aged 10–19) Total	Adolescents as a proportion of total population	Girls aged 15–19 who are currently married/in union (%)	Women aged 20–24 who gave birth before age 18 (%)	Adolescent birth rate Number of births per 1,000 girls aged 15–19	Attitudes towards domestic violence: Adolescents aged 15–19 who think that a husband is justified in hitting or beating his wife under certain circumstances (2002–2009*) (%) male	female	Secondary education (2005–2009*) Net enrolment ratio total	male	female	Net attendance ratio total	male	female	HIV knowledge: Adolescents age 15–19 who have comprehensive knowledge of HIV (2005–2009*) (%) male	female
	2009	2009	2000–2009*	2000–2009*	2000–2008*	male	female	total	male	female	total	male	female	male	female
Afghanistan	6767	24	–	–	151	–	–	27	38	15	12 x	18 x	6 x	–	–
Albania	604	19	8	3	17	37	24	74 x	75 x	73 x	78	79	77	21	36
Algeria	6698	19	2	–	4	–	66	66 x	65 x	68 x	61	57	65	–	12
Andorra	–	–	–	–	7	–	–	71	69	75	–	–	–	–	–
Angola	4411	24	–	–	165	–	–	–	–	–	21 x	22 x	20 x	–	–
Antigua and Barbuda	–	–	–	–	67	–	–	–	–	–	–	–	–	–	–
Argentina	6828	17	–	–	65	–	–	79	75	84	–	–	–	–	–
Armenia	482	16	7	3	26	31	22	86	83	88	94	93	95	7	19
Australia	2826	13	–	–	18	–	–	88	87	89	–	–	–	–	–
Austria	955	11	–	–	11	–	–	–	–	–	–	–	–	–	–
Azerbaijan	1629	18	10	4	42	63	39	98	99	97	81	82	80	2	3
Bahamas	61	18	–	–	44	–	–	85	83	87	–	–	–	–	–
Bahrain	139	18	–	–	14	–	–	89	87	92	81 x	77 x	85 x	–	–
Bangladesh	33907	21	46	40	133	–	41	41	40	43	49	46	53	–	16
Barbados	34	13	–	–	53	–	–	–	–	–	–	–	–	–	–
Belarus	1139	12	4	–	22	–	–	87	–	–	96	95	97	–	32
Belgium	1248	12	–	–	11	–	–	87	89	85	–	–	–	–	–
Belize	70	23	–	–	91	–	14	63	61	66	59	58	60	–	39
Benin	2041	23	22	23	114	12	41	20 x	26 x	13 x	34	40	27	31	17
Bhutan	150	21	15	–	46	–	–	47	46	49	–	–	–	–	–
Bolivia (Plurinational State of)	2188	22	11	20	89	–	17	70	70	70	77	78	75	24	22
Bosnia and Herzegovina	459	12	7	–	15	–	4	–	–	–	89	89	89	–	45
Botswana	432	22	–	–	51	–	–	64	62	67	40 x	36 x	44 x	–	–
Brazil	33724	17	25	16 x	56	–	–	82	78	85	77	74	80	–	–
Brunei Darussalam	70	18	–	–	26	–	–	88	87	90	–	–	–	–	–
Bulgaria	756	10	–	–	42	–	–	83	85	82	–	–	–	–	–
Burkina Faso	3634	23	24	27	131	–	68	15	18	13	16	17	15	–	18
Burundi	1955	24	10	–	30	–	–	–	–	–	7	8	6	–	30
Cambodia	3570	24	10	9	52	–	49	34	36	32	28	29	26	41	50
Cameroon	4459	23	22	33	141	–	58	–	–	–	43	45	42	–	32
Canada	4221	13	–	–	14	–	–	95 x	95 x	94 x	–	–	–	–	–
Cape Verde	123	24	8	22	92	24	23	57 x	54 x	60 x	–	–	–	36	37
Central African Republic	1014	23	57	38 x	133	–	–	10	13	8	13	16	10	26	16
Chad	2621	23	42	48	193	–	–	10 x	16 x	5 x	10 x	13 x	7 x	13 x	8 x
Chile	2861	17	–	–	51	–	–	85	84	87	–	–	–	–	–
China	206753	15	–	–	5	–	–	–	–	–	–	–	–	–	–
Colombia	8740	19	14	20	96	–	–	71	68	75	68	64	72	–	–
Comoros	142	21	–	17 x	95	–	–	15	15	15	11 x	10 x	11 x	–	–
Congo	846	23	16	29	132	–	76	–	–	–	39	39	40	18	8
Cook Islands	–	–	–	–	47	–	–	59 x	57 x	61 x	–	–	–	–	–
Costa Rica	850	19	–	–	69	–	–	–	–	–	62	59	65	–	–
Côte d'Ivoire	4784	23	20	29	111	–	63	21 x	27 x	15 x	27	32	22	30	18
Croatia	507	11	–	–	14	–	–	88	87	89	–	–	–	–	–
Cuba	1500	13	–	–	44	–	–	83	82	83	–	–	–	–	51
Cyprus	122	14	–	–	5	–	–	96	95	97	–	–	–	–	–
Czech Republic	1096	11	–	–	12	–	–	–	–	–	–	–	–	–	–
Democratic People's Republic of Korea	3971	17	–	–	1	–	–	–	–	–	–	–	–	–	–
Democratic Republic of the Congo	15938	24	23	23	127	–	74	–	–	–	27	30	24	18	14
Denmark	696	13	–	–	6	–	–	90	88	91	–	–	–	–	–
Djibouti	199	23	4	–	27	–	–	22	25	18	41	45	37	–	16
Dominica	–	–	–	–	47	–	–	68	62	74	–	–	–	–	–
Dominican Republic	2025	20	19	25	98	14	6	58	52	63	62	56	68	33	39
Ecuador	2762	20	16	–	100	–	–	62	61	62	–	–	–	–	–
Egypt	16603	20	13	7	50	–	50 y	71 x	73 x	69 x	69	72	67	16	3
El Salvador	1431	23	21	–	68	–	–	55	54	56	–	–	–	–	–
Equatorial Guinea	156	23	–	–	128	–	–	22 x	–	–	22 x	23 x	22 x	–	–
Eritrea	1113	22	29	25	85	–	70	26	30	22	22 x	23 x	21 x	–	–
Estonia	146	11	–	–	25	–	–	90	88	91	–	–	–	–	–
Ethiopia	19998	24	22	28	109	53	77	25	31	20	27	30	23	32	21
Fiji	176	21	–	–	30	–	–	79	76	83	–	–	–	–	–
Finland	641	12	–	–	9	–	–	96	96	97	–	–	–	–	–

	Adolescents population (aged 10–19)		Marital status	Age at first birth	Adolescent birth rate	Attitudes towards domestic violence		Secondary education (2005–2009*)						HIV knowledge	
		Adolescents as a proportion of total population	Girls aged 15–19 who are currently married/in union (%)	Women aged 20–24 who gave birth before age 18 (%)	Number of births per 1,000 girls aged 15–19	Adolescents aged 15–19 who think that a husband is justified in hitting or beating his wife under certain circumstances (2002–2009*) (%)		Net enrolment ratio			Net attendance ratio			Adolescents age 15–19 who have comprehensive knowledge of HIV (2005–2009*) (%)	
	Total					male	female	total	male	female	total	male	female	male	female
	2009	2009	2000–2009*	2000–2009*	2000–2008*										
France	7456	12	–	–	11	–	–	98	98	99	–	–	–	–	–
Gabon	342	23	18	35	–	–	–	–	–	–	35 x	34 x	36 x	–	–
Gambia	386	23	25	–	104	–	71	42	42	41	37	39	34	–	40
Georgia	602	14	11	–	44	–	5	81	82	79	88	89	88	–	12
Germany	8378	10	–	–	10	–	–	–	–	–	–	–	–	–	–
Ghana	5347	22	8	16	70	28	41	47	49	45	42	42	42	30	28
Greece	1092	10	–	–	11	–	–	91	91	91	–	–	–	–	–
Grenada	22	21	–	–	54	–	–	89	93	85	–	–	–	–	–
Guatemala	3310	24	18	24 x	92	–	–	40	41	39	23 x	23 x	24 x	–	–
Guinea	2305	23	36	44	153	–	.79	28	34	21	22	27	17	20	17
Guinea-Bissau	354	22	22	–	170	–	41	10 x	12 x	7 x	8	8	7	–	19
Guyana	151	20	14	22	90	–	19	–	–	–	69	66	73	–	48
Haiti	2282	23	17	15	69	–	29	–	–	–	20	18	21	34	31
Holy See	–	–	–	–	–	–	–	–	–	–	–	–	–	–	–
Honduras	1751	23	20	26	108	–	18	–	–	–	32	29	36	–	28
Hungary	1123	11	–	–	19	–	–	91	91	91	–	–	–	–	–
Iceland	46	14	–	–	15	–	–	90	89	91	–	–	–	–	–
India	243387	20	27	22	45	57	53	–	–	–	54	59	49	35	19
Indonesia	40926	18	13	10	52	–	41	68	69	68	58	57	59	2 y	6 y
Iran (Islamic Republic of)	13301	18	16	–	31	–	–	75	75	75	–	–	–	–	–
Iraq	7199	23	19	–	68	–	57	40	46	33	40	46	34	–	2
Ireland	565	13	–	–	17	–	–	88	86	90	–	–	–	–	–
Israel	1184	17	–	–	15	–	–	86	85	88	–	–	–	–	–
Italy	5676	9	–	–	7	–	–	92	92	93	–	–	–	–	–
Jamaica	568	21	5	–	60	–	6	77	75	79	90	88	92	–	59
Japan	12020	9	–	–	5	–	–	98	98	98	–	–	–	–	–
Jordan	1368	22	6	4	28	–	91 y	82	80	84	87	85	89	–	12 y
Kazakhstan	2561	16	5	6 x	31	–	7	89	88	89	97	97	97	–	22
Kenya	9058	23	12	26	103	54	57	49	50	48	41	40	42	52	42
Kiribati	–	–	–	–	39	–	–	68	65	72	–	–	–	–	–
Kuwait	415	14	–	–	13	–	–	80	80	80	–	–	–	–	–
Kyrgyzstan	1134	21	8	4 x	29	–	28	80	80	81	91	90	92	–	19
Lao People's Democratic Republic	1571	25	–	–	110	–	79	36	39	33	36	39	32	–	–
Latvia	246	11	–	–	18	–	–	–	–	–	–	–	–	–	–
Lebanon	788	19	–	–	18	–	–	75	71	79	64 x	61 x	68 x	–	–
Lesotho	515	25	17	15	98	60	56	25	20	31	21	16	27	18 x	26 x
Liberia	912	23	19	38	177	37	48	20 x	25 x	14 x	20	21	18	21	18
Libyan Arab Jamahiriya	1122	17	–	–	4	–	–	–	–	–	–	–	–	–	–
Liechtenstein	–	–	–	–	4	–	–	83	85	81	–	–	–	–	–
Lithuania	427	13	–	–	19	–	–	92	91	92	–	–	–	–	–
Luxembourg	61	12	–	–	10	–	–	84	82	85	–	–	–	–	–
Madagascar	4674	24	27	36	148	9	31	24	23	24	19 x	17 x	21 x	13 x	18 x
Malawi	3748	25	33	34	178	28	32	25	26	24	13	13	13	42	42
Malaysia	5305	19	–	–	12	–	–	68	66	70	–	–	–	–	–
Maldives	72	23	17	–	14	–	–	69	68	71	–	–	–	–	–
Mali	3101	24	50	46	190	–	69	29	35	22	20	23	17	19	18
Malta	52	13	–	–	17	–	–	82	79	85	–	–	–	–	–
Marshall Islands	–	–	–	–	88	–	–	45	43	47	–	–	–	35	27
Mauritania	738	22	25	25	88	–	–	16	17	15	19	21	17	10	4
Mauritius	214	17	–	–	35	–	–	80	79	81	–	–	–	–	–
Mexico	20991	19	12	–	90	–	–	72	71	74	–	–	–	–	–
Micronesia (Federated States of)	27	24	–	–	51	–	–	25 x	–	–	–	–	–	–	–
Monaco	–	–	–	–	–	–	–	–	–	–	–	–	–	–	–
Mongolia	530	20	4	3	19	–	17	82	79	85	88	85	91	–	32
Montenegro	86	14	3	–	17	–	6	–	–	–	91	90	92	–	29
Morocco	6277	20	11	8	18	–	64	35 x	37 x	32 x	37 x	39 x	36 x	–	12 x
Mozambique	5237	23	40	42	185	–	37	6	6	6	20	21	20	–	14
Myanmar	8911	18	–	–	17	–	–	49	49	50	49 x	51 x	48 x	–	–
Namibia	507	23	5	17	74	44	38	54	49	60	47	40	53	59	62
Nauru	–	–	–	–	84	–	–	58 x	–	–	–	–	–	8	8
Nepal	6821	23	32	23	106	27	24	–	–	–	42	46	38	45	29
Netherlands	2019	12	–	–	4	–	–	88	88	89	–	–	–	–	–

TABLE 11. ADOLESCENTS

	Adolescents population (aged 10–19)		Marital status	Age at first birth	Adolescent birth rate	Attitudes towards domestic violence		Secondary education (2005–2009*)						HIV knowledge	
	Total	Adolescents as a proportion of total population	Girls aged 15–19 who are currently married/in union (%)	Women aged 20–24 who gave birth before age 18 (%)	Number of births per 1,000 girls aged 15–19	Adolescents aged 15–19 who think that a husband is justified in hitting or beating his wife under certain circumstances (2002–2009*) (%)		Net enrolment ratio			Net attendance ratio			Adolescents age 15–19 who have comprehensive knowledge of HIV (2005–2009*) (%)	
	2009	2009	2000–2009*	2000–2009*	2000–2008*	male	female	total	male	female	total	male	female	male	female
New Zealand	616	14	–	–	32	–	–	91 x	90 x	92 x	–	–	–	–	–
Nicaragua	1338	23	22	28	109	–	19	45	42	48	41 x	35 x	47 x	–	–
Niger	3512	23	59	51	199	–	68	9	11	7	11	13	9	14	12
Nigeria	35386	23	29	28	123	35	40	26	29	22	44	45	43	28	20
Niue	–	–	–	–	53	–	–	93 x	91 x	96 x	–	–	–	–	–
Norway	642	13	–	–	9	–	–	96	96	96	–	–	–	–	–
Occupied Palestinian Territory	1023	24	13	–	60	–	–	87	85	90	–	–	–	–	–
Oman	592	21	–	–	8	–	–	78	79	78	–	–	–	–	–
Pakistan	40478	22	16	10	20	–	–	33	37	28	36	39	33	–	2
Palau	–	–	–	–	29	–	–	–	–	–	–	–	–	–	–
Panama	631	18	–	–	83	–	–	66	63	69	–	–	–	–	–
Papua New Guinea	1522	23	15	–	70	–	–	–	–	–	–	–	–	–	–
Paraguay	1368	22	11	16 x	65	–	–	58	57	60	80 x	81 x	80 x	–	–
Peru	5822	20	11	15	59	–	–	75	75	75	70 x	70 x	70 x	–	17
Philippines	19735	21	10	7	53	–	15	61	55	66	63 x	55 x	70 x	–	19
Poland	4622	12	–	–	14	–	–	94	93	95	–	–	–	–	–
Portugal	1114	10	–	–	17	–	–	88	84	92	–	–	–	–	–
Qatar	155	11	–	–	16	–	–	79	67	98	–	–	–	–	–
Republic of Korea	6682	14	–	–	2	–	–	95	97	94	–	–	–	–	–
Republic of Moldova	535	15	10	5	29	25	24	83	82	85	84	82	85	–	–
Romania	2392	11	–	–	36	–	–	73	74	72	–	–	–	1 x	3 x
Russian Federation	15491	11	–	–	29	–	–	–	–	–	–	–	–	–	–
Rwanda	2227	22	3	7	43	–	51	10	–	–	5	5	5	49	45
Saint Kitts and Nevis	–	–	–	–	67	–	–	86	87	85	–	–	–	–	–
Saint Lucia	33	19	–	–	50	–	–	80	77	82	–	–	–	–	–
Saint Vincent and the Grenadines	21	19	–	–	72	–	–	90	85	95	–	–	–	–	–
Samoa	47	26	–	–	29	–	–	71	66	75	–	–	–	–	–
San Marino	–	–	–	–	1	–	–	–	–	–	–	–	–	–	–
Sao Tome and Principe	39	24	19	–	91	–	34	38	36	40	40	39	41	–	43
Saudi Arabia	5191	20	–	–	7	–	–	73	70	76	–	–	–	–	–
Senegal	3008	24	29	22	96	–	66	25	28	22	18	20	16	21	18
Serbia	1246	13	6	–	22	–	5	88	87	89	84	81	87	–	43
Seychelles	–	–	–	–	59	–	–	92	–	–	–	–	–	–	–
Sierra Leone	1258	22	30	40	143	57	55	25	30	20	19	21	17	26	16
Singapore	688	15	–	–	5	–	–	–	–	–	–	–	–	–	–
Slovakia	674	12	–	–	21	–	–	–	–	–	–	–	–	–	–
Slovenia	203	10	–	–	5	–	–	91	91	92	–	–	–	–	–
Solomon Islands	119	23	–	–	70	73	72	30	32	29	29	29	30	26	29
Somalia	2027	22	25	–	123	–	75 y	–	–	–	7	9	5	–	3
South Africa	9985	20	4	15	54	–	–	72	70	74	44 x	41 x	48 x	–	–
Spain	4259	9	–	–	13	–	–	95	93	97	–	–	–	–	–
Sri Lanka	3063	15	9	4	28	–	54 y	–	–	–	–	–	–	–	–
Sudan	9738	23	25	17 x	–	–	–	–	–	–	19	17	22	–	–
Suriname	94	18	11	–	66	–	19	65	55	74	61	56	67	–	41
Swaziland	309	26	7	28	111	59	54	29	31	26	36	31	41	50	52
Sweden	1138	12	–	–	6	–	–	99	99	99	–	–	–	–	–
Switzerland	873	12	–	–	4	–	–	85	87	83	–	–	–	–	–
Syrian Arab Republic	4501	21	10	–	75	–	–	68	68	67	64	64	65	–	6
Tajikistan	1699	24	6	–	27	–	85 y	83	88	77	82	89	74	–	2
Thailand	10375	15	15	–	43	–	–	72	68	77	80	77	84	–	46
The former Yugoslav Republic of Macedonia	292	14	2	–	21	–	14	82	82	81	78	79	78	–	23
Timor-Leste	282	25	–	–	59	–	–	31	30	33	–	–	–	–	–
Togo	1521	23	16	19 x	–	–	54	23 x	30 x	15 x	39	45	32	–	15
Tonga	23	22	–	–	16	–	–	66	60	74	–	–	–	–	–
Trinidad and Tobago	204	15	6	–	33	–	10	74	71	76	87	84	90	–	49
Tunisia	1815	18	–	–	6	–	–	71	67	76	–	–	–	–	–
Turkey	13663	18	10	8	51	–	30	74	77	70	47 x	52 x	43 x	–	–
Turkmenistan	1065	21	5	2	21	–	37 y	–	–	–	84	84	84	–	4
Tuvalu	–	–	–	3	23	83	69	–	–	–	–	–	–	57	31
Uganda	8077	25	20	35	159	69	70	22	22	21	16	16	15	38	31
Ukraine	5163	11	6	3	30	8	3	85	84	85	92	90	93	33	39
United Arab Emirates	501	11	–	–	22	–	–	84	83	85	–	–	–	–	–

| | Adolescents population (aged 10–19) | | Marital status Girls aged 15–19 who are currently married/in union (%) | Age at first birth Women aged 20–24 who gave birth before age 18 (%) | Adolescent birth rate Number of births per 1,000 girls aged 15–19 | Attitudes towards domestic violence Adolescents aged 15–19 who think that a husband is justified in hitting or beating his wife under certain circumstances (2002–2009*) (%) | | Secondary education (2005–2009*) | | | | | | HIV knowledge Adolescents age 15–19 who have comprehensive knowledge of HIV (2005–2009*) (%) | |
| | Total | Adolescents as a proportion of total population | | | | | | Net enrolment ratio | | | Net attendance ratio | | | | |
	2009	2009	2000–2009*	2000–2009*	2000–2008*	male	female	total	male	female	total	male	female	male	female
United Kingdom	7627	12	–	–	26	–	–	93	92	95	–	–	–	–	–
United Republic of Tanzania	10009	23	21	29	139	54	60	5 x	5 x	5 x	8	8	8	39	35
United States	43532	14	–	–	41	–	–	88	88	89	–	–	–	–	–
Uruguay	529	16	–	–	60	–	–	68	64	71	–	–	–	–	–
Uzbekistan	6092	22	5	4	26	63	63	91	92	90	90	91	90	–	27
Vanuatu	54	23	13	–	–	–	–	38 x	41 x	35 x	37	38	36	–	14
Venezuela (Bolivarian Republic of)	5487	19	16	–	101	–	–	69	66	74	36 x	30 x	43 x	–	–
Viet Nam	17182	20	5	4	35	–	53	62 x	–	–	78	77	78	–	45
Yemen	5964	25	19	25 x	80	–	–	37	49	26	38	48	27	–	2 y
Zambia	3088	24	18	34	151	55	61	43	47	39	37	38	35	38	36
Zimbabwe	3314	26	21	21	101	50	55	38	39	37	45	46	43	–	51

SUMMARY INDICATORS

Africa#	227318	23	22	25	108	–	57	31	33	29	33	35	32	29	21
Sub-Saharan Africa#	194803	23	23	28	123	43	57	30	32	28	29	30	27	31	24
Eastern and Southern Africa	91042	23	19	27	118	51	60	34	35	33	23	24	22	39	31
West and Central Africa	93824	23	27	29	129	34	55	26	29	22	33	36	31	25	19
Middle East and North Africa	83589	20	15	–	38	–	–	64	66	62	53	54	51	–	–
Asia#	663166	18	24 **	19 **	36	–	48 **	–	–	–	53 **	56 **	50 **	30 **	18
South Asia	334645	21	28	22	54	56	51	–	–	–	51	55	47	35	16
East Asia and Pacific	328521	16	11 **	8 **	18	–	38 **	66 **	65 **	67 **	64 **	63 **	65 **	5 **	23
Latin America and Caribbean	107678	19	18	18	75	–	–	74	72	77	71	68	74	–	–
CEE/CIS	57595	14	7	5	34	–	30	81	82	81	–	–	–	–	–
Industrialized countries§	117594	12	–	–	23	–	–	92	91	92	–	–	–	–	–
Developing countries§	1069532	19	21 **	20 **	55	–	50 **	54 **	54 **	53 **	50 **	52 **	48 **	30 **	19
Least developed countries§	190214	23	30	31	123	–	56	31	33	29	29	30	28	31	21
World	1214488	18	21 **	20 **	51	–	49 **	61 **	61 **	60 **	51 **	53 **	48 **	–	–

For a complete list of countries and territories in the regions and subregions, see page 124.
§ Includes territories within each country category or regional group. Countries and territories in each country category or regional group are listed on page 124.

DEFINITIONS OF THE INDICATORS

Marital status – Percentage of girls aged 15–19 who are currently married or in union. This indicator is meant to provide a snapshot of the current marital status of girls in this age group. However, it is worth noting that they are still exposed to the risk of marrying before they exit adolescence.

Age at first birth – Percentage of women aged 20–24 who gave birth before age 18. This standardized indicator from population-based surveys captures levels of fertility among adolescents up to the age of 18. Because it is based on the answers of women aged 20–24, the risk of their having given birth before their 18th birthday is behind them.

Adolescent birth rate – Number of births per 1,000 adolescent girls aged 15–19.

Attitudes towards domestic violence – Percentage of women (aged 15–49) who consider a husband to be justified in hitting or beating his wife for at least one of the specified reasons. Women were asked whether a husband is justified in hitting or beating his wife under a series of circumstances, i.e., if his wife burns the food, argues with him, goes out without telling him, neglects the children or refuses sexual relations.

Secondary school net enrolment ratio – Number of children enrolled in secondary school who are of official secondary school age, expressed as a percentage of the total number of children of official secondary school age.

Secondary school net attendance ratio – Number of children attending secondary or tertiary school who are of official secondary school age, expressed as a percentage of the total number of children of official secondary school age.

Comprehensive knowledge of HIV – Percentage of young men and women (aged 15–19) who correctly identify the two major ways of preventing the sexual transmission of HIV (using condoms and limiting sex to one faithful, uninfected partner), who reject the two most common local misconceptions about HIV transmission and who know that a healthy-looking person can be HIV-infected.

MAIN DATA SOURCES

Child population – United Nations Population Division.

Marital status – Multiple Indicator Cluster Surveys (MICS), Demographic and Health Surveys (DHS) and other national surveys.

Age at first birth – Demographic and Health Surveys (DHS).

Adolescent fertility – UNFPA databases based on data for 2000–2008 (most recent year available)

Secondary school enrolment – UNESCO Institute of Statistics.

Secondary school attendance – Demographic and Health Surveys (DHS) and Multiple Indicator Cluster Surveys (MICS).

HIV knowledge – AIDS Indicator Surveys (AIS), Behavioural Surveillance Surveys (BSS), Demographic and Health Surveys (DHS), Multiple Indicator Cluster Surveys (MICS), Reproductive Health Surveys (RHS) and other national household surveys; 'HIV/AIDS Survey Indicators Database', <www.measuredhs.com/hivdata>.

NOTES

– Data not available.

x Data refer to years or periods other than those specified in the column heading, differ from the standard definition or refer to only part of a country. Such data are not included in the calculation of regional and global averages.

y Data differ from the standard definition or refer to only part of a country. Such data are included in the calculation of regional and global averages.

* Data refer to the most recent year available during the period specified in the column heading.

** Excludes China.

TABLE 12. EQUITY

Countries and territories	Birth registration (%) 2000–2009				Skilled attendant at birth (%) 2000–2009				Underweight prevalence in children (%) under five 2003–2009				Immunization Measles coverage (%) 2000–2008				Use of improved sanitation facilities (%) 2008		
	Poorest 20%	Richest 20%	Ratio of richest to poorest	Source	Poorest 20%	Richest 20%	Ratio of richest to poorest	Source	Poorest 20%	Richest 20%	Ratio of poorest to richest	Source	Poorest 20%	Richest 20%	Ratio of richest to poorest	Source	Urban	Rural	Ratio of urban to rural
Afghanistan	–	–	–		–	–	–		–	–	–		–	–	–		60	30	2.0
Albania	98	99	1.0	DHS 2008–2009	98	100	1.0	DHS 2008–2009	8	4	2.2	DHS 2008–2009	–	–	–		98	98	1.0
Algeria	–	–	–		88	98	1.1	MICS 2006	5	2	2.4	MICS 2006	–	–	–		98	88	1.1
Andorra	–	–	–		–				–				–				100	100	1.0
Angola	17	48	2.8	MICS 2001	23	67	3.0	MICS 2001	–	–	–		–				86	18	4.8
Antigua and Barbuda	–				–				–				–				98	–	–
Argentina	–				–				–				–				91	77	1.2
Armenia	93	99	1.1	DHS 2005	93	100	1.1	DHS 2005	5	3	1.4	DHS 2005	72	61	0.8	DHS 2005	95	80	1.2
Australia	–				–				–				–				100	100	1.0
Austria	–				–				–				–				100	100	1.0
Azerbaijan	92	97	1.1	DHS 2006	76	100	1.3	DHS 2006	15	2	7.0	DHS 2006	50 z	83 z	1.7 z	DHS 2006	85	77	1.1
Bahamas	–				–				–				–				100	100	1.0
Bahrain	–				–				–				–				100		
Bangladesh	6	19	3.0	MICS 2006	5	51	10.6	DHS 2007	51	26	1.9	DHS 2007	80	89	1.1	DHS 2007	56	52	1.1
Barbados	–				–				–				–				100	100	1.0
Belarus	–	–	–		100	100	1.0	MICS 2005	2	0	6.7	MICS 2005	97 z	87 z	0.9 z	MICS 2005	91	97	0.9
Belgium	–				–				–				–				100	100	1.0
Belize	93	98	1.1	MICS 2006	–				–				–				93	86	1.1
Benin	46	75	1.6	DHS 2006	52	96	1.9	DHS 2006	25	10	2.4	DHS 2006	–				24	4	6.0
Bhutan	–				–				–				–				87	54	1.6
Bolivia (Plurinational State of)	–	–	–		38	99	2.6	DHS 2008	8	2	3.8	DHS 2008	62	74	1.2	DHS 2003	34	9	3.8
Bosnia and Herzegovina	99	100	1.0	MICS 2006	99	100	1.0	MICS 2006	2	3	0.5	MICS 2005	81 z	84 z	1.0 z	MICS 2006	99	92	1.1
Botswana	–				84	100	1.2	MICS 2000	–				–				74	39	1.9
Brazil	–				–				–				–				87	37	2.4
Brunei Darussalam	–				–				–				–				–	–	
Bulgaria	–				–				–				–				100	100	1.0
Burkina Faso	52	90	1.7	MICS 2006	56	65	1.2	MICS 2006	38	18	2.1	MICS 2006	72	84	1.2	MICS 2006	33	6	5.5
Burundi	58	64	1.1	MICS 2005	25	55	2.2	MICS 2005	–	–			77	78	1.0	MICS 2005	49	46	1.1
Cambodia	59	77	1.3	DHS 2005	21	90	4.3	DHS 2005	35	19	1.8	Other 2008	70	82	1.2	DHS 2005	67	18	3.7
Cameroon	51	91	1.8	MICS 2006	23	98	4.4	MICS 2006	30	5	6.2	MICS 2006	52	83	1.6	DHS 2004	56	35	1.6
Canada	–				–				–				–				100	99	1.0
Cape Verde	–				–				–				–				65	38	1.7
Central African Republic	23	83	3.7	MICS 2006	27	89	3.3	MICS 2006	25	17	1.5	MICS 2006	–				43	28	1.5
Chad	0	37	121.7	DHS 2004	1	48	53.7	DHS 2004	–				8	38	4.8	DHS 2004	23	4	5.8
Chile	–				–				–				–				98	83	1.2
China	–	–	–		–				–				–				58	52	1.1
Colombia	72	99	1.4	DHS 2005	89	100	1.1	DHS 2005	8	2	3.5	DHS 2005	69	90	1.3	DHS 2005	81	55	1.5
Comoros	72	93	1.3	MICS 2000	49	77	1.6	MICS 2000	–				–				50	30	1.7
Congo	69 y	91 y	1.3 y	DHS 2005	40	95	2.4	DHS 2005	16	5	3.1	DHS 2005	49	84	1.7	DHS 2005	31	29	1.1
Cook Islands	–				–				–				–				100	100	1.0
Costa Rica	–				–				–				–				95	96	1.0
Côte d'Ivoire	28	89	3.2	MICS 2006	29	95	3.3	MICS 2006	21	6	3.4	MICS 2006	58	86	1.5	MICS 2006	36	11	3.3
Croatia	–				–				–				–				99	98	1.0
Cuba	–				–				–				–				94	81	1.2
Cyprus	–				–				–				–				100	100	1.0
Czech Republic	–				–				–				–				99	97	1.0
Democratic People's Republic of Korea	–				–				–				–				–	–	
Democratic Republic of the Congo	29	37	1.3	DHS 2007	59	98	1.7	DHS 2007	27	15	1.8	DHS 2007	51	85	1.7	DHS 2007	23	23	1.0
Denmark	–				–				–				–				100	100	1.0
Djibouti	–				–				–				–				63	10	6.3
Dominica	–				–				–				–				–	–	
Dominican Republic	59	97	1.6	Other 2006	95	99	1.0	DHS 2007	–				73 z	87 z	1.2 z	DHS 2007	87	74	1.2
Ecuador	79	92	1.2	Other 2004	99	98	1.0	Other 2004	–				–				96	84	1.1
Egypt	99	100	1.0	DHS 2005	55	97	1.8	DHS 2008	8	5	1.4	DHS 2008	95	97	1.0	DHS 2005	97	92	1.1
El Salvador	98	99	1.0	Other 2008	91	98	1.1	Other 2008	12 y	1 y	12.9 y	Other 2008	–	–	–		89	83	1.1
Equatorial Guinea	–				47	85	1.8	MICS 2000	–				–				–	–	
Eritrea	–	–	–		7	81	12.1	DHS 2002	–				80	95	1.2	DHS 2002	52	4	13.0
Estonia	–				–				–				–				96	94	1.0
Ethiopia	3	18	7.0	DHS 2005	1	27	38	DHS 2005	36	25	1.5	DHS 2005	25	53	2.1	DHS 2005	29	8	3.6
Fiji	–				–				–				–				–	–	

	Birth registration (%) 2000–2009				Skilled attendant at birth (%) 2000–2009				Underweight prevalence in children (%) under five 2003–2009				Immunization – Measles coverage (%) 2000–2008				Use of improved sanitation facilities (%) 2008		
	Poorest 20%	Richest 20%	Ratio of richest to poorest	Source	Poorest 20%	Richest 20%	Ratio of richest to poorest	Source	Poorest 20%	Richest 20%	Ratio of poorest to richest	Source	Poorest 20%	Richest 20%	Ratio of richest to poorest	Source	Urban	Rural	Ratio of urban to rural
Finland	–	–	–		–	–	–		–	–	–		–	–	–		100	100	1.0
France	–	–	–		–	–	–		–	–	–		–	–	–		100	100	1.0
Gabon	88	92	1.0	DHS 2000	–	–	–		15 x	4 x	4.0 x	DHS 2000	34	71	2.1	DHS 2000	33	30	1.1
Gambia	52	64	1.2	MICS 2005–2006	28	89	3.1	MICS 2005–2006	21	10	2.0	MICS 2005–2006	95	91	1.0	MICS 2005–2006	68	65	1.0
Georgia	89	98	1.1	MICS 2005	95	99	1.0	MICS 2005	2	1	2.3	MICS 2005	–	–	–		96	93	1.0
Germany	–	–	–		–	–	–		–	–	–		–	–	–		100	100	1.0
Ghana	60	88	1.5	DHS 2008	22	94	4.2	DHS 2008	19	9	2.2	DHS 2008	88	95	1.1	DHS 2008	18	7	2.6
Greece	–	–	–		–	–	–		–	–	–		–	–	–		99	97	1.0
Grenada	–	–	–		–	–	–		–	–	–		–	–	–		96	97	1.0
Guatemala	–	–	–		–	–	–		–	–	–		–	–	–		89	73	1.2
Guinea	21	83	4.0	DHS 2005	26	57	2.2	Other 2007	24	19	1.3	Other 2008	42	57	1.4	DHS 2005	34	11	3.1
Guinea-Bissau	21	61	2.9	MICS 2006	19	79	4.0	MICS 2006	17	8	2.1	MICS 2006	69	89	1.3	MICS 2006	49	9	5.4
Guyana	87	98	1.1	MICS 2006–2007	64	93	1.5	MICS 2006–2007	10	4	2.7	MICS 2006–2007	74 z	82 z	1.1 z	MICS 2006–2007	85	80	1.1
Haiti	72	92	1.3	DHS 2005–2006	6	68	10.5	DHS 2005–2006	22	6	3.6	DHS 2005–2006	50	67	1.3	DHS 2005–2006	24	10	2.4
Holy See	–	–	–		–	–	–		–	–	–		–	–	–		–	–	–
Honduras	92	96	1.0	DHS 2005–2006	33	99	2.9	DHS 2005–2006	16	2	8.1	DHS 2005–2006	85	86	1.0	DHS 2005–2006	80	62	1.3
Hungary	–	–	–		–	–	–		–	–	–		–	–	–		100	100	1.0
Iceland	–	–	–		–	–	–		–	–	–		–	–	–		100	100	1.0
India	24	72	3.1	NFHS 2005–2006	19	89	4.6	NFHS 2005–2006	57	20	2.9	NFHS 2005–2006	40	85	2.1	NFHS 2005–2006	54	21	2.6
Indonesia	23	84	3.7	DHS 2007	65	86	1.3	DHS 2007	–	–	–		63	85	1.3	DHS 2007	67	36	1.9
Iran (Islamic Republic of)	–	–	–		–	–	–		–	–	–		–	–	–		–	–	–
Iraq	–	–	–		–	–	–		–	–	–		–	–	–		76	66	1.2
Ireland	–	–	–		–	–	–		–	–	–		–	–	–		100	98	1.0
Israel	–	–	–		–	–	–		–	–	–		–	–	–		100	100	1.0
Italy	–	–	–		–	–	–		–	–	–		–	–	–		–	–	–
Jamaica	–	–	–		–	–	–		–	–	–		–	–	–		82	84	1.0
Japan	–	–	–		–	–	–		–	–	–		–	–	–		100	100	1.0
Jordan	–	–	–		98	100	1.0	DHS 2007	3	0	26.0	DHS 2009	92	96	1.0	DHS 2007	98	97	1.0
Kazakhstan	99	100	1.0	MICS 2006	100	100	1.0	MICS 2006	5	2	2.8	MICS 2006	–	–	–		97	98	1.0
Kenya	48	80	1.7	DHS 2008–2009	20	81	4.0	DHS 2008–2009	25	9	2.8	DHS 2008–2009	55	88	1.6	DHS 2003	27	32	0.8
Kiribati	–	–	–		–	–	–		–	–	–		–	–	–		–	–	–
Kuwait	–	–	–		–	–	–		–	–	–		–	–	–		100	100	1.0
Kyrgystan	94	95	1.0	MICS 2005–2006	93	100	1.1	MICS 2005–2006	2	2	0.8	MICS 2005–2006	–	–	–		94	93	1.0
Lao People's Democratic Republic	62	85	1.4	MICS 2006	3	81	27.1	MICS 2006	38	14	2.7	MICS 2006	32	60	1.9	MICS 2006	86	38	2.3
Latvia	–	–	–		–	–	–		–	–	–		–	–	–		82	71	1.2
Lebanon	–	–	–		–	–	–		–	–	–		–	–	–		100	–	–
Lesotho	24	36	1.5	DHS 2004	34	83	2.5	DHS 2004	–	–	–		82	85	1.0	DHS 2004	40	25	1.6
Liberia	1 y	7 y	6.1 y	DHS 2007	26	81	3.2	DHS 2007	21	13	1.6	DHS 2007	45	86	1.9	DHS 2007	25	4	6.3
Libyan Arab Jamahiriya	–	–	–		–	–	–		–	–	–		–	–	–		97	96	1.0
Liechtenstein	–	–	–		–	–	–		–	–	–		–	–	–		–	–	–
Lithuania	–	–	–		–	–	–		–	–	–		–	–	–		–	–	–
Luxembourg	–	–	–		–	–	–		–	–	–		–	–	–		100	100	1.0
Madagascar	58	95	1.6	DHS 2003–2004	22	90	4.1	DHS 2008–2009	40	24	1.7	DHS 2003–2004	38	84	2.2	DHS 2003–2004	15	10	1.5
Malawi	–	–	–		43	77	1.8	MICS 2006	18	12	1.6	MICS 2006	67	88	1.3	DHS 2004	51	57	0.9
Malaysia	–	–	–		–	–	–		–	–	–		–	–	–		96	95	1.0
Maldives	–	–	–		–	–	–		–	–	–		–	–	–		100	96	1.0
Mali	42	82	2.0	DHS 2006	35	86	2.5	DHS 2006	31	17	1.8	DHS 2006	68	78	1.1	DHS 2006	45	32	1.4
Malta	–	–	–		–	–	–		–	–	–		–	–	–		100	100	1.0
Marshall Islands	92	98	1.1	DHS 2007	68	99	1.5	DHS 2007	–	–	–		–	–	–		83	53	1.6
Mauritania	28	83	2.9	MICS 2007	21	95	4.6	MICS 2007	–	–	–		57	76	1.3	MICS 2007	50	9	5.6
Mauritius	–	–	–		–	–	–		–	–	–		–	–	–		93	90	1.0
Mexico	–	–	–		–	–	–		–	–	–		–	–	–		90	68	1.3
Micronesia (Federated States of)	–	–	–		–	–	–		–	–	–		–	–	–		–	–	–
Monaco	–	–	–		–	–	–		–	–	–		–	–	–		100	–	–
Mongolia	99	98	1.0	MICS 2005	98	100	1.0	MICS 2005	7	3	2.8	MICS 2005	–	–	–		64	32	2.0
Montenegro	94	99	1.0	MICS 2005–2006	98	100	1.0	MICS 2005–2006	4	1	4.1	MICS 2005–2006	–	–	–		96	86	1.1
Morocco	–	–	–		30	95	3.2	DHS 2003–2004	15	3	4.5	DHS 2003–2004	83	98	1.2	Other 2003–2004	83	52	1.6
Mozambique	20	48	2.4	MICS 2008	37	89	2.4	MICS 2008	24	8	3.1	MICS 2008	61	96	1.6	DHS 2003	38	4	9.5
Myanmar	–	–	–		–	–	–		–	–	–		–	–	–		86	79	1.1
Namibia	46	92	2.0	DHS 2006–2007	60	98	1.6	DHS 2006–2007	22	7	3.1	DHS 2006–2007	70	95	1.4	DHS 2006–2007	60	17	3.5
Nauru	71	88	1.2	DHS 2007	97	98	1.0	DHS 2007	7	3	2.7	DHS 2007	–	–	–		50	–	–

TABLE 12. EQUITY

	Birth registration (%) 2000–2009				Skilled attendant at birth (%) 2000 2009				Underweight prevalence in children (%) under five 2003–2009				Immunization – Measles coverage (%) 2000–2008				Use of improved sanitation facilities (%) 2008		
	Poorest 20%	Richest 20%	Ratio of richest to poorest	Source	Poorest 20%	Richest 20%	Ratio of richest to poorest	Source	Poorest 20%	Richest 20%	Ratio of poorest to richest	Source	Poorest 20%	Richest 20%	Ratio of richest to poorest	Source	Urban	Rural	Ratio of urban to rural
Nepal	22	47	2.2	DHS 2006	5	58	12.0	DHS 2006	47	19	2.5	DHS 2006	73	95	1.3	DHS 2006	51	27	1.9
Netherlands	–	–	–		–	–	–		–	–	–		–	–	–		100	100	1.0
New Zealand																			
Nicaragua	63	93	1.5	DHS 2001	42	99	2.4	DHS 2006–2007	9	1	6.6	Other 2006–2007	–	–	–		63	37	1.7
Niger	20	67	3.3	DHS/MICS 2006	21	71	3.3	DHS/MICS 2006	–	–	–		32 z	74 z	2.3 z	DHS/MICS 2006	34	4	8.5
Nigeria	9	62	7.0	DHS 2008	8	86	10.3	DHS 2008	32	12	2.8	DHS 2003	17	75	4.4	DHS 2008	36	28	1.3
Niue	–	–	–		–	–	–		–	–	–		–	–	–		100	100	1.0
Norway	–	–	–		–	–	–		–	–	–		–	–	–		100	100	1.0
Occupied Palestinian Territory	–	–	–		–	–	–		–	–	–		–	–	–		91	84	1.1
Oman	–	–	–		–	–	–		–	–	–		–	–	–		97	–	–
Pakistan	18	38	2.1	DHS 2006–2007	16	77	4.8	DHS 2006–2007	–	–	–		36	76	2.1	DHS 2006–2007	72	29	2.5
Palau	–	–	–		–	–	–		–	–	–		–	–	–		96	–	–
Panama	–	–	–		–	–	–		–	–	–		–	–	–		75	51	1.5
Papua New Guinea	–	–	–		–	–	–		–	–	–		–	–	–		71	41	1.7
Paraguay	–	–	–		–	–	–		–	–	–		–	–	–		90	40	2.3
Peru	–	–	–		54	100	1.9	DHS 2009	9	1	13.1	DHS 2009	81	92	1.1	DHS 2000	81	36	2.3
Philippines	–	–	–		26	94	3.7	DHS 2008	–	–	–		70	89	1.3	DHS 2003	80	69	1.2
Poland	–	–	–		–	–	–		–	–	–		–	–	–		96	80	1.2
Portugal	–	–	–		–	–	–		–	–	–		–	–	–		100	100	1.0
Qatar	–	–	–		–	–	–		–	–	–		–	–	–		100	100	1.0
Republic of Korea	–	–	–		–	–	–		–	–	–		–	–	–		100	100	1.0
Republic of Moldova	97	98	1.0	MICS 2000	99	100	1.0	DHS 2005	5	1	8.2	DHS 2005	43 z	63 z	1.5 z	DHS 2005	85	74	1.1
Romania	–	–	–		–	–	–		–	–	–		–	–	–		88	54	1.6
Russian Federation	–	–	–		–	–	–		–	–	–		–	–	–		93	70	1.3
Rwanda	82	81	1.0	DHS 2005	43	71	1.7	DHS 2007–2008	24	7	3.5	DHS 2005	85	88	1.0	DHS 2005	50	55	0.9
Saint Kitts and Nevis	–	–	–		–	–	–		–	–	–		–	–	–		96	96	1.0
Saint Lucia	–	–	–		–	–	–		–	–	–		–	–	–				
Saint Vincent and the Grenadines	–	–	–		–	–	–		–	–	–		–	–	–		–	96	–
Samoa	–	–	–		–	–	–		–	–	–		–	–	–		100	100	1.0
San Marino	–	–	–		–	–	–		–	–	–		–	–	–		–	–	–
Sao Tome and Principe	63	78	1.2	MICS 2006	70	88	1.2	MICS 2006	–	–	–		–	–	–		30	19	1.6
Saudi Arabia	–	–	–		–	–	–		–	–	–		–	–	–		100	–	–
Senegal	31	81	2.6	DHS 2005	20	89	4.4	DHS 2005	21	5	4.2	DHS 2005	71	81	1.1	DHS 2005	69	38	1.8
Serbia	98	99	1.0	MICS 2005–2006	98	100	1.0	MICS 2005–2006	4	1	3.5	MICS 2005–2006	–	–	–		96	88	1.1
Seychelles	–	–	–		–	–	–		–	–	–		–	–	–		97	–	–
Sierra Leone	43	62	1.4	DHS 2008	28	71	2.5	DHS 2008	22	12	1.8	DHS 2008	66	84	1.3	MICS 2005	24	6	4.0
Singapore	–	–	–		–	–	–		–	–	–		–	–	–		100	–	–
Slovakia	–	–	–		–	–	–		–	–	–		–	–	–		100	99	1.0
Slovenia	–	–	–		–	–	–		–	–	–		–	–	–		100	100	1.0
Solomon Islands	80	78	1.0	DHS 2007	56	88	1.6	DHS 2007	14	10	1.4	DHS 2007	–	–	–		98	–	–
Somalia	1	7	6.6	MICS 2006	11	77	7.2	MICS 2006	42	14	3.0	MICS 2006	22	42	1.9	MICS 2006	52	6	8.7
South Africa	–	–	–		–	–	–		–	–	–		–	–	–		84	65	1.3
Spain	–	–	–		–	–	–		–	–	–		–	–	–		100	100	1.0
Sri Lanka	–	–	–		97	99	1.0	DHS 2006–2007	29	11	2.6	DHS 2006–2007	–	–	–		88	92	1.0
Sudan	6	86	14	Other 2006	15	90	5.8	Other 2006	31	17	1.9	Other 2006	–	–	–		55	18	3.1
Suriname	94	98	1.0	MICS 2006	81	96	1.2	MICS 2006	9	5	1.8	MICS 2006	–	–	–		90	66	1.4
Swaziland	18	50	2.8	DHS 2006–2007	45	86	1.9	DHS 2006–2007	8	4	2.0	DHS 2006–2007	89	93	1.0	DHS 2006–2007	61	53	1.2
Sweden	–	–	–		–	–	–		–	–	–		–	–	–		100	100	1.0
Switzerland	–	–	–		–	–	–		–	–	–		–	–	–		100	100	1.0
Syrian Arab Republic	92	99	1.1	MICS 2006	78	99	1.3	MICS 2006	10	7	1.5	MICS 2006	65	89	1.4	MICS 2006	96	95	1.0
Tajikistan	89	86	1.0	MICS 2005	90	90	1.0	Other 2007	17	13	1.3	Other 2007	89 z	96 z	1.1 z	MICS 2005	95	94	1.0
Thailand	99	100	1.0	MICS 2005–2006	93	100	1.1	MICS 2005–2006	11	3	3.3	MICS 2005–2006	94	95	1.0	MICS 2005–2006	95	96	1.0
The former Yugoslav Republic of Macedonia	89	99	1.1	MICS 2005	95	100	1.0	MICS 2005	3	0	5.3	MICS 2005	49 z	77 z	1.6 z	MICS 2005	92	82	1.1
Timor-Leste	–	–	–		–	–	–		–	–	–		–	–	–		76	40	1.9
Togo	58	96	1.7	MICS 2006	30	97	3.3	MICS 2006	–	–	–		57	72	1.3	MICS 2006	24	3	8.0
Tonga	–	–	–		–	–	–		–	–	–		–	–	–		98	96	1.0
Trinidad and Tobago	94	98	1.0	MICS 2006	98	100	1.0	MICS 2006	–	–	–		91 z	72 z	0.8 z	MICS 2006	92	92	1.0
Tunisia	–	–	–		–	–	–		–	–	–		–	–	–		96	64	1.5
Turkey	89	99	1.1	DHS 2008	73	100	1.4	DHS 2008	4	1	8.4	DHS 2008	–	–	–		97	75	1.3
Turkmenistan	94	97	1.0	MICS 2006	99	100	1.0	MICS 2006	8	2	3.2	MICS 2006	91	80	0.9	DHS 2000	99	97	1.0

	Birth registration (%) 2000–2009				Skilled attendant at birth (%) 2000–2009				Underweight prevalence in children (%) under five 2003–2009				Immunization – Measles coverage (%) 2000–2008				Use of improved sanitation facilities (%) 2008		
	Poorest 20%	Richest 20%	Ratio of richest to poorest	Source	Poorest 20%	Richest 20%	Ratio of richest to poorest	Source	Poorest 20%	Richest 20%	Ratio of poorest to richest	Source	Poorest 20%	Richest 20%	Ratio of richest to poorest	Source	Urban	Rural	Ratio of urban to rural
Tuvalu	39	71	1.8	DHS 2007	99	98	1.0	DHS 2007	1	0	0	DHS 2007	–	–	–		88	81	1.1
Uganda	17	26	1.5	DHS 2006	28	76	2.7	DHS 2006	21	8	2.5	DHS 2006	49	65	1.3	DHS 2000–2001	38	49	0.8
Ukraine	100	100	1.0	MICS 2005	97	99	1.0	DHS 2007	–	–	–		–	–	–		97	90	1.1
United Arab Emirates	–	–	–		–	–	–										98	95	1.0
United Kingdom	–	–	–		–	–	–										100	100	1.0
United Republic of Tanzania	10	60	6.1	HMIS 2007–2008	26	85	3.3	DHS 2004–2005	–				65	91	1.4	DHS 2004–2005	32	21	1.5
United States	–	–	–		–	–	–						–	–	–		100	99	1.0
Uruguay	–	–	–		–	–	–						–	–	–		100	99	1.0
Uzbekistan	100	100	1.0	MICS 2006	100	100	1.0	MICS 2006	5	3	1.5	MICS 2006	97 z	98 z	1.0 z	MICS 2006	100	100	1.0
Vanuatu	13	41	3.1	MICS 2007	55	90	1.6	MICS 2007	–								66	48	1.4
Venezuela (Bolivarian Republic of)	87	95	1.1	MICS 2000	*95*	*92*	*1.0*	*MICS 2000*	–				–	–	–		–	–	–
Viet Nam	72	97	1.3	MICS 2006	53	99	1.9	MICS 2006	–	–			70	96	1.4	MICS 2006	94	67	1.4
Yemen	5	50	9.3	MICS 2006	17	74	4.3	MICS 2006	–	–			52	85	1.6	MICS 2006	94	33	2.8
Zambia	5	31	5.8	DHS 2007	27	91	3.4	DHS 2007	16	11	1.5	DHS 2007	88	94	1.1	DHS 2007	59	43	1.4
Zimbabwe	67	85	1.3	DHS 2005–2006	39	92	2.4	Other 2009	16 y	7 y	2.3 y	Other 2009	54	74	1.4	DHS 2005–2006	56	37	1.5

SUMMARY INDICATORS

	Poorest 20%	Richest 20%	Ratio	Source	Poorest 20%	Richest 20%	Ratio	Source	Poorest 20%	Richest 20%	Ratio	Source	Poorest 20%	Richest 20%	Ratio	Source	Urban	Rural	Ratio
Africa#	29	61	2.1		27	80	3.0		26	12	2.1		49	79	1.6		55	32	1.7
Sub-Saharan Africa#	23	58	2.5		24	78	3.3		28	13	2.1		45	77	1.7		44	24	1.8
Eastern and Southern Africa	23	47	2.1		21	68	3.2		28	15	1.9		51	76	1.5		55	28	2.0
West and Central Africa	25	65	2.6		26	86	3.3		28	12	2.4		40	78	2.0		35	21	1.7
Middle East and North Africa	–	–	–		46	93	2.0		14	7	1.9		–	–	–		90	66	1.4
Asia#	25	66	2.6		25 **	85 **	3.3 **		54 **	20 **	2.7 **		49 **	85 **	1.7 **		63	40	1.6
South Asia	21	62	2.9		18	83	4.6		55	20	2.7		44	84	1.9		57	26	2.2
East Asia and the Pacific	46	88	1.9		54 **	92 **	1.7 **		–				69 **	88 **	1.3 **		66	55	1.2
Latin America and the Caribbean	–	–	–		–	–	–		–				–	–	–		86	55	1.6
CEE/CIS	94	98	1.0		88	99	1.1		6	2	2.6		–	–	–		93	82	1.1
Industrialized countries§	–	–	–		–	–	–		–				–	–	–		100	98	1.0
Developing countries§	31	66	2.1		30 **	84 **	2.8 **		38 **	15 **	2.5 **		51 **	83 **	1.6 **		68	40	1.7
Least developed countries§	20	47	2.3		23	71	3.0		33	18	1.9		56	78	1.4		50	31	1.6
World	–	–	–		31 **	84 **	2.7 **		38 **	15 **	2.5 **		51 **	83 **	1.6 **		76	45	1.7

§ Includes territories within each country category or regional group. Countries and territories in each country category or regional group are listed on page 124.

For a complete list of countries and territories in the regions and subregions, see page 124.

DEFINITIONS OF THE INDICATORS

Birth registration – Percentage of children less than 5 years old who were registered at the time of the survey. The numerator of this indicator includes children whose birth certificate was seen by the interviewer or whose mother or caretaker said the birth had been registered.

Skilled attendant at birth – Proportion of births attended by skilled health personnel (doctor, nurse or midwife).

Underweight prevalence (WHO) – Percentage of children 0–59 months old who are below minus two standard deviations from median weight-for-age according to WHO Child Growth Standards.

Measles coverage – Percentage of infants who received measles-containing vaccine.

Use of improved sanitation facilities – Percentage of the population using any of the following sanitation facilities: facilities with sewer connections, septic system connections, pour-flush latrines, ventilated improved pit latrines, pit latrines with a slab or covered pit.

MAIN DATA SOURCES

Sources of data for all indicators presented in this table are included next to each data point, except for the 'Use of improved sanitation facilities' indicator, for which the data source is WHO/UNICEF Joint Monitoring Programme for Water Supply and Sanitation, 2010.

Italicized data are from different sources than the data presented for the same indicators in other tables of the report: Table 2 (Nutrition – Underweight prevalence), Table 8 (Women – Skilled attendant at birth), Table 9 (Child Protection – Birth registration).

Sources for immunization data in this table differ from the total data sources presented in Table 3, which are the WHO/UNICEF Joint Immunization estimates. Immunization coverage survey data have been excluded from selected CEE/CIS countries for which data reflect maternal recall only rather than both vaccination card and maternal recall.

NOTES	
–	Data not available.
x	Data refer to years or periods other than those specified in the column heading, differ from the standard definition or refer to only part of a country. Such data are not included in the calculation of regional and global averages.
y	Data differ from the standard definition or refer to only part of a country. Such data are included in the calculation of regional and global averages.
z	Recommended measles vaccination age in country is greater than 21 months; the coverage shown is therefore an underestimate.
**	Excludes China.

Acronyms

AIDS   acquired immune deficiency syndrome

CEDAW   Convention on the Elimination of All Forms of Discrimination against Women

DHS   Demographic and Health Surveys

FGM/C   female genital mutilation/cutting

GDP   gross domestic product

HIV   human immunodeficiency virus

IUCW   International Union for Child Welfare

MDG   Millennium Development Goal

MICS   Multiple Indicator Cluster Surveys

NGO   non-governmental organization

UN   United Nations

UNAIDS   Joint United Nations Programme on HIV/AIDS

UNDP   United Nations Development Programme

UNESCO   United Nations Educational, Scientific and Cultural Organization

UNFPA   United Nations Population Fund

UNICEF   United Nations Children's Fund

WHO   World Health Organization

World YWCA World Young Women's Christian Association

WOSM   World Organization of the Scout Movement